PSYCHIATRY

Second Edition

Michael Gelder
Emeritus Professor of Psychiatry, University of Oxford

Richard Mayou
Professor of Psychiatry, University of Oxford

John Geddes
Senior Clinical Research Fellow, University of Oxford

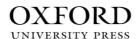

OXFORD

UNIVERSITY PRESS

OXFORD

UNIVERSITY PRESS

Great Clarendon Street, Oxford OX2 6DP

Oxford University Press is a department of the University of Oxford.
If furthers the University's objective of excellence in research, scholarship,
and education by publishing worldwide in

Oxford New York

Athens Auckland Bangkok Bogota Buenos Aires Calcutta
Cape Town Chennai Dar es Salaam Delhi Florence Hong Kong Istanbul
Karachi Kuala Lumpur Madrid Melbourne Mexico City Mumbai
Nairobi Paris São Paolo Singapore Taipei Tokyo Toronto Warsaw
with associated companies in Berlin Ibadan

Oxford is a registered trade mark of Oxford University Press
in the UK and in certain other countries

Published in the United States
by Oxford University Press Inc., New York

First published as The Concise Oxford Textbook Psychiatry 1994
Published in new edition as Psychiatry, an Oxford Core Text 1999
Reprinted (with corrections) 2000

A catalogue record for this book is available from the British Library

Library of Congress Cataloging in Publication Data

Gelder, Michael G.
Psychiatry/Michael Gelder, Richard Mayou, John Geddes.
(Oxford core texts)   (Oxford medical publications)
Rev. ed. of: Concise Oxford textbook of psychiatry/Michael
Gelder, Dennis Gath, Richard Mayou. 1994
Includes bibliographical references and index.
1. Psychiatry.   I. Mayou, Richard.   II. Geddes, John MD.
III. Gelder, Michael G.   Concise Oxford textbook of psychiatry.
IV. Title.   V. Series.   IV. Series: Oxford medical publications.
{DNLM: 1. Mental Disorders.   WM 140 G315p 1999}
RC454.G38   1999   616.89—dc21   98-22504

1 3 5 7 9 10 8 6 4 2

ISBN 0 19 262888 7

Printed in Great Britain
on acid-free paper by
The Bath Press, Avon

Preface

This text is the second edition of the book formerly titled *The Concise Oxford Textbook of Psychiatry*. This edition is shorter than that of the first, though the number of pages is little different because we have made greater use of lists and tables. Chapters 9 and 10 of the first edition have been amalgamated and shortened to form a single chapter on schizophrenia and related disorders. Some material has been separated from the text into Advanced information sections. For example, the management of patients taking lithium, which is important for practitioners but need not be known in detail by students.

Recommendations about treatment are evidence-based and Chapter 4, on aetiology, has been rewritten to describe the evidence-based approach to psychiatry. We have not thought it appropriate to provide references in a book for students. Readers who wish to review the evidence for our statements will find extensive references in the companion volume, *The Oxford Textbook of Psychiatry* (3rd edition). They may also wish to use the methods of searching the literature described in Chapter 4.

Oxford   M. G.
                                                                 R. M.
                                                                 J. G.

Contents

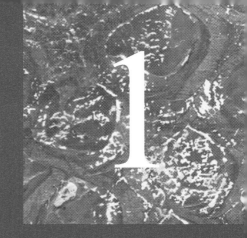

Signs and symptoms

- Signs, symptoms, and syndromes
- Description of symptoms and signs

Signs and symptoms

A sound knowledge of psychiatry is essential for all doctors because psychiatric problems are common in patients of all kinds. In general practice, for example, a quarter of the patients seen have a psychiatric problem, either alone or with a physical illness. In general hospital practice, many patients have psychiatric problems which may or may not be related to physical illness.

Students new to psychiatry often have concerns that the clinical skills required will be different from those of medicine and surgery. The skills required are in fact similar—careful history taking, systematic clinical examination, and sound clinical reasoning. The only major difference is that the clinical examination includes the mental as well as the physical state of the patient. Psychiatry also emphasizes the important clinical skill of communicating with patients—a skill that will enhance all clinical practice. However skilled a clinician may be in other ways, he will not use his skills to best effect unless he can communicate well with patients, enabling them to understand their own illness, how they can help themselves, and what the doctor can do.

Concern that psychiatric patients will behave in odd, unpredictable, or alarming ways may lead to a student avoiding talking to patients, preferring to learn only from books. This avoidance is misguided. While a small proportion of patients with the most severe disorders may behave oddly or unpredictably, only a very few behave in alarming ways. We recommend that the student should talk to as many patients as feasible. A textbook can certainly help the study of psychiatry, but talking to patients is essential for adequate learning.

All clinical medicine is part science, part art. The art is concerned with adapting scientific knowledge to the particular needs of a patient. To practise this art, the doctor must gain insight into the way that an illness affects the patient and his life. The doctor must therefore understand each patient as an individual. This understanding comes from knowledge about personality and the ways in which different people react to illness. The study of psychiatry provides the clinical student with a unique opportunity to learn about personality and individual differences. Such learning is best achieved by spending time listening to patients and their relatives.

This chapter is concerned with the description and definition of the symptoms and signs of psychiatric disorders. Chapter 2 deals with the ways of eliciting these symptoms and signs during clinical examination. Inevitably, the present chapter contains a large amount of detail, and readers may find it helpful to read it twice. During the first reading they should study the introductory sections and aim at a general understanding of the more frequent abnormal phenomena. During the second reading they should attend to the details of the abnormal phenomena, relating them whenever possible to known patients.

Signs, symptoms, and syndromes

In psychiatry, as in the rest of medicine, signs and symptoms often occur together in recognizable patterns known as 'syndromes'. It is important to identify syndromes because they give a better guide to treatment and prognosis than do individual signs or symptoms. For example, the symptom of depressed mood occurs in the syndromes of depressive disorder, dementia, and schizophrenia, which differ from one another in their prognosis and treatment. Depressed mood also occurs in people who are otherwise healthy, for example, the bereaved. The distinction between depressed mood and depressive disorder is particularly relevant in general medicine. The doctor may have to decide, for example, whether depressed mood in a cancer patient is a normal response to the prospect of dying, or whether it is part of a depressive disorder which would respond to treatment with antidepressant drugs.

The form and content of symptoms

Many psychiatric symptoms have two aspects: *form* and *content*. The distinction can be explained with an example. A patient may say that, when alone and out of hearing distance of other people, he hears voices telling him that he is a homosexual. The *form* of his experience is an auditory hallucination (a sensory perception in the absence of an external stimulus, see p. 7), and the *content* is the statement that he is a homosexual. A second patient may hear voices saying that he is about to be killed by persecutors. The form of this symptom is again an auditory hallucination, but the content is different. A third person may experience repeated intrusive thoughts that he is a homosexual but realize that these thoughts are untrue. The content of this symptom is the same as that of the first patient, but the form is different—an obsessional thought (see p. 14). In making a diagnosis, the form of the symptom is important: delusions and obsessional symptoms have a different diagnostic significance. In helping the patient, the content is important as a guide to how he may respond; for example, a deluded patient might attack someone whom he wrongly believes to be a persecutor.

Signs, symptoms, and the person

Although it is important to elicit the details of signs and symptoms of mental disorder, the doctor should never lose sight of the patient as a person. He should try to understand how the disorder affects the patient's feelings; for example, making him apprehensive or hopeless; and how it affects social roles, for example, as a parent. Thus, the doctor needs to understand what is it like for a depressed mother to have to care for small children, or for a person with schizophrenia to try to work despite experiencing hallucinations and persecutory delusions. The more the doctor can gain insight into these experiences, the more he can help his patient. A similar understanding is important when caring for patients with physical illnesses; hence, the experience gained during training in psychiatry is likely to be valuable in other clinical work.

OXFORD MEDICAL PUBLICATIONS

Psychiatry

Oxford Core Texts

Clinical Dermatology
Paediatrics
Endocrinology
Neurology
Psychiatry

Box 1.1 Association between mood and appearance

Depression

The corners of the mouth are turned down and the centre of the brow has vertical furrows. The head is inclined forward with the gaze directed downwards, and shoulders are bent. The patient's gestures are reduced.

Elation

A lively, cheerful expression. Posture and expressive movements are normal.

Anxiety

The brow is furrowed horizontally, the posture is tense, and the person is restless and sometimes tremulous. Often there are accompanying signs of autonomic overactivity, such as pale skin and increased sweating of the hands, feet, and axillae.

Anger

The eyebrows are drawn down, widening of the palpebral fissure, and a squaring of the corners of the mouth that may reveal the teeth. The shoulders are square and the body tense as if ready for action.

Description of symptoms and signs

Abnormalities of mood

Changes in mood are the most common symptoms of psychiatric disorder (Table 1.1). They are the prominent symptoms of depressive and anxiety disorders but can occur also in every kind of psychiatric disorder, and in the reactions of healthy people to stressful events and to physical illness. Sometimes the term *affect* is used instead of 'mood'; for example, 'the patient's affect is normal'. (This term is applied more commonly to syndromes in which mood change is the main feature, as in **affective disorder**.)

The terms *mood* and *affect* refer to depression, elation, anxiety, and anger. Irritability is a state in which anger occurs more readily than in normal people. Each mood state is accompanied by changes in facial expression and posture (see Box 1.1).

Abnormalities of the nature of mood

Pathological depression of mood is a pervasive lowering of mood which is accompanied by feelings of sadness and a loss of the ability to experience pleasure (*anhedonia*).

Pathological elation of mood is a pervasive raising of the mood accompanied by excessive cheerfulness or even ecstasy.

Pathological anxiety is a feeling of apprehension that is out of proportion to the actual situation. Often, there are accompanying signs of autonomic overactivity, such as pale skin and increased sweating of the hands, feet, and axillae. The term **phobia** denotes the symptom of anxiety arising in relation to a specific stimulus. The mood is identical to that of anxiety; it is the association with a particular object, event or situation that defines the phobia as a separate symptom.

Table 1.1.
Abnormalities of mood

Abnormalities in the nature of mood
- depression
- elation
- anxiety
- anger

Abnormalities in the variability of mood
- blunting, flattening
- lability
- 'incontinence'

Inconsistency between mood and thinking
- Incongruity of affect

Phobic anxiety is associated with a tendency to avoid the stimuli that evoke anxiety. A phobic person may experience anxiety when thinking about the stimulus but not in its presence (anticipatory anxiety). Phobias are common in healthy people; for example, phobias of spiders, snakes, thunderstorms, and high places. Phobias of these and other kinds are the prominent symptoms of phobic disorders (see pp. 111–17) and occur also as minor aspects of other anxiety disorders and of depressive disorders.

So-called 'obsessional phobias' are different; they are described on p. 15.

Abnormalities in the variability of mood

In healthy people mood varies from day to day. This normal variation may be disturbed in illness. Diminution of normal emotional responsiveness is called **blunting** or **flattening** of affect, while exaggerated responsiveness is called **labile mood**. When such changes are marked, the term **emotional incontinence** is sometimes used; this phenomenon occurs sometimes after strokes or as part of dementia.

Abnormalities in the consistency of mood with thinking

Mood is normally consistent with thoughts and actions. Thus, a person is likely to experience a mood of depression when recalling a sad event, or to experience a mood of elation when recalling a happy event. Sometimes (mainly in schizophrenia), mood and thinking are not consistent in this way; for example, the person may look and feel happy when thinking about a sad event. This phenomenon is called **incongruity of affect**. It has to be distinguished carefully from apparent cheerfulness that hides embarrassment. Some patients with depressive disorders fail to show the characteristic facial expression of depression even though their mood is very low (sometimes called 'smiling depression').

Depersonalization and derealization

These common symptoms are less easy to comprehend than anxiety or depression because they are less often experienced by healthy people.

Depersonalization is the experience of being unreal, detached, and unable to feel emotion. The lack of emotional responsiveness can be extremely distressing. People with this condition find it difficult to describe, and often use figures of speech such as 'it is as if I am cut off by a wall of glass'. A statement of this kind is a fanciful comparison ('as if'), and not a delusion (p. 10).

Derealization is a similar experience in relation to the environment: other people seem lifeless ('as if made of cardboard'), and objects lose their emotive quality.

Depersonalization and derealization can occur in healthy people (often when tired), and also as symptoms of any kind of psychiatric disorder, most often anxiety disorders, depressive disorders, and schizophrenia. They also occur in temporal lobe epilepsy.

Disorders of perception

Before considering abnormalities of perception, it is necessary to define two terms. **Perception** is the process of becoming aware of what is presented through the sense organs. **Imagery** is an experience within the mind, usually without the sense of reality that is part of perception. Imagery is experienced when a face is remembered or when we think in pictures. Imagery differs from perception in that it can be called up and terminated by voluntary effort, and is usually obliterated by actual perception in the same modality. Abnormalities of perception are of four kinds:

(1)   changes in the intensity of things perceived

(2)   changes in the quality of perception

(3)   illusions

(4)   hallucinations.

Each kind of abnormality will be described but with particular attention to hallucinations, which are of most significance in diagnosis. Sometimes, perception is normal in intensity and quality but has a changed **meaning** for the person who experiences it. This is a disorder of thinking, not of perception; nevertheless it is sometimes referred to incorrectly as delusional perception (see p. 11).

Changes in the intensity of perception

In mental disorder, perceptions can change in **intensity**. In mania they seem more intense, and in depressive disorder less intense.

Changes in the quality of perception

Perceptions can also change in **quality**, seeming distorted or unpleasant; for example, some schizophrenic patients report that food in general tastes unpleasant, or flowers smell acrid.

Illusions

An **illusion** is *a misperception of an external stimulus*. Illusions may occur in four circumstances:

1.   When the level of *sensory stimulation is reduced* (e.g. at dusk the outline of a bush may be misperceived as a man).

2.   When *attention is not focused* on the sensory modality (e.g. a person focusing on reading may mistakenly identify a sound as a voice).

3.   When the level of *consciousness is reduced*, during an illness (see delirium, pp. 314–15).

4.   When there is a *strong mood state* such as fear.

Illusions are experienced by healthy people, particularly when more than one of the above circumstances occur together; for example, when a frightened person is in a badly lit place. Illusions also occur with the reduced consciousness of delirium, especially when sensory stimulation is reduced (see p. 188).

Hallucinations

A **hallucination** is *a perception experienced in the absence of an external stimulus to the corresponding sense organ*; for example, hearing a voice when no one is speaking within hearing distance. A hallucination has two special qualities:

1.   It is experienced as a true perception, not as imaginary.

2.   It seems to come from the outside world (except in the rare case of somatic hallucinations, see below).

Unless the experience has these two qualities it is not a hallucination. (Experiences that possess one of these qualities, but not the other, are called **pseudohallucinations**.)

Although hallucinations are generally regarded as the hallmark of mental disorder, healthy people experience them occasionally, especially when falling asleep (**hypnagogic hallucinations**) or waking (**hypnopompic hallucinations**). These normal hallucinations are brief, and usually of a simple kind such as hearing a bell ring or a name called. Usually, the person wakes suddenly and quickly recognizes the nature of the experience. These two kinds of hallucination do not point to mental disorder.

Types of hallucination Hallucinations can occur in all sensory modalities but those of hearing and seeing are most frequent (Table 1.2).

Auditory hallucinations may be experienced as voices, noises, or music. Hallucinatory voices may seem to speak words, phrases, or sentences. The main kinds of auditory hallucination are shown in Table 1.2. Some address the patient as 'you' (*second person hallucinations*), while others talk about the patient as 'he' or 'she' (*third person hallucinations*), which are characteristic of schizophrenia (see p. 165) Sometimes, a voice seems to say what the patient is about to say; sometimes it repeats what he has just been thinking (*thought echo*).

Visual hallucinations may be experienced as flashes of light or as complex images such as the figure of man. They usually appear normal in size, but sometimes are unusually small or large. Visual hallucinations are associated particularly with organic mental disorders but can occur in other conditions.

Hallucinations of smell and taste are uncommon. They may be recognizable smells or flavours but more often they are unlike any smell or flavour that has been experienced before, and have an unpleasant quality.

Tactile hallucinations are also uncommon. They may be experienced as superficial sensations of being touched, pricked, or strangled; or as sensations just below the skin which may be attributed to insects or other small creatures burrowing through the tissues.

Hallucinations of deep sensation are also uncommon. They may be experienced as feelings of the viscera being pulled or distended, or as sexual stimulation.

Diagnostic associations of hallucinations Hallucinations may occur in all kinds of severe psychiatric disorder (affective disorders, schizophrenia, and organic disorders) and, as explained above, occasionally among healthy people. *Visual hallucinations* occur particularly in organic psychiatric disorders, but also in severe affective disorders and schizophrenia. Although not specific to organic disorder, they should always prompt a thorough search for other evidence of this diagnosis (see pp. 192–4). The finding of hallucinations does not generally point to a particular diagnosis. The uncommon hallucinations of taste, smell, and deep sensation occur mainly in schizophrenia. There are some special kinds of hallucination that characterize a particular disorder; they are explained in the chapters on clinical syndromes.

Table 1.2.

Classification of hallucination

According to sensory modality
- auditory
- visual
- of smell or taste
- of tactile sensations
- of deep sensations

Special kinds of auditory hallucination
- second person
- third person
- echoing or repeating thoughts

Disorders of thinking

The term **thought disorder** denotes five kinds of abnormality:

(1) abnormality of the amount and speed of thought (the **stream** of thought);

(2) abnormality of the ways in which thoughts are linked together (the **form** of thought);

(3) **delusions**;

(4) **overvalued ideas**;

(5) **obsessional and compulsive symptoms**.

Disorders of the stream of thought

In disorders of the stream of thought both the amount and the speed of thoughts are changed. There are three main abnormalities:

1. **Pressure of thought** Thoughts are unusually rapid, abundant, and varied. It characteristically occurs in mania but also in schizophrenia

2. **Poverty of thought** Thoughts are unusually slow, few, and unvaried. It characteristically occurs in severe depressive disorder, but also in schizophrenia.

3. **Thought blocking** The mind is suddenly empty of thoughts. Thought blocking should not be confused with sudden distraction, or the intrusion of a different line of thinking. Healthy people sometimes have the experience of losing the train of thought ('the mind going blank'). Thought blocking should be recorded only when the patient describes the characteristic experience of an abrupt and complete emptying of the mind. It occurs especially in schizophrenic patients, who may interpret the experience in an odd way, saying that their thoughts have been removed by another person (see p. 165).

Disorders of the form of thought

There are three main disorders of the ways in which thoughts are linked together:

1. **Flight of ideas** Thoughts and conversations move quickly from one topic to another, so that one train of thought is not completed before the next is taken up. Because the topics change so rapidly, the links between one topic and another may be difficult to follow, but nonetheless the links are understandable. The links are of several kinds: *rhyming*, for example, following a phrase containing the word 'chair', with another containing the word 'pear' (this sequence is sometimes called *clang association*); or *punning*, that, is using a sound that has more than one meaning (e.g. male/mail). In addition, a new train of thought may be set off by a *distracting cue* in the environment. Flight of ideas is characteristic of mania.

2. **Loosening of associations** A lack of logical connection between the parts of a train of thought, not explicable by the processes described under flight of ideas. This lack of logical association is sometimes called *knight's move thinking* (referring to the indirect move of the knight in chess). Usually, the interviewer is alerted to the presence of loosening of associations because the patient's conversation seems muddled and hard to follow. This muddled thinking differs from that due to

anxiety or low intelligence. Anxious people become more coherent when put at ease, and those of low intelligence do so when questions are simplified. When there is loosening of associations, the links between ideas cannot be made more understandable in either of these ways. Instead, the interviewer has the experience that the more he tries to clarify the patient's thinking, the less he understands it. Loosening of associations occurs most often in schizophrenia. Several specific kinds of loosening of association have been identified in schizophrenia. They are described in chapter 1 of *The Oxford Textbook of Psychiatry*.

3. **Perseveration** The persistent and inappropriate repetition of the same sequence of thought, as shown by repetition of speech or actions. It can be demonstrated by asking a series of questions; the patient gives the correct answer to the first question, but continues to give the same answer inappropriately to subsequent questions that require a different answer. Perseveration occurs most often in dementia but may occur in other disorders

Loosening of associations is often difficult to distinguish reliably from flight of ideas. It can be useful to tape-record a sample of speech and listen to it repeatedly.

Delusions

A **delusion** is *a belief that is held firmly but on inadequate grounds, is not affected by rational argument or evidence to the contrary, and is not a conventional belief that the person might be expected to hold given his cultural background and level of education.* This rather lengthy definition is required to distinguish delusions, which are indicators of mental disorder, from other kinds of strongly held belief found among healthy people. A delusion is usually a false belief but not always so (see below).

The statement that a delusion is held on inadequate grounds means that it is arrived at through *abnormal thought processes*. It is held so strongly that it is not altered by evidence to the contrary that would convince other people. For example, a patient who holds the delusion that persecutors are in the next room will not alter his belief when shown that the room is empty; instead, he may suggest that the persecutors left in some improbable way before the room was opened. The strength of a belief is not enough to define it as a delusion because some normal people have non-delusional beliefs that are impervious to evidence that would convince most other people. For example, a person who has been brought up to believe in spiritualism is unlikely to change his conviction when presented with contrary evidence that a non-believer would find convincing, but his strongly held conviction is not a delusion

Although delusions are almost always false beliefs, occasionally they are true or subsequently become true. For example, a man may develop the delusional belief that his wife is unfaithful when there is no evidence of infidelity of any kind and no other rational reason for holding the belief. Such a belief has been arrived at in an abnormal way, even if the wife is in fact unfaithful. The important point is that a belief is delusional not because it is false but because it was derived in an abnormal way. Although the point is of theoretical importance, in practice it seldom gives rise to difficulties.

Although delusional beliefs are usually odd, it is a mistake to assume that a belief is delusional simply because of its oddness. Some people express strange beliefs (e.g. attempted poisoning by a relative), which are eventually confirmed by facts. Such beliefs should therefore be investigated to determine whether they could be factually correct.

Some delusions occur as sudden and total convictions. Other delusions develop more gradually, starting from a belief that is not held with complete conviction. Similarly, delusions may weaken gradually as the amount of conviction decreases. Such less firm beliefs are called *partial delusions*—a term that should be used only when the belief is known to have been preceded by full delusional conviction, or applied with hindsight to a belief that developed later into a full delusion (but could not have been known to be a partial delusion at the time).

Although a patient may be convinced totally that his delusional belief is true, this conviction does not necessarily influence all his feelings and actions. This separation of belief from feeling and action occurs most often in chronic schizophrenia: for example, a patient may have the false fixed belief that he is a member of the Royal Family and yet live contentedly in a hostel for discharged psychiatric patients.

Primary and secondary delusions A **primary delusion** occurs *suddenly*, with *complete conviction*, and *without any other abnormal mental event* leading up to it. It is, therefore, difficult to understand how the delusion arose. For example, a patient may suddenly develop the unshakable conviction that he is changing sex, without ever having thought so before and without any event that could have prompted the idea. In practice, it is often difficult to decide whether or not a delusion is primary, because patients do not find it easy to recall and explain the exact sequence of their abnormal experiences. Primary delusions are rare, and may be too readily diagnosed by inexperienced interviewers. It is important to avoid this error, because primary delusions are important evidence for schizophrenia.

Three other terms are used sometimes to describe special kinds of primary delusions. The first is used when a delusion is preceded by a change (not an abnormality) in mood. The patient feels threatened without knowing why, searches for an explanation and then becomes convinced, for example, that he is being followed. This phenomenon is called **delusional mood** (it is really the mood preceding a delusion). The second term is used when a delusion begins as a sudden misinterpretation of the significance of something perceived. For example, a patient may suddenly believe that the arrangement of objects on a table indicates that his life is threatened. This phenomenon is sometimes called **delusional perception** (but it is really a delusional of a normal percept). The third term, **delusional memory**, is applied when a delusion misinterprets past events, usually in someone who is already deluded. For example, a patient may hold the delusion that others are trying to poison him; he may then develop the belief that poison was put in his food on a previous occasion when he felt ill, even though he did not hold this belief at the time. In fact, the memory is normal; it is the interpretation of the remembered event that is abnormal.

A **secondary delusion** arises understandably from *a preceding abnormal experience*. The preceding abnormal experience may be of various kinds such as:

- *a hallucination*: for example, a person hears a voice and believes he is being followed;
- *a mood*: for example, a person with deep depression believes that other people think he is worthless;
- *another delusion*: for example, a person with the delusion that he has no money believes he will be imprisoned for unpaid debt.

Some secondary delusions have an integrative function, making more sense of the original abnormal experience (as in the first example). Others increase the patient's distress (as in the other examples). In this way some patients develop a series of secondary delusions related to one another ('systemized delusions' which form a **delusional system**).

Shared delusions Usually, other people recognize delusional beliefs as false and they argue with the deluded person in an attempt to correct them. Occasionally, a person who lives with a deluded patient comes to share the delusional beliefs. This person is then said to have shared delusions or **folie à deux** (see p. 181). The affected person's conviction is often unshakable as long as he remains with the patient, but usually weakens quickly when the two are separated.

Delusional themes Delusions are usually grouped according to their main themes. (Table 1.3) Since there is some correspondence between delusional theme and type of disorder, which is helpful in diagnosis, the main themes will be described briefly and related to the disorders in which they occur most often. The associations are described more fully in the chapters on these disorders.

1. **Persecutory** delusions are often called **paranoid** delusions. (Strictly speaking, the word 'paranoid' refers to all kinds of false belief about relationships between people so that grandiose, jealous, and amorous delusions can also be called paranoid.) Most persecutory delusions are concerned with people or organizations that are believed by the patient to be trying to inflict harm on him, damage his reputation, or make him insane. In assessing such ideas it is important to remember that in some cultures it is normal to ascribe misfortunes to the malign activities of other people who are believed to practise witchcraft, and such ideas are not delusions. Persecutory delusions are common in **schizophrenia**, and also occur in **organic states** and **severe depressive disorders**. A patient with a depressive disorder characteristically accepts that the supposed actions of his persecutors are justified by his own wickedness; in schizophrenia he characteristically resents them.

2. **Delusions of reference** are concerned with the idea that objects, events, or the actions of people have a special significance for the patient. For example, a remark heard on television is believed to be directed specifically to the patient; or a gesture by a stranger is believed to convey something about the patient. Delusions of this kind are associated with **schizophrenia**.

3. **Grandiose and expansive delusions** are beliefs of exaggerated self-importance. The patient may think himself wealthy, endowed with unusual abilities, or

Table 1.3.
Delusional themes

1. persecutory (paranoid)
2. of reference
3. grandiose and expansive
4. of guilt and worthlessness
5. nihilistic
6. hypochondriacal
7. of jealousy
8. sexual or amorous
9. of control
10. religious
11. concerning the possession of thoughts

in other ways special. Such ideas occur mainly in **mania** and sometimes in **schizophrenia**.

4. **Delusions of guilt and worthlessness** are beliefs that the person has done something shameful or sinful. Usually, the belief concerns an innocent error that did not cause guilt at the time (e.g. a patient may be convinced that a small error in an income tax return will be discovered and lead to prosecution). This kind of delusion occurs most often in **severe depressive disorders**.

5. **Nihilistic delusions** are, strictly speaking, beliefs about the non-existence of some person or thing, but the meaning is extended to include beliefs that the patient's career is finished, that he is about to die or has no money, or that the world is doomed. Nihilistic delusions occur most often in **severe depressive disorders**.

6. **Hypochondriacal delusions** are false beliefs about illness. The patient believes, in the face of convincing medical evidence to the contrary, that he is ill. Such delusions are more common among the elderly, reflecting the increasing concerns about health in later life. Related delusions are concerned with the appearance of parts of the body, for example, the belief that the (normally shaped) nose is seriously misshapen. Patients with these delusions about their appearance may seek the help of plastic surgeons. Delusions of these kinds occur in depressive disorders and schizophrenia. (Other kinds of hypochondriacal ideas are discussed on pp. 216–18.)

7. **Delusions of jealousy** are more common among men. They may lead to dangerously aggressive behaviour towards the person who is believed to be unfaithful (see pathological jealousy, pp. 179–81).

8. **Sexual or amorous delusions** are more frequent among women. Usually, the woman believes that she is loved by a man who has never spoken to her and who is inaccessible—for example, an eminent public figure.

9. **Delusions of control** are beliefs that personal actions, impulses, or thoughts are controlled by an outside agency. This experience has to be distinguished from two others: first, hearing hallucinatory voices giving commands which are obeyed voluntarily; and second, holding culturally normal beliefs concerning the divine control of human actions. Delusions of control strongly suggest **schizophrenia**.

10. **Religious delusions** may be guilty (concerned, for example, with divine punishment for minor sins), or expansive (concerned with special powers). It is important to determine whether the belief is a true delusion or a belief that is widely held by members of a religious group, and therefore not a delusion

11. **Delusions concerning the possession of thoughts**. Healthy people have no doubt that their thoughts are their own and can be known to other people only if spoken aloud or revealed through behaviour. Some patients hold abnormal beliefs concerning the possession of thoughts, for example: (i) that some of their thoughts are not their own but have been implanted by an outside agency—the *delusion of thought insertion*; (ii) that some of their thoughts have been taken away—the *delusion*

of thought withdrawal; (iii) that their thoughts are known to other people through telepathy, radio, or some other unusual way—the *delusion of thought broadcasting*. All three symptoms are found most often in schizophrenia.

Overvalued ideas

An **overvalued idea** is an *isolated, preoccupying strongly held belief that dominates a person's life and may affect his actions but (unlike a delusion) has been derived through normal mental processes.* For example, a person whose parents developed cancer within a short time may be convinced that cancer is contagious even though his doctor presented evidence to the contrary, and may avoid visiting a friend with cancer who has asked to see him. The distinction between overvalued ideas and delusions may be difficult to make, since the two kinds of idea can be equally strongly held and the differentiation depends on a retrospective judgement by the interviewer about the way in which the idea was formed. In practice, this difficulty seldom causes problems since diagnoses are not made on a single symptom, but on the pattern of several symptoms. When there is doubt about whether a particular idea is a delusion, there are usually other ideas that are clearly delusional, or symptoms of a different kind.

Obsessional and compulsive symptoms

Obsessions are *recurrent and persistent thoughts, impulses, or images that enter the mind despite efforts to exclude them.* The characteristic feature is the subjective sense of a struggle (resistance) against the intruding mental phenomena. The person has no doubt that the intruding thoughts are produced in his own mind rather than implanted from elsewhere (a point of contrast with delusions of the possession of thoughts described above). Usually, obsessions are about matters which the person finds distressing or unpleasant. The person recognizes that the ideas are senseless and usually feels ashamed to tell other people about them.

Resistance is an important feature because it distinguishes obsessions (in which resistance is present) from delusions (in which it is absent). When obsessions have been present for a long time, resistance may decrease so that this distinction becomes difficult to make. In practice, this difficulty seldom causes diagnostic problems because by the time that resistance has diminished the diagnosis has usually been made.

Obsessions have to be *distinguished from*:

1. Ordinary preoccupations of healthy people.

2. Intrusive concerns of anxious or depressed patients (see p. 105).

3. Recurring thoughts and images associated with disorders of sexual preference (see p. 301).

4. Recurring thoughts and images associated with drug dependency.

5. Delusions.

Patients with these non-obsessional ideas do not regard them as unreasonable, and do not resist them. Obsessional symptoms are essential features of **obsessive-compulsive disorder**, and occur sometimes in many kinds of psychiatric disorder, especially anxiety and depressive disorders.

Types of obsessional symptoms

Obsessions can occur in several forms:

- *Obsessional thoughts* are repeated, intrusive words or phrases, such as obscenities or blasphemies; or thoughts about distressing occurrences (e.g. that the hands have become contaminated with bacteria which will spread disease).

- *Obsessional ruminations* are more complicated sequences of thoughts (e.g. about the ending of the world).

- *Obsessional doubts* are uncertainties about a previous action (e.g. whether or not the person has switched off an electrical appliance that might catch fire).

- *Obsessional impulses* are urges to carry out actions, which are usually aggressive, dangerous, or socially embarrassing (e.g. using a knife to stab someone, jumping in front of a moving train, or shouting obscenities in church). Whatever the urge, the person recognizes that it is irrational and does not wish to carry it out. This is an important point of distinction from delusions, which are regarded as rational by the patient, and which may lead to action, such as aggression against a supposed persecutor.

- *Obsessional phobia* is the term sometimes applied to obsessional thoughts with a fearful content (e.g. 'I may have cancer') or to obsessional impulses that arouse anxiety (e.g. the urge to stab another person). The term is confusing and is best avoided by using one of the four terms given in the preceding paragraphs.

Content of obsessional thoughts Obsessional thoughts can be about any topic but most are centred around six themes. Why this should be so is not known. The six themes are:

(1) **dirt and contamination** for example, the idea that the hands are contaminated with bacteria;

(2) **aggressive actions** for example, the idea that the person may harm another person, or shout angry remarks;

(3) **orderliness** for example, the idea that objects have to be arranged in a special way, or clothes put on in a particular order;

(4) **illness** for example, the idea that the person may have cancer (ideas of contamination may also refer to illness; e.g. that a disease may result from the feared bacterial contamination);

(5) **sex** usually thoughts or images of practices that the person finds disgusting;

(6) **religion** for example, blasphemous thoughts, or doubts about the fundamentals of belief (e.g 'does God exist?'), or about the adequacy or completeness of a religious practice such as confession.

Compulsions Compulsions are *repeated, stereotyped, and seemingly purposeful actions which the person feels compelled to carry out but resists, recognizing that they are irrational.* Compulsions are also known as *compulsive rituals*. Although compulsions are not thoughts but abnormal actions, it is convenient to describe them here. Most compulsions are associated with obsessions. In some cases the association seems under-

Table 1.4.

Obsessional and compulsive symptoms

Obsessions
- thoughts
- ruminations
- doubts
- impulses
- phobias

Compulsions (*rituals*)
- checking
- cleaning
- counting
- dressing

standable, as when handwashing is associated with ideas that the hands are contaminated. In other cases there is no obvious connection between the actions and the thoughts, as when checking the position of objects is associated with aggressive ideas. Most compulsions produce an immediate lessening of the distress associated with obsessional thoughts (e.g. handwashing) although their long-term effect is to prolong them (see p. 120). Compulsions may be accompanied by doubting thoughts that the behaviours have not been executed correctly, leading to further repetitions. In this way, the behaviour may be prolonged for hours.

Compulsions can be of any kind but there are four common themes (Table 1.4):

(1) **checking rituals**, which are often concerned with safety (e.g. checking repeatedly that a gas tap has been turned off);

(2) **cleaning rituals** such as repeated handwashing or domestic cleaning;

(3) **counting rituals** such as counting to a particular number or counting in threes;

(4) **dressing rituals** in which the clothes are set out or put on in a particular way.

Motor symptoms and signs

Abnormalities of *facial expression*, *posture*, and *social behaviour* are common in mental disorders of all kinds. Motor abnormalities such as **mannerisms, sterotypies**, and **catatonic symptoms** are briefly described in the chapter on schizophrenia (p. 167) and more extensively in the *Oxford Textbook of Psychiatry*. Here we will describe movement disorders which are not defined elsewhere:

Tics are *irregular repeated movements involving a group of muscles* (e.g. a sideways movement of the head).

Choreiform movements are *brief involuntary movements which are co-ordinated but purposeless*, such as grimacing or movements of the arms.

Dystonia is *a muscle spasm*, which is often painful and may lead to contortions.

Disorders of memory

In order to describe abnormalities of memory it is necessary to have a classification of normal memory. There are several schemes of which the following is useful in clinical practice (although it does not correspond completely with research findings). Memory can be thought of as having three kinds of 'store':

1. **Sensory stores** receive information from the sense organs and retain it for a brief period (about 0.5 second) until it has been processed.

2. **Short-term memory** stores hold information for longer (about 15–20 seconds). Information can be retained for longer by repeated rehearsal (e.g. when an unfamiliar phone number is repeated until it can be dialled).

3. **Long-term memory** receives information that has been selected for more permanent storage, and has a much larger capacity than the other two. Information is stored according to characteristics such as meaning or the sound of words. The mood state at the time of storage is important: memo-

ries stored when the person was unhappy are recalled more readily in an unhappy than in a happy state of mind. Two useful distinctions can be made about long-term memory. The first is between memory for events (*episodic memory*) and memory for language and knowledge (*semantic memory*). The second is between *recognition* of material presented, and *recall* without such a cue (the latter being more difficult).

Several terms are used to describe abnormalities of memory:

- **Anterograde amnesia** occurs after a period of unconsciousness. It is impairment of memory for events between the ending of complete unconsciousness and the restoration of full consciousness.

- **Retrograde amnesia** is loss of memory for events before the onset of unconsciousness. It occurs after head injury or electroconvulsive therapy (ECT).

- **Jamais vu** is failure to recognize events that have been encountered before, while **déjà vu** is the recognition of events as familiar when they have never been encountered. Both abnormalities may occur in neurological disorders.

- **Confabulation** is the reporting as 'memories' of events that did not take place at the time in question. It occurs in some patients with severe disorders of recent memory (see the *amnesic syndrome*, p. 195).

Memory is affected in several kinds of psychiatric disorder. In *depressive disorder* unhappy memories are recalled more readily than other kinds of memory. In *organic disorder* all aspects of long-term memory are usually affected, although the memory of earlier events is impaired less than that of more recent ones. In some organic disorders there is a differential impairment (the *amnesic syndrome*) in which the memory for recent events is most affected, and semantic memory least (see p. 195).

Disorders of consciousness

Consciousness is awareness of the self and the environment. Its level varies between the extremes of coma and alertness. Several terms are used for the intervening states of consciousness:

- **Clouding of consciousness** refers to a state of drowsiness with: incomplete reaction to stimuli; impaired attention, concentration, and memory; and slow, muddled thinking.

- **Stupor** refers to a state in which the person is mute, immobile, and unresponsive, but appears to be conscious because the eyes are open and follow external objects. (This is the usage in psychiatry: in neurology the same term often implies a degree of impairment of consciousness.)

- **Confusion** refers properly to muddled thinking but the term **confusional state** is sometimes applied to a state in which muddled thinking is associated with impairment of consciousness, illusions, hallucinations, delusions, and anxiety. *Delirium* is a better term for this syndrome.

Disorders of attention and concentration

Attention is the ability to focus on the matter in hand. *Concentration* is the ability to maintain that focus. Attention and concentration can be impaired in many kinds of psychiatric disorder but especially in anxiety disorder, depressive disorder, mania, schizophrenia, and organic disorder. Detection of impaired attention or concentration does not help in diagnosis but is important in assessing the patient's disability; for example, poor concentration may prevent a person from working effectively in an office.

Insight

As a technical term **insight** means *a correct awareness of one's own mental condition.* Insight is not simply present or absent, but a matter of degree. It is described best in terms of four criteria:

1. Awareness of oneself as presenting phenomena that other people consider abnormal (e.g. being unusually active and elated).

2. Recognition that these phenomena are abnormal.

3. Acceptance that these abnormal phenomena are caused by one's own mental illness (rather than, for example, poison administered by a persecutor).

4. Awareness that treatment is required.

In general, insight is lost to a greater extent in psychosis than in non-psychotic disorders. Assessment of insight is extremely important in determining a patient's likely cooperation with treatment: for example, a patient who believes that he is being persecuted may not accept that his beliefs are a sign of illness, and may not be willing to accept treatment. None the less he may be aware that he is distressed and sleeping badly, and agree to accept help with these problems (which he ascribes to the persecution).

Further reading

Sims, A. C. P. (1995). *Symptoms in the Mind* (2nd edn). W. B. Saunders, London. *A comprehensive textbook of the symptoms and signs of psychiatric disorder.*

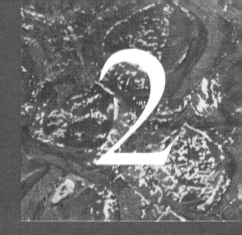

Interviewing and clinical evaluation

- General advice about interviewing

- Interviewing an informant

- Taking a psychiatric history

- Brief interviews for screening

- Mental state examination

- Some difficulties in mental state examination

- Physical examination

- Special investigations

- Psychological assessment

- Interviewing relatives

- Interviews in an emergency

- Risk assessment

- The formulation

Interviewing and clinical evaluation

The clinical interview is very important in psychiatry because it is the main method used to:

- obtain the necessary information to make a diagnosis;
- understand the person with the illness;
- understand the circumstances of the patient;
- form a therapeutic relationship with the patient;
- provide the patient with information about the illness, treatment recommendations, and prognosis.

In practice, these functions may occur during the same interview. However, by keeping the aims of the interview clearly in mind, the clinician can modify the interview for specific clinical situations.

A successful interview (in which accurate information is obtained for diagnosis, a good relationship is formed between patient and doctor and the patient understands the doctors recommendations) is more likely when the clinician has good interviewing skills.

This chapter contains advice about diagnostic interviewing, and about the evaluation of information obtained from interviews. The main aim of such an interview is to obtain the information required to formulate a treatment plan. In psychiatry, interviews are also used **as treatment**: advice about psychological treatment is given in Chapter 17.

Interviewing is a practical skill, which can be learnt effectively only when reading is supplemented both by watching experienced interviewers at work and by practising under supervision. The reader will need this practical training as well as the advice presented in this chapter.

General advice about interviewing

This section applies to interviewing in any medical interview.

Putting the patient at ease

This initial step need not take long but requires attention to small details of the arrangements for the interview.

- If possible, interviewing should be carried out in a place where the conversation cannot be overheard. Privacy may be difficult to obtain when the patient is seen in a medical ward or crowded home; if at all practicable a move should be made to more private surroundings, such as a side room on a medical ward or another room in the home.

- The arrangements for seating are important. If possible, sit at an angle to the patient rather than immediately opposite, so that the patient does not feel under constant scrutiny. (For a right-handed interviewer, it is best if the patient sits on the interviewer's left, since in this way it is easier to attend to the patient while taking notes.) When interviewing at the bedside, sit beside the patient rather than stand over him.

- Greet the patient by name. Most patients prefer to be greeted formally initially using Mr/Mrs/Miss.

- Introduce yourself with your own name and your role (doctor, locum doctor, medical student, etc.).

- Explain how the interview will proceed, how long it will last, and why it is necessary to take notes.

Starting the interview

Begin the interview with a general question which encourages the patient to express the problem in his own words: for example, 'tell me about your problem'; or 'tell me what you have noticed wrong'.

During the reply, observe whether the patient appears at ease, cooperative, and able to express himself coherently. Several problems may occur at this early stage. Often, the patient is anxious despite the interviewer's efforts to put him at ease. If this occurs, try to find out the cause of the anxiety and, if possible, reassure the patient. For example, the patient may be worried that his statements may be passed to someone else without his permission; or he may have come to the interview reluctantly at someone else's insistence (as often happens, for example, if the patient has an alcohol problem). If present, these concerns should be discussed and appropriate assurance should be given before the interview continues.

If the patient responds to the initial request for information in a muddled way, try to find out the reason. A muddled response may be due to:

- anxiety;

- low intelligence;

- cognitive impairment because of a confusional state or dementia.

If cognitive impairment seems possible, brief tests of concentration and memory (see pp. 35–7) should be given. If the test results are abnormal, consider whether it may be better to stop the interview and obtain a clearer history from an informant. These problems may arise, for example, when an elderly demented patient is interviewed at home by the general practitioner, or when a patient with an acute organic disorder is interviewed in a medical ward.

When the patient has completed an initial account of the problem, make a systematic enquiry about the complaints. For such an enquiry, it is important to *avoid closed questions and leading questions*. A closed question allows only a brief answer, usually 'yes' or 'no'; a leading question suggests the answer. Thus, 'do you wake early?' is a closed leading question; 'at what time do you wake?' is an open, non-leading question. Sometimes, the interviewer must ask a leading question in order to check an important point. Such a question should be followed by a request for an example. Thus, the question 'have you ever felt that your actions were being controlled by another person?' is a leading question about an important symptom of schizophrenia. When this question is answered affirmatively, the interviewer should ask the patient to provide examples of the experience, and should record the symptoms as present only if the examples are convincing.

If it is difficult to establish the exact dates of an event, a useful method is to relate the event in question to another event that is more likely to be fixed in the patient's mind, for example, family birthdays and holidays.

Proceeding with the interview

As the interview progresses, the interviewer's task is to keep the patient to relevant topics, while letting him talk freely. The skill is to achieve the optimal balance.

If too many questions are asked unselectively, irrelevant information may be obtained at the expense of unexpected relevant information (e.g. about an extra-marital affair). If the interviewer asks too few questions, he may miss important details, for example, the exact order in which events and symptoms occurred. The decisions which questions to use and when to interrupt depend on whether the clinician is getting the relevant information to test the specific diagnostic hypotheses. This requires good knowledge about what clinical information is important and also becomes easier with increasing clinical experience.

Non-verbal communication

As well as questions, the interviewer's non-verbal cues are important in guiding the interview. To encourage the patient to speak more, the interviewer may show increased concern, for example, by leaning forward to attend more closely, or by nodding to indicate that a point has been noted. To curb a flow of irrelevant talk, the interviewer can temporarily withhold these expressions of concern. If this is not effective, the interviewer may need to wait until a break in the patient's flow of words and may then explain the need to cover certain points systematically.

Finishing the interview

At the end of the interview, ask the patient whether he wishes to raise any questions or points that have not been mentioned.

Interviewing an informant

It is always valuable to interview another **informant** as well as the patient. An informant can provide essential information:

• when the patient is unaware of the extent of his abnormality (e.g. a disinhibited manic patient, or a demented patient with poor memory);

• when the patient knows the extent of the problem but does not reveal it (e.g. a patient with an alcohol problem);

• about the patient's premorbid personality.

It is best to see the patient first alone, then the informant alone and then both together. The patient and informant should be interviewed alone because the presence of the other person frequently inhibits the interviewee. For example, the wife of a patient may be reluctant to talk about her husband's delusions in front of him because he will become angry.

For out-patients, it is good practice to ask the patient for permission to speak to anyone accompanying him, and if appropriate, to arrange to see this person later. For in-patients or intensive management in the community, it is usually appropriate for the multidisciplinary team to ensure that the appropriate carers and relatives are interviewed and involved in treatment planning.

Taking a psychiatric history

A psychiatric history has the basic structure shown in Box 2.1. Several of the items require systematic enquiries which will be explained below. Clinical students should enure that they can take a full history by repeated practice. Once they have developed their knowledge of psychiatric disorders and gained more experience, they can move to a more selective hypothetical–deductive approach which is more likely to be useful in hospital emergency departments or in general practice.

The priorities in the initial diagnostic interview are not only to identify whether a specific diagnosis can be reached, but also to identify other problems which the patient may have and to provide a context for the diagnosis. This is important in planning treatment and estimating prognosis.

Below, we present the conventional psychiatric history which is a useful format to use when starting to learn psychiatry and remains a useful way of organizing information even for the experienced clinician.

The presenting problem

The patient's description of the problem should be given in his own words, with adequate time and without interruption. If the interviewer asks systematic questions too early, important problems may not be revealed. For example, a patient who begins by describing depression may have an associated obsessional disorder; or a patient who presents with anxiety may also have an eating disorder. In each case, the second problem may be missed if the interviewer starts questioning too soon. Also, when the patient has finished his account, the interviewer should summarize the problems and ask if there are others: for example, 'you have told me about your problems with anxiety and depression; are there any other problems?'. The patient might then reveal abuse of alcohol.

The nature of the problem
Questions should then be asked to clarify the **nature** of the problem. For example, a patient who complains of worrying excessively could be describing anxiety, obsessional symptoms, or the intrusive thoughts that occur in a depressive disorder.

The severity of the problem
Next, assess symptoms in terms of their intensity, the degree of distress caused, and the resultant interference with day-to-day activities.

Other relevant problems and symptoms
The sort of information that is relevant about other problems and symptoms depends on the presenting problem. Asking the right questions requires knowledge of the clinical syndromes described in subsequent chapters. For example, if the presenting problem is poor sleep, questions will be asked about the symptoms

Box 2.1 **The psychiatric history**

Name, age, and address of the patient; name of any informants, and their relationship to the patient

History of present condition	• Patient's description of the problem
	• Details of the nature of the problem and present severity of the symptoms
	• Systematic enquiry about other relevant problems and symptoms
	• Onset and course of symptoms, and problems
Family history	• Parents: age (now or at death), occupation, personality, and relationship with the patient
	• Similar information about siblings
	• Social position; atmosphere of the home
	• Mental disorder in other members of the (extended) family, and abuse of alcohol and drugs
Personal history	• Mother's pregnancy and the birth
	• Early development
	• Childhood separations, emotional problems, illnesses
	• Schooling and higher education
	• Occupations
	• Sexual relationships
	• Menstrual history
	• Marriage
	• Children
	• Social circumstances
	• Forensic history
Past illness	• Past medical history
	• Past psychiatric history
Personality	• Relationships
	• Leisure activities
	• Prevailing mood
	• Character
	• Attitudes and standards
	• Habits

Drugs, alcohol, tobacco

of syndromes that can cause poor sleep (see p. 237). Such questions will be concerned with depressive symptoms, anxiety symptoms, excessive use of alcohol or caffeine, or painful physical conditions, all of which could be relevant. For each presenting problem there is a repertoire of relevant questions. If an inexperienced interviewer is uncertain what questions to ask, he should obtain information by asking the patient to recount his experiences in more detail.

The onset and course of the problems

The onset and course of the problems and symptoms are considered next. The onset may be sudden or gradual, and it may be spontaneous or provoked by events. The course may be continuous or intermittent; the severity may increase gradually or stepwise. The onset of different groups of symptoms should be compared: for example, it is important to find out whether obsessional symptoms began before or after depressive symptoms, since this information is important in the choice of treatment. The same applies to problems: for example, whether abuse of alcohol began before or after marital difficulties. A record should be made of any treatment already received.

If these enquiries are systematic, they need not take long. When they are complete, the interviewer should explain that he is interested in learning next about the patient's background, starting with questions about the family.

The family history

This part of the history concerns the family in which the patient grew up: it is an account of the patient's father, mother, siblings, and if appropriate, other relatives. Enquiries about the patient's spouse and children are made later in the history. The family history is important for three reasons:

1. Some psychiatric disorders have *genetic causes*, and the finding of mental disorder in other members of the family may be relevant to this kind of cause.

2. The family is usually the *environment* in which the patient grew up, and circumstances, such as the separation or divorce of parents, or rivalry between siblings, may be relevant to the patient's psychological development.

3. *Events happening currently* to members of the family, such as the recent death of an elderly parent or the illness of a sibling, may act as stressors to the patient, or may explain some of his concerns (e.g. the recent discovery of a brain tumour in a brother may explain the patient's excessive concerns about headaches).

The amount of detail required will depend on the likely diagnoses: for example, if time is limited it is unlikely to be profitable to make detailed enquiries about the childhood environment of an elderly patient seeking help for poor memory, although it could be highly relevant to obtain this information about a young adult who is behaving in an abnormal way.

A useful introduction is: 'I would like to ask about the family into which you were born. Let us start with your father: is he still alive'? If the father has died, the cause of death, his age, and that of the patient at the time should be determined. If the father is alive, his age, state of health, and job are recorded. The father's occupation is important mainly for the light it throws on the circumstances of the family. The father's personality and relationship with the patient can be elicited by asking 'what was your father like when you were a child; what is he like now; how did you get on in childhood; how do you get on now?' Similar enquiries are made about the mother, siblings, and other important figures in the patient's early life such as a step-father or a grandmother living in the house. The social position of the family and the atmosphere in the home are the background to the patient's childhood development (which is enquired about in the personal history—see below). The reasons for enquiring about mental illness in other family members has been explained above.

Personal history

The personal history provides information about events that may have shaped the patient's personality, and determined how he reacts to the present circumstances of life. For example, sexual abuse in childhood may partly explain a woman's sexual difficulties in adult life; being the unwanted child of a cold and unaffectionate mother may partly explain a man's difficulty in forming close relationships with women in adult life. The aim in taking the personal history is to identify major stressful circumstances, to find out how the patient reacted to them, and to form a picture of influences in his earlier life which explain how he came to be as he is now. The amount of detail required varies from patient to patient, and with growing experience the interviewer will be more able to decide what is appropriate to a particular patient. The personal history can be considered in several sections.

Maternal health during pregnancy and the circumstances of the patient's delivery

With the exceptions mentioned below, this information is seldom highly relevant and seldom reliable. When it is important (e.g. in child psychiatry and many cases of mental handicap), information should be sought from the mother herself and from hospital records. In most other cases, it is necessary to know only about large deviations from the normal.

Early development

The comments above about the relevance and reliability of information about pregnancy and delivery apply equally to developmental milestones, which are seldom important except when the patient is a child or an adult with mental handicap. A record should be made of prolonged *separation* from either parent for whatever reason. The effects of this experience vary considerably, so it is important to find out whether the patient was distressed at the time and for how long. If possible, this information should be checked with the parents. Serious and prolonged *childhood illnesses* may have affected the patient's emotional development. Diseases of the central nervous system may be relevant to mental retardation.

Educational history

The educational history gives an indication of intelligence and achievements, and contributes to an understanding of personality development. Information is sought concerning friendships, shyness, leadership in activities outside the classroom, and relationships with teachers.

Occupational history

The occupational history concerns both achievements and personality. Frequent changes of job, lack of promotion, or arguments with senior staff, may reflect awkward or aggressive traits or lack of self-confidence (although there are, of course, many other reasons for these events).

Sexual relationships

The history of sexual relationships includes enquiry about the success and failure of relationships, and enquiries about sexual behaviour. Although detailed enquiries are not needed in every case, the interviewer should be able to discuss these sexual issues in a matter-of-fact but sympathetic way. Judgement should be used in deciding how much to ask in a particular case. Detailed questions about sexual behaviour are likely to be relevant when the problem is sexual dysfunction; otherwise it is usually enough simply to enquire whether there are any sexual problems. Similarly, judgement should be used in asking questions about homosexuality. If the patient is sexually active, questions about contraception are often relevant.

Menstrual history Women of should be asked about menstrual problems appropriate for their age, including symptoms of the premenstrual syndrome and the menopause.

Marital history Information about the marital history which will often be relevent includes: whether the marriage is happy; how long it has lasted; the spouse's work and personality; and the sex, age, health, and development of the children. Similar enquiries are made about any previous marriage. If the marriage is unhappy, further questions should be asked about: the nature and causes of the unhappiness; the way in which the marriage has developed; and any periods of separation or plans for future separation or divorce. The history of the marriage is a further source of insight into the patient's personality.

Social circumstances

Information required about a patient's social circumstances includes:

- **Housing and living circumstances** The size and quality of the patient's home; is the home owned or rented? Who else lives with the patient, and how they relate to one another, including the patient?

- **Finances** Does the patient have any financial problems?

Forensic history

The forensic history concerns behaviour that breaks the law. It is important in cases of alcohol or drug abuse; in other cases common sense should be used to judge its relevance. If the patient has a criminal record, it may be useful to note the charge and the penalty, and to find out whether similar behaviour has occurred previously without coming to the notice of the police.

Past illness

Previous illnesses, both medical and psychiatric, should be asked about routinely in case they are relevant directly or indirectly to the present problem. (Specific associations between medical and psychiatric disorders are discussed in Chapter 11.)

Personality

The assessment of personality is important because longstanding personality traits need to be separated from episodes of illness and they may also interact with the illness.

Personality assessment is discussed in detail in Chapter 5 and only the salient points will be mentioned here. It begins with the patient's description of his own personality. Further assessment is made by combining information from the history of education, work, and marriage (see above), with further information elicited directly about social relationships, leisure activities, prevailing mood, character, attitudes, and habits (alcohol and drug use is recorded under 'habits'). It is usually helpful to interview an informant, since few people can give a wholly objective account of their own personality. Sometimes, the interviewer's impressions of the patient at interview give additional information about personality, but these impressions can be misleading when the patient is emotionally disturbed or has a psychiatric disorder. On the other hand, general practitioners can build up an assessment of their patients' personalities over years of occasional medical contacts. Information about this assessment is valuable in any letter of referral to a psychiatrist who has not met the patient.

Brief interviews for screening

In general practice and general hospital medicine, if a patient complains of symptoms of physical illness it is often appropriate to make sure whether there are also symptoms of psychiatric disorder. For this purpose, the full psychiatric history and mental state examination are too long, and so a brief screening interview is required. Although brief, a screening interview should not be rushed; if the patient feels under pressure of time, he may not reveal important facts. However short the time, the patient should feel that he has the interviewer's undivided attention and an opportunity to say what is important.

The screening questions deal with: general well-being, anxiety, depression, memory, and use of alcohol and drugs. The following points are considered:

- *Well-being*: fatigue, irritability, poor concentration, poor sleep, and a feeling of being under pressure.

- *Anxiety* tension, sweating frequency, palpitations, repeated worrying thoughts. If replies are positive, go on to systematic questions about anxiety disorder (p. 105–7).

- *Depression*: persistent low mood, low energy, loss of interest, loss of confidence, and hopelessness. If these questions are answered positively go on to questions concerning depressive disorder (including suicidal ideas) (see pp. 127–31).

- *Memory*: enquiries should be made about difficulties in recall of recent events. If difficulties are reported (and sometimes if they are not) the interviewer should give simple tests of memory (see pp. 35–7).

- *Alcohol and drugs*: the extent of use of alcohol and drugs is noted and in appropriate cases the CAGE (Box 13.2, p. 270) or the Alcohol Use Disorders Identification Test should be used (see Box 1.13, p. 269).

Mental state examination

In taking the history (Box 2.2) the interviewer will have learnt about the patient's symptoms up to the time of the consultation. In some cases, symptoms on the day of the interview are no different from those recorded in the history of the last few

Box 2.2 Examination of mental state

Appearance and behaviour	• General appearance
	• Facial expression
	• Posture
	• Movements
	• Social behaviour
Speech	• Rate
	• Amount
	• Continuity
Mood	• Prevailing mood and associated symptoms
	• Variations of mood
	• Appropriateness of mood
Depersonalization and derealization thinking	• Preoccupations
	• Obsessional or compulsive symptoms
	• Delusions
Perception	• Illusions
	• Hallucinations
Cognitive function	• Estimate intelligence
	• Orientation (time, place, person)
	• Attention and concentration (digit span, serial 7s)
	• Memory (name and address; remote personal events)
Insight	

days. However, they may have changed and it is important therefore to examine the present mental state. The mental state examination consists of a systematic enquiry into symptoms and signs at the time of the interview combined with a structured record of observations about the patient's appearance and behaviour during the interview. Like a physical examination, the mental state examination should be orderly and systematic. As with physical examination, the beginner in psychiatry should carry out a complete mental state examination with every patient, but with increasing clinical experience and knowledge, the interviewer will focus more selectively on points judged from the history to be of particular relevance. However, even the experienced clinician should classify symptoms noted during the history according to psychopathological criteria and specifically enquire about the presence of particularly important symptoms, such as suicidal ideation or hallucinations. The ways of eliciting some signs and symptoms that occur rarely are not described here (most are features of schizophrenia); they will be found in the corresponding chapter of the *Oxford textbook of psychiatry*. The signs and symptoms referred to below have been described in Chapter 1 of this book. Like history taking, mental state examination is a practical skill which can be learnt only by watching experienced interviewers and by practising under supervision. The following account will prepare the reader for this training but cannot replace it.

Appearance and behaviour

Much can be learnt from observing a patient's appearance and behaviour. Note should be taken of the general appearance, facial expression, posture, voluntary or involuntary movements, and social behaviour.

General appearance includes physique, hair, make-up, and clothing. Signs of self-neglect include a dirty unkempt appearance and stained crumpled clothing. Self-neglect suggests alcoholism, drug addiction, dementia, and chronic schizophrenia. Manic patients may dress incongruously in brightly coloured or oddly assorted clothes.

An appearance of *weight loss* is important in psychiatry as in general medicine, suggesting especially physical illness, anorexia nervosa, depressive disorder, or chronic anxiety.

Facial expression requires close attention, particularly as a guide to mood. Turning down of the corners of the mouth and vertical furrows on the brow suggest *depression*. Horizontal furrows on the brow, wide palpebral fissures, and dilated pupils suggest *anxiety*. An unchanging 'wooden' expression may result from a *parkinsonian syndrome*, either primary or caused by antipsychotic drugs. Posture also reflects mood. A depressed patient characteristically sits leaning forward, with shoulders hunched, and with the head and eyes cast downwards. An anxious patient typically sits upright, with the head erect and the hands gripping the chair.

Movements are affected in several ways. Manic patients are overactive and restless, depressed patients inactive and slow. Some depressed patients become completely immobile and mute, a condition known as *stupor*. Anxious or agitated patients are restless, and sometimes tremulous. Any involuntary movements should be noted, including tics, choreiform movements, dystonia, or tardive dyskinesia.

Social behaviour is disturbed in manic patients, who may be unduly familiar or may break social conventions in other ways. Some demented and schizophrenic patients are disinhibited, others are withdrawn and preoccupied. In describing these behaviours, a clear description of what is done or not done is more useful than general terms like 'disinhibited' or 'bizarre'.

Relevant features should be *summed up* in a few phrases that would give a clear picture to someone who has not met the patient. For example: 'a tall, gaunt, stooping, and dishevelled man with a sad countenance who looks much older than his 40 years'.

Speech

How the patient speaks comes under this heading: the thoughts he expresses are recorded later. The interviewer should note the **rate** of speaking. Speech may be slower than usual in depressive disorder, or faster than usual in mania. The **amount** spoken is considered next. Depressed patients talk less than usual, manic patients more than usual. Occasionally a patient does not speak at all ('mutism'). Abnormalities of the **continuity** of speech should be noted, including sudden interruptions, rapid shifts of topic, and lack of a logical thread.

Mood

As noted above, the first clues to mood may be detected in expression and posture. Questions should be asked about the **prevailing mood** and about symptoms associated with particular mood states. Questioning begins with an enquiry such as: 'how are your spirits?' or 'what is your mood like?' If *depressed* mood is reported, the associated symptoms may include a feeling of being ready to cry, lack of interest and enjoyment, and pessimistic thoughts including thoughts of suicide (see p. 244). **Ideas of suicide** should be asked about in stages, for example: 'have you felt that you have lost hope for the future?'; 'have you thought life is not worth living?'; 'have you wished you could die?'; 'have you thought of ending your life?'; 'have you thought how you might do this?' Some doctors are reluctant to ask about suicide, in case the questions might suggest the idea to the patient. Questions of this kind do not suggest suicide to people who have no suicidal inclination, and they should be asked whenever relevant.

If *anxiety* is reported, associated symptoms include palpitations, dry mouth, tremor, sweating, and worrying thoughts (see pp. 105–7 for a full list).

If *elevated mood* is reported, associated symptoms include excessive self-confidence, grandiose plans, and an inflated assessment of the person's own ability (see pp. 132–3 for a full list). Of course, these symptoms have to be elicited indirectly, for example, by asking the patient about his plans and his own abilities.

Sometimes there are **variations** of mood ('labile' mood) with dejection giving way quickly to normal mood or elation, and vice versa. Sometimes there is unusually little variation in mood, a condition known as *blunted* or *flattened* mood.

Finally, the **appropriateness** of mood is noted. Normally mood and thinking go together: a sad person thinks of sad things, and an elated person thinks of happy or grandiose things. Sometimes this link is lost, so that a person can appear cheerful when describing sad things. Such *incongruity* of mood is sometimes observed in schizophrenia (see p. 164).

Depersonalization and derealization

These symptoms are described on p. 6 if present they are recorded immediately after the record of mood.

Thought

Preoccupations are themes that recur frequently in thinking but can be put out of mind by an effort of will. Preoccupations often come to notice during history taking; during mental state examination it is appropriate to find out if there are other preoccupations by asking 'what sort of things do you worry about?'; 'what sort of thoughts occupy your mind?'. A knowledge of the patient's preoccupations is always important, but particularly so in three conditions: (1) depressive disorders, where preoccupations about suicide should be explored particularly carefully (see p. 148); (2) anxiety disorders, where preoccupations may prolong the disorder (see p. 109); and (3) in sexual disorders (see p. 303).

Obsessional phenomena (see pp. 14–16) involve both thinking and behaviour, and it is convenient to consider both at this point. To elicit *obsessional thoughts* an appropriate question is 'do any thoughts keep coming repeatedly into your mind, even when you try hard to get rid of them?' If the patient says yes, he should be asked for an example. Patients are often ashamed of the content of obsessional thoughts (especially those with aggressive or sexual themes), so questioning needs to be patient and sympathetic. The interviewer should make certain that the patient regards the thoughts as his own, because some schizophrenic patients have similar intrusive thoughts which they believe to have been implanted from outside ('thought insertion', see p. 13).

Compulsive rituals (see p. 15) may be observed during mental state examination, although more often they are revealed during history taking. Although not disorders of thinking, they are conveniently recorded under obsessional phenomena. The following questions can usefully be asked: 'do you ever have to repeat actions over and over which most people would do only once?' or 'do you have to go on repeating the same action when you know this is unnecessary?'.

Delusions (see pp. 10–14) often come to notice during the taking of the history, either from the patient or from an informant. Delusions may be difficult to elicit because the patient does not regard them as abnormal, and because he may be suspicious or afraid. A good way of starting the enquiry is to ask for an explanation of any unusual statements, unpleasant experiences, or unusual events that the patient has mentioned. For example, a patient may say that his headaches started when his neighbours caused him trouble; when asked why the neighbours should do this, he may say there is a conspiracy to harm him. Patients may hide delusions, and the interviewer should be alert to evasions, vague replies, or other hints that information is being withheld.

Having discovered an unusual belief, the interviewer has to decide: (1) whether it is false; (2) how strongly it is held despite evidence to the contrary; and (3) whether it is culturally determined (see p. 10). It is important to consider carefully whether the belief *could be true*. Some beliefs are clearly false; for example, that persecutors are damaging the patient's brain by beaming radio-waves on him. Other beliefs need to be checked—for example, that neighbours are mounting a campaign against the patient.

Tact is required when finding out *how strongly* the beliefs are *held*. The patient should feel that he is having a fair hearing, and that the interviewer's response is enquiring, not argumentative. The interviewer can say that, in order to help the patient, he needs to know how the problem has been caused; he can then challenge, gently but persistently, the patient's reasons for the belief. At the same time the interviewer has to judge whether the beliefs could be *culturally determined* ideas, that is, ideas accepted by others sharing the patient's culture. Such ideas may be shared by members of an unusual religious sect, or by societies in which ideas about evil forces or witchcraft are widespread. Any doubt can usually be resolved by finding another person from the same religion or country, and by asking whether the patient's ideas could be shared by people from the same background.

Direct questions may be needed to elicit several kinds of delusion that occur in schizophrenia, namely, *delusions of thought broadcasting, thought insertion, thought withdrawal* or *control*. If there are reasons for suspecting schizophrenia, the interviewer can ask questions such as: 'do you ever think that other people can tell what you are thinking, even though you have not told them'?; or 'do you ever think that thoughts have been put into your mind?' If the answer is yes, a detailed example should be obtained, to make sure that the patient has not answered positively for the wrong reason. For example, he may have answered the first question above positively, simply because he thinks that it refers to a general tendency for facial expression to reveal what a person is thinking.

Since questions about such delusions may antagonize a patient with a minor psychiatric problem, they should be reserved for cases in which schizophrenia enters the differential diagnosis.

At this point, the reader may wish to refer to the various categories of delusion described in Chapter 1 (pp. 12–13 and Table 1.3).

Perception

Illusions occur when sensory input is restricted, for example in poor light or low levels or audibility. They are not necessarily evidence of mental abnormality, but visual illusions occur particularly in acute organic mental disorders. Illusions may come to notice when the history is taken, or when the patient is being observed, for example in a medical ward. Visual illusions can be elicited with a question such as 'have you seen anything unusual?' (or frightening if the patient seems afraid). If the answer is positive, the interviewer needs to find out whether the visual experience is based on an actual visual stimulus (e.g. mistaking a shadow for a threatening person).

Hallucinations can occur in any sensory modality: visual and auditory hallucinations are the most common, but hallucinations of smell, taste, touch, and deep sensation occur as well. Enquiries about hallucinations should be made tactfully, lest the patient takes offence. With experience, the interviewer will be able to judge when it is safe to omit these enquiries. If enquiry is indicated, questions can be introduced by saying: 'when their nerves are upset some people have unusual experiences'. Questions can then be asked about hearing voices or sounds when there is nobody within earshot, or about seeing unusual things. If the patient says 'yes' to either of these questions, he should be asked whether the voice, sound, or vision appeared to be inside or outside his head. When the history makes it relevant, similar questions should be asked about other kinds of hallucinations. If the patient describes *auditory hallucinations*, further questions should be asked, to determine whether they are of a kind which is characteristic of schizophrenia (see p. 168). He should be asked whether he hears sounds or voices; if the latter, whether one voice or more; and whether the voices talk to him or to each other. Hallucinations of voices discussing the patient (*third person hallucinations*, see p. 8) should be distinguished from the delusion that people at a distance are discussing the patient (*a delusion of reference*, see p. 12). If the hallucinatory voices talk to the patient (*second person hallucinations*, p. 8), the interviewer should find out whether they give commands, and if so, what kind of commands, and whether the patient feels impelled to obey them. The reasons for these distinctions are explained in Chapter 9. Other kinds of hallucinations, found mainly in schizophrenia, are described on pp. 7–9.

Cognitive function

Orientation

Orientation is assessed by asking about the patient's awareness of time, place, and personal identity. Questions begin with the time, day, month, year, and season.

In assessing responses to questions about time, the interviewer should remember that many people do not know the exact time of day (although they usually know it to the nearest hour) or the exact date (though they are usually accurate to a few days). Orientation in place is assessed by asking the patient to name the place in which the interview is held. If the answer is inaccurate, further questions are asked about the kind of place (e.g. his home, a hospital ward, or a home for the elderly), and the name of the town.

Personal orientation is assessed by asking about other people in the same place (e.g. relatives in the home, or the staff in a hospital ward). If the patient gives wrong answers, he should be asked about his own identity—his name, occupation, and role in life.

Disorientation is an important symptom which indicates impairment of consciousness.

Attention and concentration

Attention is the ability to focus on the matter in hand. Concentration is the ability to sustain that focus. While taking the history, the interviewer should look out for evidence of impaired attention and concentration. In the mental state examination, specific tests are given. It is usual to begin with the 'serial 7s test'. The patient is asked to subtract 7 from 100 and then to take 7 from the remainder repeatedly until it is less than seven. The interviewer assesses whether the patient can concentrate on this task. If it seems that poor performance could be due to lack of skill in arithmetic, the patient should be asked to do a simpler subtraction, or to say the months of the year in reverse order. If mistakes are made with these tests, he can be given the less demanding task of naming the days of the week in reverse order. Tests of attention are given before tests of memory because poor attention can lead to poor performance on memory tasks, even when there is no memory defect.

Memory

Difficulties in remembering may come to light during history taking, when questions can be asked about everyday difficulties in remembering. During the examination of mental state, tests are given to assess immediate, recent, and remote memory. None of these tests is wholly satisfactory, and the results should be assessed cautiously and in relation to other information about the patient's ability to remember. If there is doubt, standardized psychological tests can be given by a clinical psychologist.

Short-term memory is assessed by asking the patient to repeat sequences of digits immediately after they have been spoken slowly enough for him to register them (the 'digit span test'). An easy sequence of three digits is given first to make sure that the patient understands the task. Then a new sequence of four digits is presented. If the patient can repeat four digits correctly, five, six, and then seven are given. If he reaches a level at which he cannot repeat the digits, the test is repeated with a different sequence of the same length. A normal person of average intelligence can repeat seven digits correctly; five or less suggests impairment. (The test involves concentration and therefore—as noted above—cannot be used to assess memory when tests of concentration are abnormal.)

Next, the interviewer assesses the patient's ability to take in and *remember new information*. By convention, the new information is a name, an address, and the name of a flower. Common names and addresses likely to be familiar to the patient should be avoided. It is important to ask the patient to reproduce the task straight away to make sure it has been registered correctly, and then to remember the information. If the material is not registered correctly, the task is repeated until there is accurate immediate recall. Other topics are then discussed for five minutes, at which time recall is tested. The patient's response should be recorded verbatim and the number of errors noted. A healthy person of average intelligence should make only minor errors in this task.

Memory for recent events is assessed by asking about news items from the last day or two, or about recent events in the patient's life that are known with certainty to the interviewer (do not ask the traditional question about what the patient had for breakfast unless you know the answer). Questions about news items should be adapted to the patient's interests, and should have been widely reported in the media.

Long-term memory can be assessed by asking the patient to recall personal events or well-known public events from some years before. Personal events could be the birth dates of the patient's children or grandchildren (provided these dates are known with certainty by the interviewer); public events could be the names of earlier political leaders, sportsmen, or musicians. Awareness of the sequence of events is as important as the recall of individual items.

Observations by others. When a patient is in a general hospital, important information about memory is available from **observations made by nurses**. These observations include how rapidly the patient learns the daily routine of the ward, and the names of staff and other patients; and whether he forgets where he has put things, or cannot find his way about (though the latter may indicate spatial disorientation rather than poor memory). When the patient is at home, relatives may report comparable observations about the patient's ability to learn and remember.

Special tests. Among elderly patients, these questions about memory do not distinguish well between those who have cerebral pathology and those who do not. For cases of doubt there are standardized ratings of memory for recent personal events, past personal events, and general events, which allow a better assessment of severity. Standardized tests of learning and memory can help also in the diagnosis of organic mental disorder, and can be used for quantitative assessments of the progression of memory disorder. These tests are usually administered by a clinical psychologist.

Intelligence

During history taking, the interviewer should be alert to the possibility that the person is of low intelligence. If this seems possible and the impression is confirmed during mental state examination, a test of intelligence can be arranged.

Insight

By the end of the history taking and mental state examination, the interviewer should have a provisional estimate of the patient's awareness of the morbid nature of his experiences. Direct questions should then be asked to assess this awareness further. First, questions are asked about the patient's awareness of the nature of individual symptoms; for example, whether or not he believes that extreme feelings of guilt are justified. Second, the interviewer finds out whether the patient believes himself to be ill (rather than, say, persecuted by his enemies); if so, whether he thinks that the illness is physical or mental; and whether he sees himself as needing treatment. The answers are important because they suggest how far the patient is likely to collaborate with treatment. The answers to all questions should be noted. It is of little value to record merely 'partial insight' or 'no insight'.

Some difficulties in mental state examination

Apart from the obvious problem of examining patients who speak little or no English—a problem that requires the help of an interpreter—difficulties can arise with patients who are unresponsive, or overactive, or confused.

Unresponsive patients

When patients are mute, or stuporous (conscious but not speaking or responding in any way) it is only possible to make observations of behaviour; however, these observations can be useful if done properly.

It is important to remember that stuporous patients sometimes become suddenly violent and so it is wise to be accompanied when examining such a patient. Before deciding that the patient is mute, it is important that the interviewer:

- speaks the language of the patient;
- has allowed adequate time for reply;
- has tried a variety of topics;
- has assessed whether the patient will communicate in writing.

As well as making the observations of behaviour described on p. 31, note whether the patient's eyes are open or closed: if open, note whether they follow objects, move apparently without purpose, or are fixed; if closed, whether they are opened on request, and if not, whether attempts at opening them are resisted.

A physical examination including neurological assessment is essential in all such cases. A specialist will also seek certain uncommon signs found in catatonic schizophrenia (*waxy flexibility* of muscles and *negativism*, see p. 167) but these are difficult to assess for a clinician who has little experience of them.

In all such cases it is essential to interview an informant to discover the onset and course of the condition.

Overactive patients

When the patient is overactive (e.g. because of mania) questions have to be limited to a few that seem particularly important, and conclusions have to be based mainly on observations of behaviour and spontaneous utterances. Some of the overactivity may be in response to efforts at restraint, and a quiet confident approach by the interviewer may calm the patient and allow a more adequate examination.

Patients who appear confused

When the patient gives the history in a muddled way, and especially if he appears perplexed or frightened, test cognitive functions early in the interview. If consciousness is impaired, try to orientate the patient and reassure him before starting the interview again in a simplified form. In such cases every effort should be made to interview another informant.

Physical examination

As in the rest of medicine, the extent of the physical examination is judged on the diagnostic possibilities in each case. In case of doubt, a physical examination should be performed. When an organic syndrome is suspected, it is essential to carry out a relevant neurological examination. In selected cases this should include assessment of language, constructional apraxias, and agnosias. The methods of examination are described in textbooks of neurology, and taught to medical students during neurology training. Those who have not had this training are advised to study the summary of salient points in chapter 2 of *The Oxford Textbook of Psychiatry*, to consult a textbook of neurology, and to obtain supervised practice of the relevant clinical skills.

Special investigations

Special investigations are chosen according to the patient's symptoms and the differential diagnosis: no single set of routine investigations is essential for every patient.

Psychological assessment

This kind of assessment requires special training; it is carried out usually by a clinical psychologist. In most cases it is not necessary to have a precise assessment of *intelligence*. If a patient seems to be of low intelligence, or if his psychological symptoms could be a reaction to work beyond his intellectual capacity, intelligence tests are essential. In child psychiatry, tests of intelligence are often supplemented by tests of *reading ability* (see Chapter 19).

Specific neuropsychological tests are available for assessing dysfunction of the frontal or parietal cortex. Brain imaging methods are now more useful in diagnosis, but the tests have some value in following the progress of disease.

Personality tests contribute little to the assessment of an individual patient, where more can be learnt from the clinical assessment described earlier in this chapter. Personality tests are more useful in research with groups of patients.

Rating-scales of behaviour are used occasionally to follow the progress of a disorder, and often during behavioural treatment see p. 369.

Interviewing relatives

When assessing psychiatric problems, interviews with one or more close relatives of the patient are important, both to obtain information about the patient's condition, and to involve relatives in the treatment plan. A history from a relative (or close friend) is essential when the patient is suffering from a mental disorder or personality disorder severe enough to impair his ability to give an unbiased and accurate account. In less severe disorders, a relative can help by giving another view of the patient's illness and personality. For example, a relative may be more able than the patient to date the onset of illness accurately, especially if it was gradual; or to describe how the disorder affects other people. When it is important to know about the patient's childhood, an interview with a parent or older sibling may be helpful.

With few exceptions, the patient's permission should be obtained before interviewing a relative. Exceptions occur when the patient is a child, and when an adult patient is mute, stuporose, confused, violent, or extremely retarded. Apart from these cases, the doctor should explain to the patient that he wishes to interview a relative to obtain additional information needed for diagnosis and treatment. He should emphasize that confidential information given to the doctor by the patient will not be passed to the relative. If any information needs to be given to a relative (e.g. about treatment), the patient's prior permission should be obtained.

Adequate time should be allowed for the interview; the relatives may be anxious, and time may be needed to put them at ease, gather facts, and provide any necessary information. Sometimes, relatives misunderstand the purpose of the interview, thinking that demands are about to be made on them to help in treatment. Others fear that they may be blamed for the patient's illness; for example, the parents of a young schizophrenic may worry that they have failed as parents. The interviewer should be sensitive to such ideas and should discuss them in a reassuring way.

If the relatives are having problems as a result of the patient's illness, the interviewer should discuss how they can obtain help. If appropriate, he may offer to help them himself; but if this offer would conflict with his primary duty to the patient, he should seek an alternative. For example, a general practitioner could ask a partner to share in the management, or could obtain the help of a social worker or psychiatrist.

If a relative reveals something which the doctor could usefully discuss with the patient, the relative's permission should be obtained before the doctor raises the subject with the patient. For example, a wife might report that her husband drinks heavily, although he has denied heavy drinking to the doctor. The wife may be unwilling that the information be passed on, because of fear of retaliation. The wife's wish must be respected. The doctor can only try to help the husband by tactfully giving him an opportunity to disclose the information later.

Problems may arise when someone other than a known nearest relative telephones the doctor about the patient. Information should not be given over the telephone, even when the doctor is certain of the caller's identity. Instead, the patient should be consulted and, if he agrees, an interview arranged. The clinician should avoid a conspiratorial atmosphere in which he conceals conversations with family members or take sides in their disputes.

Interviews in an emergency

When urgent action is required, the interview may have to be brief. Nevertheless, it is important to collect the information needed to make a provisional diagnosis or differential diagnosis and to formulate a plan of action. This information includes, at least, the presenting symptoms or behaviours, together with their onset, course, and present severity; other relevant symptoms, with their onset, course, and severity; any stressful circumstances around the time of onset and at the present time; recent or current physical illness; past mental disorder; the use of alcohol and drugs; the social circumstances, and the possibilities of support.

Table 2.1.

Risk factors for harm to others

Demographic risk factors
Previous violence to others
Male
Living alone
Divorced/separated
Unemployed
Recent life crisis
Social restlessness
Illness related risk factors
Psychotic illness
Poor compliance or engagement with services
Recent discontinuation of medication
Substance abuse
Mental state related factors
Irritability, anger, hostility, suspiciousness
Specific threats made by the patient
Hallucinations commanding violence to others
Suicidal ideas in a severely depressed patient (see p. 247)
Paranoid delusions
Delusional jealousy

An account of previous personality is also valuable, although it may be difficult to obtain in the time available. Family and personal history can be covered quickly with a few salient questions. Throughout, the interviewer should be thinking which questions need to be answered at once and which can be deferred until later.

Risk assessment

One of the most important clinical skills in psychiatry is **risk assessment**. *Risk* is the probability that an adverse event will occur: risk assessment involves a clinical assessment of the likelihood of a specific adverse event. In psychiatry, the main adverse events in the context of risk assessment are **self-harm** (including suicide) and **harm to others** (including homicide).

In this section we describe the general approach to the assessment of risk. The assessment of suicide risk is described more fully in Chapter 12.

The aims of risk assessment are to:

- Identify the possible adverse events for the patient
- Identify and quantify the *risk factors* which increase the likelihood of the event
- Identify and quantify the *protective factors* which decrease the likelihood of the event
- Identify which of these factors can be modified
- Estimate the current likelihood of the adverse event.

The assessment of risk is based on a normal, thorough psychiatric assessment. It is important to obtain information from other relevant sources as well as the patient (including an informant, medical records, social services, the police). In the assessment, particular attention should be paid to the presence of risk or protective factors. The risk factors for suicide and deliberate self-harm are described in Chapter 12. The main risk factors for harm to others are shown in Table 2.1. The strongest predictor of future violence is a past history of violence. It is best to consider these factors as acting cumulatively although we currently have little evidence on which to base quantitative assessments of risk.

When the risk assessment is complete, the findings should be fully documented in a **management plan**. This should include a **formulation of risk** which starts with a description of which potential adverse events have been considered. This should be followed by a description of any risk or protective factors for the adverse event and an estimate of how likely the event is, both in the short and longer term. Finally, consideration should be made of what can be done to reduce the risk. Risk assessment is the first part of the process of **risk management**, the aims of which are to reduce the level of risk to an acceptable level and to set up a system for **risk monitoring**. The possible interventions to reduce the risk will depend on which risk factors have been identified, but may include involvement of the police, appropriate treatment of mental illness (including compulsory admission to hospital if necessary), and provision of community support and monitoring.

Finally, the management plan should be adequately **communicated to others** involved in the case and regularly **reviewed**. It is important to note that if a person is identified as being at risk of harm, the need to warn this person may override patient confidentiality.

The formulation

Formulations are concise assessments of diagnosis, aetiology, treatment, and prognosis. Relevant information from the summary is used, but the formulation is not just a summary in another form; it is an exercise in clinical reasoning. Since this way of thinking about a case is useful also in general practice and general hospital medicine, an outline will be given here. Readers requiring a more detailed discussion are referred to *The Oxford Textbook of Psychiatry*.

As shown in Table 2.2, a formulation begins with a *brief statement of the problem*, for example: a 35-year-old mother of three children complains of depression and is drinking excessively. The *differential diagnosis* is considered next. In this case the depressive symptoms may be part of a depressive disorder, with the excessive drinking secondary; or the main problem may be alcohol abuse with secondary depressive symptoms; or there may be a third condition accounting for both the depressive symptoms and the alcohol abuse, such as a severe anxiety disorder. A note is made of the evidence for or against each diagnosis (e.g. which problem began first; or whether there are other symptoms supporting a diagnosis of depressive disorder, see pp. 128–31). Then, the most likely diagnosis is chosen.

Next the *aetiology is* discussed, with reference to predisposing, precipitating, and maintaining factors. Only convincing evidence should be included. For example, if this patient's diagnosis is depressive disorder, a strong family history of manic-depressive disorder would suggest genetic causes; part-time employment as a barmaid might predispose her to abuse alcohol when depressed; a bout of influenza might precipitate the depressive disorder; and marital conflict might maintain it.

If appropriate, a list is then given of any *further investigations* required.

The *treatment plan* should mention drug treatment, psychological treatment, and social measures. For example, this patient might require antidepressant drugs, counselling with her husband about their problems, and help with the care of her children until she is less depressed. The treatment plan should also consider the needs of the children themselves, with an assessment of the care they have been receiving including the possibilities of neglect or abuse.

Assessment of the *prognosis is* usually the most difficult part of the formulation. It depends on factors that are, in turn, difficult to predict: for example, in this case whether the marital problems will be resolved. Even if there is uncertainty, consideration of the prognosis helps the clinician to think about the patient's future needs as well as the immediate ones.

An example of a full formulation is given in *The Oxford Textbook of Psychiatry,* chapter 2.

Problem lists

A problem list is another useful way of summarizing a complicated case. It is particularly useful in cases with both medical and psychiatric aspects, and is therefore valuable in general practice and general hospital medicine. An example of a problem list is shown in Table 2.3. The problem list makes these steps clear to anyone who sees the patient when the original doctor is unavailable, and serves as a reminder of times to review progress. Thus, the patient's response to antidepressants was to be checked weekly for three weeks by the family doctor, and then reviewed; the mother's progress was also to be reviewed in three weeks to find out whether her

Table 2.2.
The formulation

- Statement of the problem
- Differential diagnosis
- Aetiology
- Further investigations
- Plan of treatment
- Prognosis

Case study

A 54-year-old woman consulted her general practitioner because of mixed anxiety and depressive symptoms. The diagnosis was depressive disorder, and the immediate cause was evidently the stress of caring for an elderly debilitated mother (also the general practitioner's patient), whose condition had worsened in the last two months. Important contributory factors were menorrhagia and chronic agoraphobia which prevented the patient from visiting friends and relatives. The immediate plan was to treat the patient's depressive disorder with amitriptyline, and to obtain respite care for her mother. In the longer term, the agoraphobia would be treated with behaviour therapy, and a gynaecological opinion would be obtained about the menorrhagia.

Table 2.3.

Example of a problem list

	Problem	Action	Agent	Review
1	Anxiety and depression	Amitriptyline rising to 150 mg at night. Check response weekly for 3 weeks then review	GP	
2	Caring for elderly mother	Obtain respite care for mother	Geriatrician	3 weeks
3	Chronic agoraphobia	Behaviour therapy	Clinical psychologist	3 months
	Menorrhagia	Gynaecological opinion	GP	1 month

condition has improved, and to discuss future management with the geriatrician. An appointment was to be made for a clinical psychologist to treat the agoraphobia; the progress of this arrangement was to be checked in three months, when some plan of treatment would be in place though probably not completed. The progress of gynaecological referral was to be checked in one month to make sure it had taken place and to integrate the results into the developing plan of treatment.

The life chart

A life chart is a way of summarizing the relationships between stressful events and episodes of physical and psychiatric illness. It is useful when the history is long and complicated. There are five columns: the year, the patient's age, life events, physical illness, and psychiatric disorder. The second column shows the years of the patient's life.

The example in Table 2.4 is of a woman with a depressive disorder. In the past she has had three episodes of actual or suspected physical illness, two periods of emotional disturbance in childhood (bed-wetting; school refusal), and one at the age of 18 (adjustment reaction), and a previous depressive disorder at age 37. The events in her life are recorded, and the chart shows how they relate to one another. None of the episodes of psychiatric disturbance closely followed physical illness or

Table 2.4.

Example of a life chart

Year	Age	Events	Physical illness	Psychiatric disorder
1953	Born			
4	1			
5	2			
6	3			
7	4			
8	5	Started school		Bed-wetting
9	6			
1960	7			
1	8			
2	9			
3	10	Grandmother died		School refusal
4	11			
5	12			
6	13	Father's illness	Unexplained	
7	14		abdominal pain	
8	15			
9	16			
1970	17			
1	18	Started at university		Adjustment reaction
2	19			
3	20			
4	21			
5	22	Married		
6	23			
7	24	First child born		
8	25			
9	26	Second child born (Caesarean section)		
1980	27			
1	28			
2	29		Cone biopsy	
3	30			
4	31			
5	32			
6	33			
7	34	Mother died		Depressive disorder
8	35			
9	36		Intestinal obstruction	

Table 2.4.

(cont.)

Year	Age	Events	Physical illness	Psychiatric disorder
1990	37			
1	38			
2	39	Husband's illness		Depressive disorder
3	40			
4	41	First son depressed starting university		
5	42			
6	43			
7	44	Husband died		
8	45			Depressive disorder

childbirth. The episodes are, however, related to life events which have common themes of separation (starting school and going to university) and of loss (the deaths of the patient's grandmother and mother). The present illness fits into this pattern since it began when the husband died. These relationships, which can be seen clearly in the chart, are less easy to discern from the history alone.

Letters of referral to psychiatrists

When a letter of referral is written to a psychiatrist it is important to include several items of information that will assist in the assessment and may not be obtained easily by the psychiatrist at the first interview. These items include:

- the course and development of the disorder, with the dates at which problems began or changed;

- the recent mental state;

- any abnormal behaviour that may be denied by the patient (e.g. excessive use of alcohol) or not recognized by the patient (e.g. lapses of memory in a patient who may be demented);

- relevant points in the past medical history;

- details of any *treatment given* together with a note of the therapeutic response and side effects; *family relationships*, including marital problems and difficulties between parents and children; the patient's *personality* as known to the referring doctor from his previous contacts with the patient.

(Letters from consultant psychiatrists to general practitioners are discussed in *The Oxford Textbook of Psychiatry*, chapter 2.)

Further reading

Goldberg, D. (ed.) (1997). *The Maudsley Handbook of Practical Psychiatry*. Oxford University Press.
A practical guide to psychiatric examination in a range of clinical situations—including advice on managing difficult interviews.

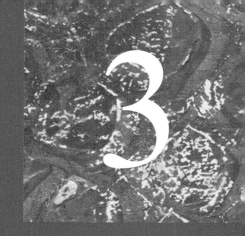

Classification

Classification

In psychiatry, as in the rest of medicine, classification helps to bring order to the great diversity of phenomena met in clinical practice. Its purpose is to identify clinical features that occur together regularly and help to predict outcome and response to treatment. Classification is concerned with disorders; patients have to be understood as individuals.

The diagnostic approach has been criticized as: (1) failing to recognize the uniqueness of the individual patient; and (2) stigmatizing patients. However, used properly diagnosis is accompanied by an understanding of the ill person and stigma is reduced by better public understanding of mental disorder.

The basic classification in psychiatry should be known by all doctors. It is elaborated in two widely used diagnostic systems: the International Classification of Diseases (ICD) produced by the World Health Organization, and the Diagnostic and Statistical Manual (DSM) developed by the American Psychiatric Association. The few differences between these systems are not important except for doctors specializing in psychiatry.

Some commonly used terms

Illness, disease, and disorder

In general medicine, the entities in a classification are known as diseases and the term *disease* denotes the presence of physical pathology. A distinction is made between disease and *illness*, a term that denotes a state of subjective distress. Disease and illness usually occur together but not always. Some patients have a disease but do not feel ill, for example in the early—'silent'—stage of a carcinoma. Some patients feel ill but have no disease, they have medically unexplained symptoms (see p. 216).

In psychiatry, the entities in the classification are known as *disorders* rather than diseases. This term is chosen because only a minority of psychiatric conditions have an identified physical pathology so that the term *disease*, as used in general medicine, is not strictly appropriate. Instead, the causes include biochemical abnormalities and the effects of faulty learning (see Chapter 4). The term *disorder* indicates that the symptoms are caused by an abnormality although this is not necessarily the organic pathology implied by the term *disease*. Thus, the entities in the classification have names such as *anxiety disorder* or *depressive disorder*.

In psychiatry, the term *illness* is used as in the rest of medicine to denote the patient's state of distress. However, in the English and some other legal systems the term *illness* is used differently and corresponds approximately to the psychiatric term *disorder*. Thus, a doctor who uses the legal procedures of English law to arrange the involuntary admission of a patient to hospital has to state whether the patient has a *mental illness*. In practice, the doctor answers by deciding whether, in medical terms, there is a psychiatric disorder.

Organic and functional

Disorders with a definite structural pathology are called organic and disorders without such pathology are called functional. The term *functional psychosis* is sometimes used to refer to schizophrenia and manic-depressive disorder so as to contrast them with psychosis due to structural brain disease. Also, anxiety and obsessional disorders are sometimes referred to as functional disorders. This distinction is used less often now because modern methods of investigation have revealed previously undiscovered structural changes in some conditions previously thought to be functional (e.g. schizophrenia, see p. 162).

Psychosis and neurosis

Psychiatric disorders are sometimes grouped into *psychoses* and *neuroses* although this grouping are no longer employed in the official systems of classification.

Psychosis is a collective term for the more severe forms of psychiatric disorder in which hallucinations and delusions may occur and insight is lost. Schizophrenia, manic-depressive disorder, and the dementias are psychoses. The term *psychosis* has been criticized because it groups together conditions that have little in common, and is generally less useful than a specific diagnosis such as schizophrenia. However, some clinicians continue to use the term especially when it is difficult to make a more precise diagnosis, for example, to decide whether a patient who has hallucinations and delusions has schizophrenia or mania. Used in this way psychosis is a provisional category to be replaced by a more precise one when further evidence has accumulated.

Neurosis is a collective term for psychiatric disorders in which, irrespective of severity, there are no hallucinations or delusions and no loss of insight. The objections to the term *neurosis* are the same as those for *psychosis*: it embraces conditions that have little in common, and it is less informative than a more specific diagnosis such as anxiety disorder. Like psychosis, however, neurosis continues to be used in clinical practice as a convenient term for disorders that cannot be assigned to a more precise diagnosis.

Some criticisms of the diagnostic approach

Classifying disorders and understanding patients

The use of classification in psychiatry has sometimes been criticized as inappropriate or even harmful on the grounds that it fails to recognize the uniqueness of the individual patient. To make this criticism is to misunderstand the purpose of classification which is concerned only with those aspects of the patient's problems that fall into a pattern that has been observed regularly in other patients. When these common features have been identified, there remain the particular features of the individual patient. The doctor's task is not only to diagnose the disorder but also to understand the person who is ill. The individual factors determine how the patient copes with the disorder and complies with treatment, and they influence prognosis.

It might appear that the diagnosis of personality disorder is an exception to this line of reasoning. However, even the diagnosis of personality disorder is concerned only those aspects of personality that are observed regularly in other people; when these have been identified there remain the many aspects of the person which reflect his unique upbringing and experience. (Types of classification are in *Additional information.*)

Diagnosis and stigma

It has been said that diagnosis stigmatizes patients. It is true that the diagnosis of schizophrenia may cause social stigma, as do some medical diagnoses such as AIDS. This is not a reason to avoid the diagnosis of schizophrenia—as some of the objectors have suggested—but a reason to inform the public about the nature of psychiatric disorder so that unfavourable attitudes can change. Failure to diagnose schizophrenia deprives patients of the treatment and other help that they need.

Basic classification in psychiatry

The various diagnostic systems contain the same basic categories. The few differences are in nomenclature and in the details of the criteria fore diagnosis. The categories (listed in Table 3.1.) are:

- **Mental disorders**: abnormalities of behaviour or psychological experience with a recognizable onset after a period of normal functioning.
- **Adjustment disorder and reactions to stress**: conditions that are less severe than mental disorders and occur in relation to stressful events or changed circumstances.
- **Personality disorder**: dispositions to behave in certain abnormal ways—present continuously from early adult life.
- **Other disorders**: conditions that do not fit into the previous groups; for example, abnormalities of sexual preference.
- **Disorders starting in childhood.**
- **Mental retardation**: impairment of intellectual functioning present continuously from early life.

Mental disorders are classified further into the main categories shown in Table 3.2. Most of these main categories are divided further in ways that are explained in subsequent chapters.

Reliability of diagnosis

Diagnosis is of little value unless doctors agree with one another about the same patient. Good agreement depends on:

1. **Interviewing technique** Doctors vary in the information they elicit from the same patient, and they may interpret the information differently. These variations can be reduced by using standardized interviews in which predetermined questions are asked and rules are used to define whether particular symptoms are present.

Table 3.1.
The basic classification

- Mental disorder
- Adjustment disorder
- Personality disorder
- Other disorders
- Disorders starting in childhood
- Mental retardation

Table 3.2.
Classification of mental disorders

- Delirium, dementia, and related disorders
- Psychoactive substance use disorders
- Anxiety and obsessional disorders
- Affective (mood) disorder
- Schizophrenia and related disorders
- Somatoform disorders
- Dissociative disorders
- Factitious disorders
- Disorders starting in childhood
- Developmental disorders
- Conduct disorders

Additional information **Types of classification**

Classification by cause and by syndrome

In general medicine, most conditions can be classified on the basis of aetiology (e.g. viral pneumonia) or structural pathology (e.g. pulmonary embolus). Some general medical conditions cannot be classified in this way (e.g. migraine and trigeminal neuralgia) and are classified instead on the pattern of symptoms. Most psychiatric disorders have to be classified on the pattern of symptoms. The exceptions are the few disorders with a structural pathology (e.g. Alzheimer's disease).

Categorical and dimensional classifications

Medical classifications use categories. These work well when there is a clear dividing line between normality and disease (e.g. a cerebral neoplasm). A categorical classification is less appropriate when there is a continuum between normal and abnormal (e.g. essential hypertension) because any dividing line separates cases that are little different one from another. The alternative is to employ a dimensional classification in which cases are described by their positions on the dimension rather than categorized as normal or abnormal.

Many psychiatric disorders are on a continuum. Thus there is no sharp dividing line between anxiety disorders and normal anxiety and it has been suggested therefore that such disorders should be classified along dimensions. Although this approach has been used by psychologists to classify personality it is not used for clinical work in which it is generally more useful to categorize conditions as disordered or not.

Hierarchies and co-morbidity

Some patients have more than one disorder. When this happens one of two approaches can be followed. The first, is to use a hierarchy in which some diagnoses take precedence over others. For example, when symptoms of schizophrenia and dementia occur together, only the latter would be diagnosed since the brain disorder that caused dementia could have caused the schizophrenia-like symptoms. The alternative is to diagnose all conditions that meet diagnostic criteria; in the foregoing example, dementia and schizophrenia would be diagnosed. This approach is used in the American classification, DSM-IV.

The international classification, ICD-10, adopts an intermediate position. Clinicians are advised to make as many diagnoses as they consider necessary to describe the case completely. When this advice is followed, not all co-morbid conditions are recorded; for example, simple phobias occur so often in agoraphobia that they may be regarded as part of the clinical picture. Simple phobia would not be recorded as a diagnosis unless these phobias were exceptionally severe.

Multiaxial classification

In a multiaxial classification several kinds of disorder are considered in every case and recorded on 'axes'. The usual axes are: clinical syndrome, personality disorder, physical disease, severity of stressors, and disability. In everyday practice only the first three axes are used commonly—psychiatric disorder, personality, and physical disease. These three diagnoses can, of course, be recorded without assigning them to separate axes, but the axial system ensures that they are considered in every case. Multiaxial classification is used more often in child than in adult psychiatry with intelligence taking the place of personality.

2. Diagnostic criteria Reliability can be increased by providing a clear definition for each diagnosis, and by specifying discriminating symptoms. *Discriminating symptoms* occur commonly in the defined syndrome but rarely in other syndromes. They are important in diagnosis but may not be important in planning treatment. An example is the delusion that thoughts are being inserted into the mind, a discriminating symptom for schizophrenia. *Characteristic symptoms* occur frequently in the defined syndrome but may also occur in other syndromes. Such symptoms do not help in diagnosis, but may be important to the patient and relevant in planning treatment. An example is thoughts of suicide, which do not help in diagnosis because they occur in several kinds of disorder, but which are very important in planning care.

Diagnostic criteria can be general descriptive statements or more precise inclusion and exclusion criteria called an **operational definition**. For example, in the diagnostic system known as DSM (see below), the category of major depressive disorder requires five current symptoms from a list of nine, together with the exclusion of organic causes, schizophrenia, and bereavement reaction. Operational criteria lead to more reliable diagnoses but they leave more patients without a diagnosis because they just fail to meet the criteria.

Systems of classification

The International Classification of Diseases (ICD)

This system of classification was developed by the World Health Organization. It is now in its tenth edition generally referred to as ICD-10. The section on psychiatry is used in all countries of the world for the compilation of statistics for international comparisons, and in most countries for clinical purposes. To facilitate its wide use ICD-10 has been translated into all the widely spoken languages of the world. The section on psychiatry is available in three forms, one for *clinical practice*, another for *research*, and a third for use in *primary care*. The clinical version uses descriptions of the features of typical cases as the criterion for diagnosis. The *research version* uses operational criteria.

The version for *primary care* includes only the diagnoses seen most often in this branch of practice and provides case descriptions as criteria for diagnosis. These diagnoses are listed in Table 3.3. As well as common psychiatric disorders, the list includes tobacco use disorder, since this problem is common among patients in primary care. The primary care version of ICD-10 is accompanied by concise advice about criteria for diagnosis and also about the management of the disorders in primary care and the indications for seeking the help of a psychiatrist.

The Diagnostic and Statistical Manual (DSM)

This classification was developed by the American Psychiatric Association. It is now in its fourth edition known as DSM-IV. Although developed as the US national classification it is used in other countries, especially for research. It differs from ICD-10 mainly in the use of operational criteria for clinical work as well as for research. Most of these criteria are the same as those in the research version of ICD-10 and the few differences are of more concern to psychiatrists than to other doctors.

Table 3.3.

ICD-10 Primary care version

Dementia
Delirium

Alcohol use disorders
Drug use disorders
Tobacco use disorders

Chronic psychotic disorders
Bipolar disorders
Depression

Phobic disorders
Panic disorder
Generalized anxiety
Mixed anxiety and depression

Adjustment disorder

Dissociative (conversion) disorder
Unexplained somatic complaint

Eating disorders
Sleep problems
Sexual problems

Diagnosis and classification in everyday practice

In principle, a diagnostic classification is made after the history and examination of mental state have been completed. In practice, an experienced clinician begins to consider possible diagnoses in the early stages of the interview As the interview progresses the diagnostic possibilities are narrowed progressively as the interviewer compares the findings with his knowledge of the diagnostic guidelines in ICD-10 or DSM-IV. Although the classification contains a large number of diagnoses, in most cases only a few need be considered the rest being obviously inapplicable.

Occasionally, all but one or two of the clinical features fit a particular diagnosis but the others are seen more often in a different disorder. For example, a patient may have depressed mood, morbid self-blame, early morning waking, and diurnal mood variation—all symptoms typical of a depressive disorder. In addition, the patient may have the delusion that people talk about him on television—a typical symptom of schizophrenia. When this kind of incongruity occurs, the clinician should search for other evidence of the alternative syndrome. If only one or two incongruous symptoms are found it is usual to record the diagnosis that fits most of the symptoms. In such cases it is important to re-examine the patient regularly to find out whether there is any additional evidence for the 'minority' diagnosis.

Diagnosis requires more than a consideration of the present state of the patient (a cross-sectional assessment). It is also important to take into account the course of the disorder (longitudinal assessment). If, in the previous example, the patient had two previous affective disorders and no previous schizophrenia, the current atypical symptom (the delusion of being talked about on television) would be discounted further.

Further reading

Diagnostic and Management Guidelines for Mental Disorders in Primary Care ICD-10, Chapter V. Primary Care Version. WHO/Hogrefe and Huber Publishers, Göttingen.
A version of the ICD-10 classification designed for use in primary care and including guidelines on management and information for patients.

Cooper, J. E. (1994). *Pocket Guide to ICD-10 Classification of Mental and Behavioural Disorders with Glossary and Diagnostic Criteria for Research DCR-10.* Churchill Livingstone, Edinburgh.
An accessible reference to the WHO ICD-10 classification of psychiatric and behavioural disorders.

Ustun, T. B., Bertelsen, A., Dilling, H., Van Drimmelen, J., Pull, C., Okasha, and A., Sartorius, N. (1996). *ICD-10 Casebook The Many Faces of Mental Disorders.* American Psychiatric Press, Washington DC, 1996.
Case studies which illustrate the use of ICD-10.

The Quick Reference Guide to DSM-IV (1994). American Psychiatric Press, Washington DC.
A concise guide to the DSM-IV criteria.

Spitzer, R. L., Gibbon, M., Skodol, A. E., and Williams, J. B. W. (1994). *DSM-IV Casebook.* American Psychiatric Press, Washington DC.
Case studies which illustrate the use of DSM-IV.

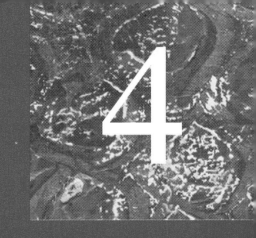

Aetiology and the scientific basis of psychiatry

- Aetiology

- Methodological approaches

- Keeping up-to-date: evidence-based medicine

Aetiology and the scientific basis of psychiatry

Doctors need to be able to combine scientific knowledge with an empathic understanding of the patient to form a coherent account of patients, their illness and their predicament. In this chapter, we will initially describe how this can be achieved for the aetiological formulation. We will then review ways of finding out the most up-to-date evidence for all kinds of clinical question (but particularly methods of identifying the best treatments for specific clinical situations) by using the strategies of evidence-based medicine.

Aetiology

A knowledge of the causes of psychiatric disorders is important for two main reasons. First, in everyday clinical work it helps the doctor to evaluate possible causes of an individual patient's psychiatric disorder. Second, it adds to the general understanding of psychiatric disorders which may contribute to advances in diagnosis, treatment, or prognosis. In this section we will only deal with the first of these—the *assessment of the causes of disorder* in the individual patient. The aetiology of specific disorders is considered when these conditions are reviewed in subsequent chapters.

Aetiology and the individual patient

The causes of psychiatric disorder in an individual patient can be assessed properly only if certain conceptual problems are understood. These problems are illustrated in the *case study*.

Case study: causes of psychiatric disorder

For four weeks a 38-year-old married man became increasingly depressed. His symptoms had started soon after his wife left him to live with another man. The following points in the history were potentially relevant to aetiology. The patient's mother had received psychiatric treatment on two past occasions, once for a severe depressive disorder, and once for mania; on neither occasion was there any apparent environmental cause for the illness. When the patient was 14 years old, his mother went to live with another man, leaving her children with their father. For several years afterwards the patient felt rejected and unhappy but eventually settled down. He married and had two children, aged 13 and 10 at the time of his illness. Two weeks after leaving home, the patient's wife returned saying that she had made a mistake and really loved her husband. Despite her return the patient's symptoms persisted and worsened. He began to wake early, gave up his usual activities, and spoke at times of suicide.

In assessing the causal significance of these events, the clinician can draw first on his knowledge of scientific studies of depressive disorders. Genetic investigations have shown that a predisposition to depressive disorder is probably genetically transmitted (see p. 138). It is possible, therefore, that this patient inherited this kind of predisposition from his mother. Is the separation from his mother likely to have been significant? There have been several studies of the long-term effects of separating children from their parents, but they refer to people who were separated when younger than the patient was at separation. So this body of knowledge does not help here. Nonetheless, extrapolation from this evidence and clinical experience suggests that his mother's departure is likely to have been important. It is also understandable that a man should feel depressed when his wife leaves him; this particular man is likely to be especially affected by the experience because the event recapitulates the similar distressing separation in his own childhood. Empathy and common sense would also suggest that the patient should have felt better when his wife came back, but he did not. This lack of improvement can be explained, however, by evidence that distressing events can induce a depressive disorder which then runs an independent course and requires treatment.

This case study illustrates several important issues concerning aetiology in psychiatry: the interaction of different causes in a single case; the need to distinguish different kinds of cause; the concept of stress and of psychological reactions to it; and the roles of scientific evidence and of evaluation based on empathy and common sense.

Explaining and understanding

There are two ways of trying to make sense of the causes of a patient's problems. Both are useful but it is important to distinguish between them. The first approach is quantitative and based on research findings; for example, a person's aggressive behaviour may be explained as the result of an injury to the frontal cortex sustained in a road accident. This statement draws on results of scientific studies of the behaviour of patients with damage to various areas of the brain. It is conventional to refer to this kind of statement as **explaining** the behaviour.

The second approach is qualitative and is based on an empathic understanding of human behaviour. We use this approach when we decide, for example, that a person was aggressive because his wife was insulted by a neighbour. The connection between these two events makes sense; it is convincing even though no quantitative study has shown a statistical association between aggression and this kind of insult. It is conventional to refer to this kind of statement as **understanding** the cause of the behaviour.

In every branch of medicine doctors need to explain and to understand their patients' problems; in psychiatry understanding is often a particularly important part of the investigation of aetiology.

Remote causes and multiple causes

In psychiatry, certain events in childhood are associated with psychiatric disorder in adult life. For example, subjects who develop schizophrenia are more likely than controls to have been exposed to complications of pregnancy and labour.

One cause can lead to several effects; for example, lack of parental affection in childhood has been reported to predispose to suicide, antisocial behaviour, and depressive disorder. Conversely, a *single effect* can have *several causes*, which act singly or in combination; for mental handicap can be caused by any one of several distinct genetic abnormalities, whilst a depressive disorder can be caused by the combined effects of genetic factors and recent stressful events.

The classification of causes

When there are multiple causes it is useful to group them into predisposing, precipitating, and perpetuating factors (Fig. 4.1 and Table 4.1).

Predisposing factors determine vulnerability to other causes that act close to the time of the illness. Many predisposing factors act early in life, for example: genetic endowment; the environment *in utero*; trauma at birth; and social and psychological factors in infancy and childhood.

Precipitating factors are events that occur shortly before the onset of a disorder and appear to have induced it. They may be physical, psychological, or social. Physical precipitating causes include diseases such as cerebral tumour, and the effects of drugs taken for treatment or used illegally. An example of *a psychological cause* is bereavement; while moving home is *a social cause*. Some causes may act in more than one way; for example, a head injury may induce a psychiatric disorder through physical changes in the brain and through psychological effects.

Perpetuating factors prolong a disorder after it has begun. Sometimes a feature of a disorder makes it self-perpetuating (e.g. some ways of thinking commonly prolong anxiety disorders, see p. 109). Social factors are also important (e.g. overprotective attitudes of relatives). Awareness of perpetuating factors is particularly important in planning treatment because they may be modifiable even when little can be done about predisposing and precipitating factors.

Models in aetiology

In discussions of aetiology the word 'model' is often used to mean a way of ordering information. Like a theory, a model seeks to explain certain phenomena and to show the relationships between them. Unlike a theory, it does so in a broad and comprehensive way that cannot be proved wrong by carrying out an experiment. Darwin's ideas of natural selection are an example of a successful model in the biological sciences. Freudian theory is an example of a model that was widely used in the past in psychiatry.

- **Reductionist models** seek to understand causation by tracing back to simpler, earlier stages. This kind of model, which is familiar in science, is exemplified in psychiatry by the supposition that schizophrenia is caused by disordered neurotransmission in certain areas of the brain.

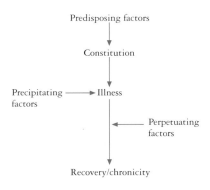

Fig. 4.1 Predisposing, precipitating, and perpetuating factors (see also Table 4.1).

Table 4.1.

Predisposing, precipitating, and perpetuating factors

Predisposing factors
Genetic endowment
Environment *in utero*
Trauma at birth
Social/psychological factors in development

Precipitating factors
Physical diseases; drugs
Psychological stressors
Social changes

Perpetuating factors
Intrinsic to the disorder
Social circumstances

- **Non-reductionist models** seek to understand causation in terms of a wider (rather than a narrower) set of issues. This kind of model, which is familiar in the social sciences, is exemplified in psychiatry by the supposition that the cause of a patient's neurosis is in his family, and that his symptoms are only one aspect of a disordered family life.

The medical model is an approach to research in which psychiatric disorders are investigated in ways that have proved useful in general medicine: for example, by identifying regularly occurring patterns of symptoms (syndromes) and relating them to pathological findings. This model has proved particularly useful in investigating organic psychiatric disorders, and in studying schizophrenia and severe affective disorders. It is less useful, although not without value, in the study of neuroses and personality disorders.

The behavioural model This term refers to an approach to research in which psychiatric disorders are explained in terms of factors that determine normal behaviour; for example drives and reinforcements, attitudes and beliefs, and cultural influences. This model has been most useful in investigating neuroses and personality disorders. Behavioural models can be either reductionist (e.g. explanations in terms of conditioning), or non-reductionist (e.g. explanations in terms of social influences).

Methodological approaches

In this section, it is not our intention to provide an extensive review of the aetiology of psychiatric disorders. Current knowledge about the causes of specific disorders is presented in the relevant chapters. Here, we provide a brief summary of the kinds of approach which have been, and are being, used in investigating the causes of psychiatric disorder. We suggest that the reader first reads the aetiology sections in the following chapters, using this section as a guide to allow them to keep up-to-date with advances in knowledge.

Epidemiology

Epidemiology is the study of the distribution of diseases in space and time within a population, and of factors that influence this distribution. In psychiatry, epidemiology is used to provide information about prevalence (which is useful for planning services) and about causation. Information about the epidemiology of particular psychiatric disorders is given in other chapters in this book. Some terms used in epidemiology are defined in Box 4.1.

In psychiatry, the best method of *case definition* is usually by reference to the definitions in a standard system of classification, such as DSM-IV or ICD-10 (see Chapter 3). The types of study designs used in psychiatric epidemiology are shown in *additional information*.

Box 4.1 **Epidemiology: definitions**

Case A person in the population or study group identified as having the disorder. In psychiatry, the *case definition* is usually a set of agreed criteria or a cut-off point on a continuous scale

Rate The ratio of the number of cases to the number of people in a defined population.

Prevalence The rate for all cases, new and old. Prevalence may be determined on a particular occasion (*point prevalence*), or over a period of time (e.g. one-year prevalence).

Incidence is the rate for *new* cases *Inception rates* represent the number of people who were healthy at the beginning of a defined period but became ill during it. *Lifetime expectation* represents the number of people who could be expected to develop a particular illness in the course of their whole life.

Additional information **Study designs used in psychiatric epidemiology**

- A **case-control study** is an observational study comparing the frequency of an exposure in a group of persons with the disease of interest (*cases*) with a group of persons without the disease (*controls*). Case-control studies are commonly used to look for *risk factors* for psychiatric disorders. For example, a finding that a group of patients with schizophrenia had a higher rate of exposure to birth complications than a non-schizophrenic control group could be interpreted as meaning that birth complications predisposed to schizophrenia. Case-control studies are quick to do and relatively cheap, but are susceptible to bias.

- A **cohort study** is an observational study in which a group of persons without the disorder are followed up to see which of them get the disorder. For example, a cohort of newly delivered babies could be followed through childhood and adolescence to see which of them developed schizophrenia—and if any birth characteristics were associated with a higher risk for the disorder. Cohort studies are potentially less susceptible to bias—but take a long time to do and are expensive.

- A **prevalence** (or **cross-sectional**) **study** is an observational study in which the presence or absence of a disorder and any other variable of interest is measured in a defined population. For example, a sample of homeless people could be surveyed to estimate the prevalence of schizophrenia.

- **Ecological studies** examine the rates of disorder in the population and relate them to other population rates of factors in the environment. For example, in the UK, it was observed that there was a reduction in the suicide rate following the change from coal gas to natural gas. This was interpreted as showing that reducing the availability of methods could prevent suicide.

Genetics

Genetic studies in psychiatry are concerned with three issues:

1. The relative contributions of genetic and environmental contributions to aetiology.

Additional information **Epidemiological study designs used in genetics**

- **Family risk studies** The affected people (probands) are identified, rates of disorder are determined among various classes of relatives, and these rates are compared with those in the general population. From the observed prevalence, estimates are computed of the numbers of people likely to develop the condition subsequently. These corrected figures are called *expectancy rates* or *morbid risks*. Rates higher than those expected in the general population show that a familial cause is likely. Family studies can show whether a condition is familial but they do not distinguish between the effects of inheritance and those of family environment.

- **Twin studies** Comparisons are made between concordance rates in uniovular (monozygotic, or MZ) twins and in binovular (dizygotic, or DZ) twins. If concordance is significantly greater among uniovular twins than among binovular twins, a significant genetic component is inferred. A more precise estimate of the contributions of heredity and environment can be made by comparing the rates of disorder among the rare cases of MZ twins reared apart, with the rates among MZ twins reared together. If rates are the same in those reared apart and those reared together, this indicates an important genetic component to aetiology.

- **Adoption studies** Children who, since early infancy, have been reared by unrelated adoptive parents are studied. Two comparisons can be made. The first is between adopted persons with a biological parent who had the disorder under investigation, and adopted persons with biological parents free from the disorder. A higher rate of the disorder among the former indicates a genetic cause. The second comparison is between the biological parents and the adoptive parents of adopted persons who have the disorder. A higher rate of the disorder among the biological parents indicates a genetic cause. Such studies can be affected by several biases; for example, adoptees may be assigned to adoptive parents on the basis of the socioeconomic status of the biological parents. In psychiatry, adoption studies have been applied to schizophrenia (see p. 161) and affective disorder (see p. 138), and the findings point to genetic causes in both conditions.

- **Mode of inheritance** This is assessed by using statistical methods to test the closeness of fit between the rates of disorder in various classes of relatives of the probands, and the rates predicted by various models of inheritance (e.g. dominant, recessive, sex-linked). When applied to psychiatric disorders such studies have generally given equivocal results, suggesting that the mode of inheritance is not simple.

2. The mode of inheritance of disorders that have a genetic basis.

3. Biochemical mechanisms involved in hereditary disease.

Some progress has been made with answering the first two questions, but little with the third.

Three methods have been used to study these problems:

- *Epidemiological* methods to studying populations and families can evaluate the contribution of genetic factors to aetiology, and throw light on the mode

Additional information Study designs used in cellular and molecular genetics

- **Cytogenetic studies** aim to identify abnormalities in the structure or number of chromosomes. *Karyotyping* is a commonly used techniques in which chromosomal spreads are examined with a microscope. Cytogenetic abnormalities have been identified as causes of learning disabilities (e.g. Down's syndrome, in which there is a trisomy of chromosome 21). Chromosomal abnormalities have not been identified as a primary cause of functional psychiatric disorders although, occasionally, such abnormalities may give indirect clues to the aetiology of some disorders. For example, subjects with **the velo-cardio-facial syndrome** (associated with a deletion on chromosome 22) have a high incidence of bipolar affective disorder.

- **Linkage studies** These studies seek to identify the chromosomal region likely to be carrying the genes responsible for a disorder in a family or group of families. Linkage studies have been successful in identifying the genes causing Huntington's disease and familial Alzheimer's syndrome. Their role is limited in disorders which are not due to single major genes, such as most psychiatric disorders. There are also problems in using linkage studies in psychiatric disorders due to uncertain phenotypes and statistical complexities. To date, no confirmed linkage has been found between a common psychiatric disorder and a specific chromosomal region.

- **Association studies** These are case-control studies (see p. 59) in which the frequency of a genetic variant (or polymorphism/allelic variant) in a group of subjects with a disorder is compared to the frequency of the variant in a group of subjects without the disorder. The *advantages* of association studies compared to linkage studies are that they are easier to perform in complex disorders, they do not need familial samples, and they make fewer statististical assumptions. The *disadvantages* are that they require a *candidate gene* (a genetic marker which is close to or part of a gene which is suspected of being involved in the disorder) and that they are susceptible to *confounding* (a situation when an observed association with a gene or other cause is simply due to other differences between the cases and controls). So far, although encouraging, association studies have not produced unequivocal results in psychiatric disorders.

of inheritance (e.g. whether dominant or recessive). The main study designs are shown in *Additional information*.

- *Cytogenetics* and *molecular genetics* provide information about chromosomal and genetic abnormalities and the mechanisms of inheritance (see *Additional information*).

Biochemical studies

Biochemical studies in psychiatry are difficult to carry out because:

1. The living brain is inaccessible to direct study and post-mortem tissue is not often available (since most psychiatric disorders do not lead to death). To overcome this problem, indirect approaches have been made through more

accessible sites; their value has been limited because concentrations of substances in cerebrospinal fluid, and especially in blood and urine, have uncertain relationships to their concentrations in the brain.

2. Animal studies are of limited use because there are no obvious parallels in animals to the mental disorders found in man. (Animal studies are useful, howevers, in the study of the actions of drugs on the brain.)

3. It is difficult to prove that any biochemical abnormalities detected are causal and not secondary either to changes in diet or in activity induced by the mental disorder, or to the effects of drugs used in treatment.

Despite these problems, *biochemical studies of post-mortem brain* tissue have been moderately informative in Alzheimer's disease, schizophrenia, and affective disorder. In Alzheimer's disease there is a widespread decline of transmitter function: however, this decline could be no more than a consequence of the loss of cells in this disorder. In schizophrenia, the density of dopamine receptors is increased in the caudate nucleus and nucleus accumbens; but this increase could be the result of treatment with antipsychotic drugs, which block dopamine receptors and so might lead to a compensatory increase in their density. In severe affective disorder, some studies have found reduced 5-HT (serotonin) function in the brainstem; but these findings were based on patients who had died by suicide, and they could result from terminal anoxia or the drugs used for suicide.

More recently, *brain imaging methods* have been used to study biochemical function in living brain tissue (see Table 4.2).

Pharmacology

If a drug alleviates a disorder, and if the mode of action of the drug is known, then it might be possible to infer the biochemical abnormality underlying the disorder. This line of argument must be pursued cautiously, however, since effective drugs do not always act directly on the biochemical abnormality underlying the disorder; for example anticholinergic drugs are effective in Parkinson's disease but the symptoms of this disorder are caused by a defect in dopaminergic transmission, not by an excess of cholinergic transmission.

Endocrinology

In psychiatric patients tests of endocrine function have been used to:

• determine how hormonal activity changes in psychiatric disorder; for example, it has been shown that cortisol is produced at an increased rate in depressed patients.

• to use changes in endocrine function as indirect measures of other processes. This usage is possible because many endocrine functions are controlled through neurotransmitters that could be involved in causing psychiatric disorder. Thus, if an abnormality in endocrine function is due to disordered function of a particular neurotransmitter in one brain system, it is possible that the same neurotransmitter could be functioning abnormally in another brain system, and that this second malfunctioning could be the cause of the psychiatric disorder. For example, endocrine abnormalities indicating reduced 5-HT function have

Table 4.2.

Brain imaging techniques

Structural imaging techniques	
Computerized tomography (CT scan)	X-rays taken of brain from many different angles combined to produce a series of images of 'slices' through the brain. Demonstrated lateral ventricular enlargement in schizophrenia.
Magnetic resonance imaging (MRI scan)	Non-ionizing radio-waves directed at brain in presence of a strong magnetic field. Asymmetric nuclei align and resonate, producing signals which are converted into an image by a computer. Demonstrated more subtle brain abnormalities in schizophrenia.
Functional imaging techniques	
Positron emission tomography (PET scan)	Radiolabelled short-living isotopes (produced in a cyclotron) injected and emit radiation which is detected by a scanner and converted to an image by a computer. Used to measure regional cerebral blood flow and ligand binding.
Single photon emission tomography (SPET scan)	Simpler than PET, does not require a cyclotron. Photons emitted by injected radiochemicals are detected by a rotating gamma camera. Used to measure regional cerebral blood flow and ligand binding.
Functional magnetic resonance imaging (fMRI)	Based on the sensitivity of MRI to magnetic effects caused by the variation in the oxygenation of haemoglobin, which is induced by local changes in blood flow during task activation. Because it does not involve radiation, may be used repeatedly in the same subject.

been found in depressive disorder, and it has been proposed that more widespread reduction of 5-HT is a cause of this disorder.

Neuropathology

Post-mortem brain studies have been carried out for over a century, yielding useful information about dementias and other organic disorders, but until recently have shown no consistent abnormalities in the functional psychoses. Modern quantitative methods have demonstrated abnormalities in the medial temporal lobes and other brain areas of patients with schizophrenia, and these abnormalities could be relevant to the aetiology of this disorder. Advances in brain imaging techniques have provided a method on invetisgating the structure and function of the brain pre-mortem (see Table 4.2).

Electrophysiology

Electrophysiological recordings made with electrodes on the skull surface (as in electroencephalography) do not give precise information about the nature and site of abnormal brain activity and have contributed little to the understanding of psychiatric disorders, except for those related to epilepsy.

Psychology

Psychology is the study of normal behaviour, and is therefore highly relevant to the study of abnormal behaviour in mental disorders. Psychological studies have contributed to the understanding of causes of anxiety disorders (see p. 181); but their main importance is not in relation to the onset of psychiatric disorder but to the factors that maintain the disorders once started. The most relevant psychological mechanisms concern conditioning, social learning, and cognitive processing. (Readers who have not studied these concepts should consult a textbook of psychology or behavioural science.)

Classic conditioning: learning through association, explains, for example, the development of situational anxiety in phobic patients following an initial attack of anxiety in the situation (see p. 115).

Operant conditioning: the reinforcement of behaviour by its consequences, explains, for example, the maintenance of disruptive behaviour in some patients by the extra attention that is provided by staff or relatives when this behaviour occurs.

Cognitive processes are concerned with aspects of the ways in which patients select interpret and act on the information from the sense organs and memory stores. Some disorders are maintained, in part, by the ways that patients think about the physical symptoms associated with emotional arousal. For example, patients with panic disorder think that palpitations are a precursor of a heart attack and so become more anxious (see p. 181). Knowledge of these psychological mechanisms has led to new methods of treatment known as and cognitive-behaviour therapies (see Chapter 17).

Coping mechanisms are ways in which people attempt to deal with stressors. The term is used in both a wide and narrow sense. The *wide sense* includes any way of responding to stressors, whether or not the response reduces the stress reaction. The *narrow sense* refers only to ways of responding that reduce the stress reaction. To avoid confusion it is useful to apply the terms *maladaptive* or *ineffective* to responses that fail to reduce the stress reaction. Coping mechanisms have two components: (1) internal processes, and (2) observable behaviour. For example, after bereavement, a person's coping mechanisms might include thinking about religious beliefs (an internal process), and joining a social club to combat loneliness (observable behaviour). Another internal coping mechanism is to change the meaning attached to an event; for example, an imposed alteration of job may be regarded at first as a threat but later as a challenging opportunity. Examples of maladaptive coping mechanisms are avoiding the problem, or consuming alcohol to relieve distress.

Ethology

Ethology, which is concerned with the observation and description of behaviour, has contributed usefully to research into behaviour disorders of children. The methods provide quantitative observations that allow comparisons of an individual's behaviour with that of other people, and with relevant behaviour in animals. Thus, the effects of separating human infants and infant monkeys from their mothers have been shown to be similar in certain ways; for example, infants of both kinds are distressed and active at first, and then call less and adopt a hunched posture. Such parallels help to distinguish between innate and culturally determined aspects of behaviour.

Sociology

Clinical observations indicate that psychiatric disorder may be provoked or influenced by factors in the social environment. Sociology, the study of human society, is therefore a potentially valuable source of information about the causes of psychiatric disorder. The main sociological concepts which have been applied to psychiatric disorders are listed below.

Social role Behaviour that develops as a result of other people's expectations of or demands on a person. Each individual takes more than one role (e.g. as worker, father, husband, and so on).

Sick role Behaviour expected and required of an ill person. It includes exemption from some responsibilities, the right to expect help from others, the expectation of a wish to recover, and an obligation to seek treatment.

Illness behaviour The behaviour of the person in the sick role. It includes seeking help, consulting doctors, taking medicines, and giving up responsibilities. A person may adopt the sick role and show illness behaviour without having any illness, or may show illness behaviour that is out of proportion to the degree of ill-health (see Chapter 11).

Social class Status within society, determined usually on the basis of job or income. There is an association between schizophrenia and low social class (see Chapter 9).

Life event A stressful aspect of living which may be associated with changes in health status. Life events have been shown to contribute to the onset and maintenance of schizophrenia, affective disorder, and some other psychiatric disorders.

Culture The way of life shared by a group of human beings. A *subculture* is the way of life shared by a subgroup within a wider cultural group. Culture affects the ways people behave when ill (the sick role and illness behaviour mentioned above), as well as the routines and values of carers and families. The presentation and course of mental disorders may be influenced by cultural factors.

Social mobility A change of role or status in a society. Schizophrenia may lead to downward social mobility (decline to a lower social class), while upward mobility may be a stressful experience provoking an adjustment disorder.

Migration Movement between societies. Migration can be a stressful experience and it has been suggested as a cause of mental disorder.

Social institution An established social organization (e.g. the family, school, or hospital). The roles taken by the mother and father, and in the relationships between the 'nuclear' family of parents and children, and the 'extended' family of grandparents, aunts, and uncles may differ between cultures. These family differences are important in understanding the impact of one member's illness on other family members.

Total institution An institution in which the inmates spend all their time in the one place and have little freedom to choose their way of life: long-stay psychiatric hospitals can be total institutions. If life in the institution is unduly ordered, repetitive, and restrictive, the people living there may lose initiative, withdraw into fantasy, or rebel. In this way, institutional living can add further handicaps ('institutionalization') to those of the mental disorder.

Keeping up-to-date: evidence-based medicine

Although every effort is made to ensure that textbooks (including this one!) are accurate, comprehensive, and up-to-date, inevitably as knowledge increases, they become out-of-date. For example, questions about treatment arise frequently in clinical practice. Although the doctor will have learned about treatments during his training, it is in this area of practice that the most rapid advances occur and so it is most difficult to keep up-to-date. New drugs, other kinds of treatment, and other clinical procedures of being introduced all the time and it can be difficult for a doctor to find unbiased information about them. For example, at the time of writing, there is considerable uncertainty about the role of new anti-Alzheimer's disease drugs such as donepezil. Imagine being a general practitioner faced with a 70-year-old woman who is beginning to dement, and whose family are very keen that she should be prescribed donepezil. Should the general practitioner prescribe the drug?

The doctor needs a way of quickly accessing the best available information—and also needs to know how to combine it with his understanding of the patient and their preferences. In the past, the doctor had to rely on potentially out-of-date or biased sources of information such as textbooks, authoritative reviews, promotional materials or, most commonly, the opinions of colleagues. Recently, a number of techniques derived from advances in clinical epidemiology and information science have been introduced. Collectively, these strategies are often called **evidence-based medicine (EBM)** and they are helpful for answering frequently arising clinical questions and keeping up-to-date. In this section we will review some of the basics of EBM, although we would recommend that the reader consults a book dealing specifically with the subject.

Table 4.3.
Types of clinical question

Type of question	Form of the question	Best study design
Diagnosis	How likely is a patient who has a particular symptom, sign or, diagnostic test result to have a specific disorder?	A *cross-sectional study* of patients suspected of having the disorder comparing the proportion of the patients who **really** have the disorder who have a positive test with the proportion of patients who do **not have** the disorder who have a positive test result.
Treatment	Is the treatment of interest more effective in producing a desired outcome than an alternative treatment (including no treatment)?	A *randomized controlled trial* (RCT) in which the patients are randomly allocated to receive either the treatment of interest of the alternative.
Prognosis	How likely is a specific outcome in this patient?	A study in which an *inception cohort* (patients at a common stage in the development of the illness, especially first onset) are followed up for an adequate length of time.
Aetiology	What has caused the disorder?	A study which compares the frequency of an exposure in a group of persons with the disease (*cases*) of interest with a group of persons without the disease (*controls*) – this may be an RCT, a case-control study, or a cohort study (see Box 4.1).

EBM breaks the process of answering clinical questions down into four stages:

1. Forming a precise, structured clinical question.

2. Searching for the best kind of evidence to answer the question.

3. Critically appraising the evidence.

4. Applying the evidence to the clinical problem.

Table 4.3 summarizes the main kinds of question that arise in clinical practice and the best study design for answering each kind of clinical question. When the best sort of evidence is not available, the clinician moves down a **hierarchy of evidence** and searches for the best available evidence. Study designs at the top of the hierarchy are more likely to be trustworthy and free from bias than those further down. The hierarchy of evidence is best worked out for treatment studies:

(1)   a well-executed systematic review of two or more randomized controlled trials comparing treatments for the disorder of interest. The key difference

between a systematic review and a non-systematic review is that the former has a methods section in which the search strategy is described explicitly.

(2) a single randomized controlled trial.

(3) a well-designed non-randomized study (e.g. cohort study, case-control study).

(4) respected authorities, expert committees, clinical experience.

Searching for the evidence

The process of answering the question should start with a search for the highest quality of evidence, moving down the hierarchy if no systematic review is found. Box 4.2 provides *sources* of evidence and Fig. 4.2 provides an *approach* to searching for evidence based on this hierarchy.

In the example, the doctor searches the Cochrane Database, Best Evidence, and Medline, but finds no systematic reviews. He therefore goes on to search for a

Box 4.2 Sources of evidence

The Cochrane Library This is published quarterly on CD-ROM, floppy disk, and the World Wide Web (http:\\update.cochrane.co.uk). It contains:

• *The Cochrane Database of Systematic Reviews (CDSR)*. This is a continually updated database of high quality systematic reviews maintained by the Cochrane Collaboration. The reviews are published in a uniform format. The CDSR is probably the best place to start searching. At present, it contains relatively few reviews, although the number is rapidly increasing.

• *The Database of Abstracts of Reviews of Effectiveness (DARE)*. This is a database of critically appraised non-Cochrane reviews maintained by the UK National Health Service Centre for Reviews and Dissemination.

• *The Cochrane Controlled Trials Register*. This is a database of controlled clinical trials identified by the Cochrane Collaboration. Many of them are not indexed on MEDLINE or other bibliographic databases.

• *The Cochrane Review Methodology Database*. This is a comprehensive database of methodological articles.

MEDLINE The computerized index of biomedical journals maintained by the National Library of Medicine in the USA and available on CD-ROM disk and on-line. It contains about 45% of relevant articles and is best at covering articles published in English. Use of MEDLINE requires some experience.

PsycLIT An electronic database similar to MEDLINE, but maintained by the American Psychological Association and specifically covering psychology and psychiatry journals.

EMBASE A European equivalent of MEDLINE, good for searching for drug trials.

Evidence-Based Medicine; Evidence-Based Mental Health. These are regularly published journals publishing systematically selected abstracts of the best research as it is published. The contents of these journals is published cumulatively on the CD-ROM, *Best Evidence*.

1. **Search for an evidence-based clinical practice guideline**

2. **Search for a good quality systematic review of randomized controlled trials of the intervention**

   Cochrane Database of Systematic Reviews

   Database of Abstracts of Reviews of Effectiveness

   Evidence-Based Mental Health

   Medline, EMBASE, or PsycLIT

3. **Search for a single randomized controlled trial**

   Cochrane Controlled Trials Register

   Evidence-Based Mental Health

   Medline, EMBASE, or PsycLIT

4. **Search for the next level of evidence**

   Medline, EMBASE, or PsycLIT

Fig. 4.2 Searching for evidence about treatment.

single randomized controlled trial. By entering the word 'Donepezil' and restricting publication type to 'Randomized Controlled Trial', he identifies one paper:

Example

Rogers, S. L. and Friedhoff, L. T. (1996). The efficacy and safety of donepezil in patients with Alzheimer's disease: results of a US multicentre, randomized, double-blind, placebo-controlled trial. *Dementia*, **7**,293–303.

Critical appraisal of the evidence

The article reported a study comparing donepezil (1,3, or 5 mg) with placebo in 161 patients with at least a 12-month history of mild to moderate Alzheimer's disease (diagnosed according to DSM-IIIR—the forerunner of DSM-IV). The main outcome measures were the change from baseline score on the cognitive subscale of the Alzheimer's Disease Assessment Scale and the clinician's overall impression of whether the patient had deteriorated after the 12-week period of the trial. In order to assess the scientific validity of the study, it is helpful to use a checklist:

- Was the assignment of patients to treatments randomized?—and was the randomization list concealed?

- Were all patients who entered the trial accounted for at its conclusion?— and were they analysed in the groups to which they were randomized?

- Were patients and clinicians kept 'blind' to which treatment was being received?

- Apart from the experimental treatment, were the groups treated equally?
- Were the groups similar at the start of the trial?

The donepezil study appears to meet these criteria.

Deciding if the results are important and if they apply to your own patient

Patients in randomized control trials (RCTs) differ from those in normal clinical practice in several ways. The subjects are often selected—they may be only one sex or from a restricted age distribution. Compared to real-life patients, they may be less likely to have multiple problems and may be more likely to comply with treatment. This is a particular issue in psychiatry where co-morbidity is very common. Unless the RCT has been designed to approximate as closely as possible to normal clinical practice (a *pragmatic* trial), the results of the study often represent the treatment (both experimental and control) under 'ideal' conditions. Before using the results to help you decide on what treatment to use for your patient, you need to assess how much your patient resembles the subjects in the study.

- Is this patient so different from those in the trial that the results do not apply?
- How great would the benefit of therapy be for this particular patient?

The next step is to estimate how effective donepezil is compared to placebo. In the study, clinical deterioration over the 12-week period, according to the clinician's overall impression, occurred in 20% of patients on placebo and 11% of patients taking donepezil, 5 mg per day. From these figures, several useful measures of effectiveness can be calculated (see Table. 4.3). Perhaps the most useful of these is the number needed to treat (NNT), which indicates the number of patients who need to be treated with donepezil as opposed to placebo, to prevent one from deteriorating over a 12-week period. In the case of donepezil, the NNT is 11. Donepezil also produced a small improvement in cognitive functioning score. However, there was no improvement in the quality of life scores. The general

Table 4.3
Clinically useful measures of the effect of treatment

Event rates (proportion clinically deteriorating over 12-week period)		Relative risk reduction (RRR)	Absolute risk reduction (ARR)	Number need to treat (NNT)
Control event rate (CER)	Experimental event rate (EER)			
Placebo	Donepezil 5mg/day	= (CER-EER)/CER	= (CER-EER)	= 1/ARR
0.20	0.11	= (0.2–0.11)/0.2 = 0.45 = 45%	= (0.20–0.11) = 0.09 = 9%	= 1/0.09 = 11

practitioner decides that, although the study provides evidence of some benefit in the short term, there is no evidence that donepezil confers benefit in the long term—or that it produces improved quality of life. He therefore advises the patient and her relatives that the benefit of the drug is still uncertain and that he would not recommend it at the present time. New research may have changed this conclusion by the time this chapter is read.

Evidence-based medicine in psychiatry

It is sometimes thought that there is little evidence on which to base treatment decisions in psychiatry—and that psychiatry is too complex to be susceptible to this approach. Both of these assumptions are wrong. In fact, there is a great deal of evidence in psychiatry, probably as much as in any other branch of medicine. The aim of EBM is to allow the doctor to access the best available evidence as quickly as possible and to integrate it with his clinical expertise to best help a particular patient. EBM also helps answer questions regarding diagnosis, prognosis, and aetiology.

As we hope we have illustrated in this chapter, clinical decisions need to be based on other factors as well as sound scientific evidence. These factors involve an understanding of the patient and their circumstances and preferences. They also include an awareness of the costs of new treatments. Limited resources mean that there is an increasing requirement for new treatments to be both at least as effective existing treatments, but also to confer some additional added value, such as fewer adverse effects or reduced costs.

Further reading

Sackett, D. L., Richardson, S., Rosenberg, W., and Haynes, R. B. (1997). *Evidence-based Medicine: How to Practise and Teach EBM*. Churchill Livingstone, Edinburgh.
How to search for, critically appraise and use research evidence in everyday clinical practice.

Henderson, A. S. (1988). *An Introduction to Social Psychiatry*. Oxford University Press.
Chapters 2, 3, and 4 describe the social causes of psychiatric disorders and the methods which have been used to investigate them.

Johnstone, E. C. (ed.) (1996). Biological psychiatry. *British Medical Bulletin*, 52 (No. 3).
Reviews findings from studies investigating the biological causes of psychiatric disorders (including chapters on psychopharmacology, genetics, neuroimaging, and neuropathology).

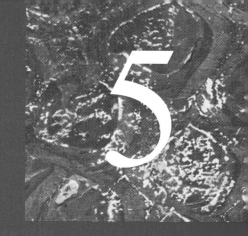

5

Personality and its disorders

- Assessment of personality
- Types of personality disorder
- Epidemiology
- Aetiology
- The prognosis of personality disorder
- The management of personality disorder

Personality and its disorders

In their day-to-day work doctors meet many patients whose personality is abnormal. They need to understand these personalities for four reasons. First, they may react in unusual ways to physical illness or its treatment, for example by becoming either overdependent or untrusting and non-compliant. Second, when personality is abnormal the clinical picture of psychiatric disorder changes, making diagnosis more difficult. Third, abnormal personalities may react differently to stressful events, for example, with aggressive or histrionic behaviour instead of anxiety. Fourth, abnormal personalities may behave in ways that are stressful or even dangerous to other people, for example, a husband who is persistently aggressive may cause his wife to become depressed or act violently towards her.

After completing this chapter, readers should have a general understanding of the ways in which personality may be abnormal and the distinction between this and personality disorder, and the ways in which these conditions are classified. They should know how to: (1) assess personality; (2) distinguish abnormal personality from mental disorder; and (3) manage abnormal personalities in everyday practice. They should have a general understanding of specialized treatments, and know when to refer to a psychiatrist.

What is personality?

The term 'personality' refers to the enduring characteristics of an individual as shown in ways of behaving in a wide variety of circumstances. Personality can be thought of as being made up of more circumscribed characteristics known as traits, such as sociability, aggressivity, and impulsivity. When describing abnormal personality it is usually better to list the principal traits, rather than attempt to apply a diagnostic label. However, some abnormal personalities are dominated by a single trait and for these a single descriptive term is useful, as will be explained later. However, even for abnormal personalities it is important to note other features, especially those positive features that might be developed further in treatment.

What is personality disorder?

Extreme deviations of personality can be recognized as disordered but it is difficult to define a dividing line between normal and abnormal. If personality could be measured like intelligence, a statistical cut-off could be used (e.g. two standard deviations from the population mean). However, although psychologists have devised measures of some aspects of personality there are no reliable and valid measures of the aspects of personality that are most important to clinical practice. In the absence of such measures, a simple pragmatic criterion is used: *a personality is disordered when it causes suffering to the person or to other people*. This definition may appear simplistic but it is useful in clinical practice, and leads to reasonable agreement between those using it.

Assessment of personality

Sources of information

In everyday life we build a picture of the personality of people we know by observing how they respond in various circumstances. General practitioners do the same with patients who they see over many years, but they and other doctors have to be able to assess the personality of patients whom they have not met before. To do this they can use four sources of information:

(1) patients' own descriptions of their personality;

(2) patients' behaviour during the interview with the doctor;

(3) patients' accounts of their behaviour in a variety of past circumstances;

(4) the views of relatives or friends.

In a job interview, the applicant's behaviour in the interview is often considered a useful guide to personality. When assessing patients, however, interview behaviour can be highly misleading because it is affected by temporary factors relating to illness as well as by personality. Thus, anxiety or depression can make patients appear more irritable or less self-confident than they generally are. Depression is particularly important since it affects a second source of evidence, namely patients' accounts of their own personality: depressed patients tend to underestimate their strengths and exaggerate their weaknesses. It is important, therefore, to check the evaluation of personality formed from patients' own accounts and from their behaviour during the interview by comparing it with the other two sources of information listed above: their record of past achievements and difficulties and, whenever possible, the accounts of relatives and friends.

General practitioners get to know well many of their patients over many years and it is helpful, when writing a referral letter to a specialist who has not met the patient before, to include relevant points about personality. The information should be given in a factual way that would not distress patients were they to read the letter.

Information required

An outline of the assessment of personality was given in Chapter 2. The reader may wish to refer to this again before continuing with the rather more detailed account given here. The headings for a systematic scheme of enquiry are shown in Table 5.1 and each requires some further explanation. Although a large number of points are considered in this account, with experience, the interviewer can focus on the relevant matters so that the enquiry need not last long. When time is short, only the most relevant points need be covered in the first interview, leaving the others to a subsequent occasion.

In assessing personality, attention should be given not only to traits that lead to difficulties but also to those that are strengths. Sometimes a trait that is a strength in one situation leads to difficulty in others; for example, obsessional traits enable people to be reliable and set high standards at work but often lead to excessive worry when they are ill. Before starting the specific enquiries listed

Table 5.1.

A scheme for assessing personality

- Social relationships
- Mood
- Personality traits
  (see Table 5.2)
- Attitudes and standards
- Habits

below, it is useful to ask a general question; for example: 'How do you think your friends would describe your personality?'

Social relationships

This section is concerned with *relationships at work* (with colleagues, people in authority, and junior staff); *friendships* with the same and the opposite sex; and *intimate relationships*. The interviewer asks whether the patient makes friends easily, has few friends or many, has close friends in whom he can confide, and has lasting friendships. The interviewer also asks whether, in company, the person is sociable and confident, or shy and reserved.

Habitual mood

The aim here is to discover the person's habitual mood, not the present or recent mood. The interviewer asks whether mood is generally cheerful or gloomy, stable or changeable. If the mood is changeable, the interviewer asks how long the changes last, and whether they occur spontaneously or in relation to events. Finally, the interviewer asks whether the person shows his feelings or hides them.

Personality traits

When enquiring about personality traits it is useful to keep in mind the list of qualities in Table 5.2. Each characteristic has a positive as well as a negative side and it is appropriate to ask patients where they lie between the extremes; for example, some people are placid, others get into arguments—where do you fit in? Characteristics such as jealousy or lack of feeling for others may not be revealed because the person is ashamed of them or does not recognize their presence. When there is doubt the patient's previous record and the account from an informant usually help to resolve it. It is useful also to check answers by asking for examples from the patient's recent life. When the observations are noted, pejorative and imprecise terms such as 'immature' or 'inadequate' should not be used: instead, the interviewer should record in what ways the person has difficulty in meeting the demands of adult life.

Attitudes, beliefs, and standards

Relevant points include attitudes to illness, religious beliefs, and moral standards. Usually, these become apparent when the personal history is being taken, but they can be explored further at this point in the interview.

Habits

Although not strictly part of personality, it is usual to ask at this point in the interview, about the use of tobacco, alcohol, and illicit drugs since their use relates in part to personality—although there are other important influences.

Is there personality disorder?

The interviewer decides whether to diagnose a personality disorder by reviewing evidence from the clinical history to decide whether the patient or others has suffered as a result of the patient's personality. This judgement is subjective and it may be difficult to decide how much the patient's problems have been caused by personality and how much by circumstances. Despite these difficulties a judgement about personality disorder is useful in planning management.

Table 5.2.

Common personality traits

(For brevity, only negative attributes are listed. Corresponding positive features should also be noted)

- Prone to worry
- Strict, fussy, rigid
- Lacking self-confidence
- Sensitive
- Suspicious, jealous
- Untrusting, resentful
- Impulsive
- Attention seeking
- Dependent
- Irritable, quarrelsome
- Aggressive
- Lacking concern for others

Table 5.3.

Classification of personality disorders in DSM-IV and ICD-10

(Generally, the same terms are used in DSM-IV and ICD-10. Where there are differences the ICD term is shown in parentheses)

Anxious, moody, and prone to worry
- Avoidant (ICD: anxious)
- Obsessive-compulsive (ICD: anankastic)
- Depressive
- Hyperthymic
- Cyclothymic

Sensitive and suspicious
- Paranoid
- Schizoid
- Schizotypal

Dramatic and impulsive
- Histrionic
- Borderline (ICD: impulsive)
- Dependent

Aggressive and antisocial
- Antisocial (ICD: dissocial)

Note: personalities lacking self-esteem and self-confidence are not classified separately in DSM-IV or ICD-10.

Table 5.4.

Anxious, moody, and prone to worry

- Persistently anxious
- Worry about problems and health
- Inflexible and obstinate
- Indecisive
- Persistently gloomy
- Unstable moods

Types of personality disorder

As explained above, psychiatrists who treat people with highly abnormal personalities find it useful to employ the formal classification of personality disorder provided in ICD-10 and DSM-IV. Other doctors, who mainly treat people with less abnormal personalities, require a simpler scheme. The following scheme is useful outside specialist psychiatric practice and compatible with the more complex specialist classification:

- Anxious, moody, and prone to worry.
- Lacking self-esteem and confidence.
- Sensitive and suspicious.
- Dramatic and impulsive.
- Aggressive and antisocial.

Each of these groups will be described further. At the end of each description there is a note in parenthesis showing how the group relates to the more elaborate specialist classification which is summarized for reference at the end of the chapter (*Additional information*, p. 84) and shown in outline in Table 5.3.

Anxious, moody, and prone to worry personalities (Table 5.4)

Some of these people are persistently anxious and fearful, others are persistently gloomy and pessimistic. Others have fluctuating moods, in which periods of mild elation and overconfidence alternate with low mood and self-deprecation. Worry may be about everyday problems of the patient or the family, or be a persistent concern about illness (hypochondriasis, see p. 218). People with the obsessional traits of inflexibility, obstinacy, and indecisiveness are included in this group. This group corresponds with the dependent, anxious-avoidant and obsessive-compulsive (anankastic) groups in the specialist classifications (see *Additional information*, p. 84.)

Personalities lacking self-esteem and confidence (Table 5.5)

This group does not appear as a separate entity in the specialist classifications of personality disorder; these patients could appear under several of the headings. It is nevertheless common and important among the less severe derivations of personality seen in primary care and general medical practice. These people lack confidence in their abilities, feel inferior to others, and expect criticism. These inner uncertainties may lead to shyness, social withdrawal, and failure to achieve, or to inappropriate efforts to please other people, or forced attempts at sociability. These personality features are associated with recurrent depressive moods, eating disorders, and self-harm and are often seem among young people who seek help for these disorders.

Sensitive, and suspicious personalities (Table 5.6)

Some people in this group see rebuffs where none exist and may be suspicious, mistrustful, touchy, and irritable. Others are cold and detached, show little concern for others, and reject help when it is offered. Still others appear eccentric, with unusual ideas about topics such as telepathy and extrasensory perception. People in this group are difficult to engage in treatment and often distrust their doctors. This group corresponds with the paranoid, schizoid and schizotypal groups in the specialist classifications (see *Additional information*.)

Dramatic and impulsive personalities (Table 5.7)

These people seek the limelight and dramatize their problems. They make unreasonable demands on other people and may use 'emotional blackmail'. They have brief enthusiasms but lack persistence. Some have a great capacity for self-deception and a lack of awareness of the impression they make on others. They react impulsively, sometimes with ill-judged behaviour including self-harm. This group corresponds with the histrionic, borderline (impulsive), and narcissistic groups in the specialist classifications (see *Additional information*, p. 84.)

Aggressive and antisocial personalities (Table 5.8)

These people have low tolerance of frustration, behave impulsively, and tend to be violent. They lack guilt and fail to learn from experience. They are unloving and unconcerned with the feelings of others. When severe, these features are referred to as antisocial personality disorder (Box 5.1) and the people are often called 'psychopaths' (although this term is no longer used in classification). Such people have an unstable work record and may be involved in violence, family problems, and offences against the law. The difficulties are often increased by abuse of alcohol or drugs. This group corresponds with the dissocial or antisocial groups in the specialist classifications (see *Additional information*, p. 84.)

Epidemiology

The overall prevalence of personality disorder in community surveys is about 10%. Overall rates are higher in men than women and decrease with age.

Table 5.5.
Personalities lacking self-esteem

- Lack confidence
- Feel inferior
- Expect criticism
- Strive to please others

Table 5.6.
Sensitive, and suspicious personalities

- Sensitive
- Suspicious
- Mistrustful
- Self-sufficient
- Lacking concern

Table 5.7.
Dramatic and impulsive personalities

- Vain, self-centred
- Demanding of others
- Acts a part; self-deceiving
- Impulsive; short-lived enthusiasms
- Unrestrained emotional display

Box 5.1 Antisocial personality disorder

'Antisocial' personality is the term used in DSM-IV; in ICD-10, the term is 'dissocial'. These people fail to sustain loving relationships and disregard the feelings of others. They may act with callousness, as in the infliction of painful, cruel, or degrading acts on other people. They may have superficial charm but lack tender feelings so that their relationships are shallow and unsustained. Marriage may be marked by violence towards the partner, or neglect of or violence to the children. Many marriages end in separation or divorce.

Impulsive behaviour and lack of consistent striving towards a goal may be reflected in an unstable work record. Impulsivity, low tolerance of frustration, and tendency to violence, often lead to repeated offences against the law. These offences may begin with petty acts of delinquency, but go on to callous and violent crime. Lack of guilt and failure to learn from experience result in behaviour that persists despite serious consequences and legal penalties.

Table 5.8.
Aggressive and antisocial personalities

- Impulsive behaviour
- Low tolerance of frustration
- Tendency to violence
- Lack of guilt
- Failure to learn from experience
- Failure to sustain relationships
- Disregard of the feelings of others

Antisocial personality disorder is more common in men, histrionic and borderline personality disorders are more common in women. Personality disorders often coexist with mental disorders. A particularly important association is between antisocial personality disorder and alcohol and substance abuse.

Aetiology

Personality and it disorders result from the interaction of genetic factors and upbringing. It is not certain what is the relative contribution of these two causes and it is difficult to make progress in answering the question because of the complexity of human upbringing and the difficulty of recording accurately factors in early life and relating them to personality features assessed many years later.

The scientific knowledge that has been accumulated concerns mainly antisocial personality disorders and it is the only aspect that will be considered here. Despite this lack of scientific data, in clinical practice it is often possible to achieve an intuitive understanding of the probable childhood origins of personality. For example, when frequent criticism and lack of affection from parents are the antecedents of a personality marked by low self-esteem.

Genetic factors The children of parents with antisocial personality disorder have greater rates of antisocial behaviour than children of parents with other kinds of personality. This excess has been reported also among adopted children of biological parents with antisocial personality indicating a genetic cause but this evidence needs to be confirmed.

The importance of **childhood experience** is supported by reports that separation from parents in early childhood is more frequent among people with antisocial personality disorder than among controls. This association could be due to parental disharmony preceding the separation, rather than to the separation itself, or to one of the consequences of separation such as upbringing in an institution.

Since **injury to the brain** at birth is sometimes followed by impulsive and aggressive behaviour, such injury has been suggested as a cause of antisocial personality disorder but without convincing evidence. Similarly, a **disorder of brain development** has been suggested, but the only indirect evidence is the finding among adults of non-specific abnormalities in the electroencephalogram (EEG) of a type characteristic of adolescents' EEG. These findings could reflect delay in the maturation of the brain in people with antisocial personality.

Recent studies have found an association between **low levels of brain 5-HT** (measured indirectly by neuroendocrine challenge tests) and aggressive behaviour. However, this interesting observation is not confined to the aggression in antisocial personality disorder.

The prognosis of personality disorder

Clinical experience indicates that abnormal features of personality including aggressive traits, tend to become less abnormal as the person grows into middle age, but there are no reliable follow-up studies to confirm this observation. In old age, abnormal features of personality may again become more intense, causing difficulties for patients and carers (see p. 325).

The management of personality disorder

Doctors need to take account of personality when assessing and treating their patients, and to know how to manage those with abnormal personalities. People with anxious personalities and those lacking self-esteem can often be helped. Suspicious and antisocial people are much less likely to respond to treatment but an understanding of their personality can improve relationships between patient and doctor, improve compliance with treatment, and reduce problems in the family.

Assessment

A scheme for assessing personality has been described on p. 76 where it was explained that to obtain a reliable picture it is usually necessary to interview an informant as well as the patient. To plan management, the assessment has to be extended in five ways (see Table 5.9). Diagnosis focuses on the deficits and unfavourable features of personality. Management requires an assessment of the **positive features** of personality to discover any that could be developed further, and to identify skills that could be increased by training to enhance self-esteem.

Provoking factors for emotional disturbance or abnormal behaviour are assessed next; for example the circumstances that lead to anxiety in an anxious personality or to anger in an aggressive person. Sometimes the link between the provoking factor and the response may reveal a previously overlooked aspect of personality; for example aggression may be provoked by social rejection by other people but the rejection may be their response to the patient's lack of social skills. To assess provoking factors, it is useful to ask the patient to keep a *daily record of the behaviour* in question and the situations in which it occurs. Most patients co-operate with this practical approach.

Use of alcohol and drugs is assessed next. Alcohol may be used for its immediate effect of reducing feelings of tension or unhappiness but its disinhibiting effects can release histrionic or aggressive behaviour, or self-harm.

The effect on the family is important, particularly on any children living with the patient. Although these considerations are most important when the person is aggressive, people who are anxious, histrionic, or suspicious can also cause difficulties for their family. The stressful effect of the patient's personality on other family members may first become evident when one of them complains of physical symptoms for which no cause can be found.

With antisocial personalities, additional enquiries should be made about aggressive acts, including those that break the law. It may be necessary to proceed to an assessment of risk (see Chapter 2).

General aspects of management (Table 5.10)

The general approach should be to help the person *gain confidence* and *learn from mistakes*. To achieve these aims, setbacks should be discussed with the patient as opportunities to find out more about the problem, not as signs of failure. The aim is to help the patient to take a series of small steps over a long time, not to bring about a rapid change. The plan should be realistic, clearly understood by the patient, and carried out consistently. The aim is to help patients solve their own

Table 5.9.

Assessment for management of personality disorder

1. Type of disorder
2. Potential strengths
3. Provoking factors
4. Alcohol and drug use
5. Effects on the family

Table 5.10.

Management of personality disorder

- Modest aims, achieved slowly
- Assist learning from experience
- Set limits
- Build on strengths
- Reduce provoking factors
- Reduce alcohol/drug intake
- Help the family

problems, not to remove responsibility from them. Also, the doctor should recognize that progress will be slow and punctuated by failures. Patience is needed when managing personality disorders.

The *relationship* between patient and doctor is particularly important when treating personality disorder. The patient should feel valued as a person, and able to trust and confide in the doctor. At the same time, the relationship should not become too intense or dependent. When more than one person is involved in treatment, their respective roles should be defined and made clear to the patient. Any attempt to play one off against the other should be discussed between the professionals and with the patient.

Great care is needed in *setting limits* for some patients with personality disorder, especially for those with overdependent histrionic or aggressive personalities. These limits should be agreed by all those involved in the patient's care and explained to the patient. These patients may seek help at inappropriate times, attempt to impose unreasonable conditions on treatment, behave in a seductive way, or threaten overdoses if their demands are not met. Once established, these behaviours can be very difficult to control, so the doctor should be alert for their first signs and explain clearly and firmly that such behaviour cannot be accepted.

Building on strengths. Management should not focus exclusively on defects in the personality. Whenever possible patients should be encouraged to recognize and develop their talents and skills by obtaining further training, changing to a job better suited for their skills or interests, or by developing more satisfying leisure activities. Such actions improve low self-esteem, which is a frequent problem among people with all kinds of personality disorder.

Provoking factors. The patient should be helped to identify and find new ways of dealing with any situations that regularly cause problems. If the patient cannot learn to respond to the situations differently he should be helped to rearrange his life so that he encounters that situations less often. These rearrangements may require patients to give up some of their previous goals and accept new ones more in keeping with the structure of their personalities.

Abuse of alcohol and drugs. When abnormal behaviour is provoked by the use of alcohol or drugs, help should be given to limit the use of these substances. Among prescribed drugs, benzodiazepines can have disinhibiting effects similar to those of alcohol. They should be avoided when prescribing for patients with abnormal personalities.

Help for the family. This may be needed, especially when the personality disorder is of the aggressive or antisocial kind. When the mother has a personality disorder, the health and development of the children should be assessed and appropriate steps taken.

Specific treatment methods

Drug treatment has little general value in treating personality disorder but there are a few specific uses:

- *Antipsychotic* drugs may be calming at a time of increased stress especially for aggressive and antisocial personalities.

- *Lithium carbonate* has been claimed to benefit some people with recurrent mood changes; a specialist opinion should be obtained before prescribing.
- *Antidepressants* are of value when there is an associated depressive disorder. It has been claimed that, in the absence of a depressive disorder, SSRIs (specific serotonin reuptake inhibitors) diminish impulsive behaviour and repeated self-harm but their long-term value is uncertain at the time of writing.
- *Carbamezapine* has been claimed to reduce aggressive behaviour in some patients. The value is uncertain and, if real, applies to a minority of such patients. Specialist opinion should be sought before prescribing.
- *Anxiolytic* drugs should generally be *avoided* because although they may improve well-being they may produce disinhibition and dependency.

Psychotherapy may help for people with low self-esteem and difficulties in social relationships. Sensitive and suspicious and antisocial and aggressive personalities seldom benefit. Cognitive-behaviour methods are generally more appropriate than dynamic therapy since they focus on current behaviour and the patient's own role in changing this.

Therapeutic community methods These methods (see p. 378) have been used to assist people with antisocial personality to learn from experiences of their relationships within the community, and from the frequent and intensive discussion of problems that takes place. Good results have been claimed for a minority of such patients but these have not been supported by randomized controlled trials, and there are no agreed criteria for selecting the minority who may be helped.

Treatment of personality types

Anxious, moody, and worrying type. These patients are generally helped most by a cognitive-behaviour treatment designed to identify and change maladaptive ways of dealing with situations that the patient finds stressful, and recognize the relation between thinking and emotion. In this group, patients with obsessional traits are least likely to change.

Sensitive and suspicious personalities. These patients seldom benefit from any kind of psychological treatment. The aim is to establish a gradually greater degree of trust with the patient. These patients may provoke strong negative feelings in their doctors who should to recognize these reactions at an early stage and ensure that such feelings do not affect their clinical judgement.

Dramatic and impulsive personalities. It is particularly important to set limits for this group. A problem-solving approach should be used to help the patient cope better with the stressful events that provoke abnormal behaviours. Dynamic psychotherapy often leads to intense transference problems (see Chapter 17, p. 365) that are difficult to manage.

Aggressive and antisocial behaviour. The approach should be practical and should take account of the patient's sensitivities. Rude or aggressive behaviour should be accepted tolerantly; at times, much effort will be needed to restrain angry responses to the patient's behaviour. Patients who are irritable and impatient should not be kept waiting without prior explanation. Potentially aggressive patients should be seen in a place in which help is within reach.

Often the most practical aim is to prevent the accumulation of secondary problems resulting from rash decisions, antagonism of potential helpers, and the abuse of drugs and alcohol. A problem-solving approach should be taken to situations that regularly provoke aggressive and antisocial behaviour. Anger-management techniques can help patients find ways of responding more appropriately. As noted above, time is sometimes spent most usefully in helping the family, especially any dependent children.

Lack of self-esteem and confidence. These patients are helped by a trusting relationship in which they are encouraged to see the positive side of their personality and gain confidence. A cognitive-behaviour approach can help patients understand the relationship between their ways of thinking and their response to situations in which they feel defeated or inferior. Assertiveness training helps people who are unduly submissive.

Additional information Specialist classifications

The scheme for personality disorders in the International Classification of Diseases, tenth edition (ICD-10) and the Diagnostic and Statistical Manual of the American Psychiatric Association, fourth edition (DSM-IV) are similar in both but with details important only to specialists. Most of the differences are in the terms used, rather than the concepts or criteria for diagnosis. All but one of these categories, are described here for reference. Antisocial personality disorder has been described on p. 79 because of its wider importance.

The specialist classification of personality disorder is shown in Table 5.3. These disorders are described briefly for reference; some of the points repeat those mentioned above when the simplified classification was described. Where the terminology in DSM-IV and ICD-10 differs, this is noted by indicating the origin of the less preferred term, for example, 'obsessive-compulsive' (ICD: 'anankastic') indicates that the DSM term is 'obsessive-compulsive', the ICD term for the same personality is 'anankastic', and the DSM term is preferred by the authors.

Group A   Anxious, moody, and prone to worry personalities
Anxious (DSM: avoidant) personality disorder
These people are persistently anxious, ill at ease in company, and fearful of disapproval or criticism. They feel inadequate and are timid. They avoid taking new responsibilities at work or new experiences generally. This tendency to avoid is recognized in the DSM term 'avoidant personality disorder'

Obsessive-compulsive (ICD: anankastic) personality disorder

These people are inflexible, obstinate, rigid in their opinions, and they focus on unimportant detail. They are indecisive and having made a decision they worry about its consequences. They are humourless and judgemental while worrying about the opinions of others. Perfectionism, rigidity, and indecisiveness can make employment impossible. Such people appear outwardly controlled but may have violent feelings of anger especially toward those who disturb their carefully ordered routine.

Dependent personality disorder

These people are passive and unduly compliant with the wishes of others. They lack vigour and self-reliance, and they avoid responsibility. Some achieve their aims by persuading other people to assist them, while protesting their own helplessness. Some are supported by a more self-reliant spouse; left to themselves, they have difficulty in dealing with the demands and responsibilities of everyday life.

Affective personality disorder

This category appears in both DSM and ICD although not among the personality disorders; instead, it is grouped with the affective disorders because it is thought to be related closely to the latter. Despite this convention, affective personality disorder is described here for convenience.

These people have lifelong abnormalities of mood regulation which can take three forms:

1. *Depressed personality disorder*. The person is persistently gloomy and pessimistic with little capacity for enjoyment.

2. *Hyperthymic personality disorder*. The person is in a persistent state of mild elation, over-optimistic, and prone to make rash judgements.

3. *Cyclothymic* (or *cycloid*) *personality disorder*. In this disorder, which is the most important of the three, mood alternates between gloomy and elated states over periods of days to weeks with a characteristic frequency for each person. This instability is particularly disrupting to work and social relationships.

Group B   Sensitive and suspicious personalities

Paranoid personality disorder

These people are sensitive and suspicious; they mistrust others and suspect their motives, and are prone to jealousy. They are touchy, irritable, argumentative, and stubborn. Some of these people have a strong sense of self-importance and a powerful conviction of being unusually talented, though unable to fulfil their potential because let down or deceived by other people.

Schizoid personality

These people are emotionally cold, self-sufficient, and detached. They are introspective and may have a complex fantasy life. The show little concern for the opinions of others, and pursue a solitary course through life. When this personality disorder is extreme, the person is cold, callous, and insensitive.

Schizotypal personality disorder

These people are eccentric and have unusual ideas (e.g. about telepathy and clairvoyance), or ideas of reference. Their speech is abstract and vague, and their affect may be inappropriate to the circumstances. It has been suggested that this kind of personality is related to schizophrenia and in ICD it is classified with schizophrenia and not as one of the personality disorders.

Group C   Dramatic and impulsive personalities

Histrionic personality disorder

These people appear sociable, outgoing, and entertaining but at the same time they are self-centred, prone to short-lived enthusiasms, and lacking in persistence. Extreme displays of emotion may leave others exhausted while the person recovers quickly and without remorse. Sexually provocative behaviour is common but tender feelings are lacking. There may be astonishing capacity for self-deception and an ability to persist with elaborate lies long after others have seen the truth.

Borderline personality disorder

The term 'borderline' refers to a combination of features seen also in histrionic and antisocial personalities. The term originates in a former and now abandoned idea that the condition was related to (on the borderline with) schizophrenia. These people have a wide variety of problems, most of which can be part of other personality disorders. They include: inability to make stable relationships; persistent feelings of boredom; damaging behaviour such as reckless spending, uncontrolled gambling, or stealing; variable moods; unwarranted outbursts of anger; uncertainty about personal identity; and recurrent suicidal threats or behaviour. They are impulsive and unable to tolerate stressful events.

Narcissistic personality disorder (included only in DSM)

Narcissism is morbid self-admiration. Narcissistic people have a grandiose sense of self-importance and are preoccupied with fantasies of success, power, and intellectual brilliance. They crave attention, exploit others, and seek favours but do not return them.

Group D   Aggressive and antisocial personalities

Antisocial personality disorder

This disorder is described in Box 5.1 (p. 79).

Further reading

Tyrer, Peter (ed.) (1996). *Personality Disorders: Diagnosis, Management and Course.* Wright/Butterworth Scientific, London.
Reviews the clinical features, diagnostic classification, treatment and prognosis of personality disorders.

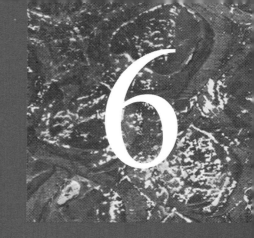

6

Reactions to stressful experiences

- General psychological response to stressful experiences

- Classification of reactions to stressful experiences

- Reactions to severe stressful events

- Normal and abnormal adjustment reactions

- Special forms of normal and abnormal adjustment

Reactions to stressful experiences

Doctors see many patients whose psychological symptoms are reactions to stressful experiences. Most of these reactions are not severe or prolonged enough to meet the criteria for an anxiety, depressive, or other disorder and yet they are distressing and require help.

Reactions to stressful experiences can be separated into: normal reactions to stress, acute stress disorder, post-traumatic stress disorder, and adjustment disorders. Normal reactions to stress involve anxiety and depression, together with psychological mechanisms which reduce the initial response to tolerable limits. These mechanisms are both voluntary ('coping strategies') and involuntary ('defence mechanisms'). Such responses are seen in patients who are physically ill or who are undergoing surgery, as well as in response to other life events. All doctors should understand this normal response and how to prevent it from becoming abnormal.

Acute stress disorder is similar to the normal stress response but the emotional response is more intense and the effects of coping and defence are more obvious, appearing as a sense of detachment, as emotional numbing, as avoidance of reminders of the stressful events.

Post-traumatic stress disorder is an abnormal response to extremely stressful events such as a serious accident or a natural disaster. There is extreme arousal, intense detachment and numbing, with transient breakdown of these mechanisms in the form of intrusive memories and dreams of the traumatic events. Post-traumatic stress disorder does not develop in every person involved in the same severe stressful events but it is not certain what predisposes some people to react in this way.

Adjustment disorders are abnormal psychological reactions to changed circumstances. Adjustment disorders may be provoked by, for example, separation, the birth of a handicapped child, or a move from home to university. There may be anxiety and depression with avoidance and denial as in the other reactions to stressful events. The condition is a response to more gradually developing events than those in acute stress disorder or post-traumatic stress disorder and the symptoms develop more slowly than in these other two disorders. All doctors should understand the normal and the abnormal forms of adjustment to: serious physical illness, terminal illness, and bereavement ('grief reaction').

General psychological response to stressful experiences

There are three components to a stress response: (1) an emotional response; (2) a somatic response; and (3) psychological changes that reduce the emotional impact of the experience. The *emotional* and *somatic responses* are of two main kinds (Table 6.1). The emotional response to danger is fear, and the response to threatening events is anxiety. The somatic reactions to danger or threat are autonomic arousal, with increased heart rate and blood pressure, etc., increased muscle tension, and dry mouth. The emotional response to separation or loss is depression,

Table 6.1.

Components of the psychological response to stressful circumstances

Emotional responses
- to threat: fear
- to loss: depression

Somatic responses
- to threat: autonomic arousal
- To loss: reduced physical activity

Coping strategies (Table 6.2)
Mechanisms of defence (Table 6.3)

Table 6.2.

Coping strategies

Potentially adaptive	•	Avoidance
	•	Working through problems
	•	Coming to terms with situations
Maladaptive	•	Excessive use of alcohol or drugs
	•	Histrionic or aggressive behaviour
	•	Deliberate self-harm

and the bodily reactions are tiredness and reduced physical activity. The third component of the stress response consists of psychological mechanisms that reduce the effect of stressful experiences, so that normal performance can continue. These psychological mechanisms, called *coping strategies* and *mechanisms of defence,* will be described next.

Coping strategies and mechanisms of defence

The term 'coping strategy' is applied to activities of which the person is aware; the term 'mechanism of defence' refers to unconscious mental processes.

Coping strategies (Table 6.2) may be adaptive or maladaptive. Both reduce the immediate response to the stressor but maladaptive strategies are unhelpful in the longer term. *Adaptive coping strategies* include avoidance of situations that cause distress, working through problems, and coming to terms with situations. *Maladaptive coping strategies* include excessive use of alcohol or drugs, histrionic or aggressive behaviour, and deliberate self-harm. The strategies listed above as adaptive can become maladaptive if used for too long. For example, avoidance is an appropriate early response to a stressful situation but if maintained for a long time it prevents the process of solving or coming to terms with problems.

Mechanisms of defence (Table 6.3) are of several kinds, described originally by Freud. Those occurring most often in response to stressful circumstances are regression, repression, denial, and displacement. They are *unconscious* processes.

Regression is the adoption of behaviour appropriate to an earlier stage of development; for example, dependence on others. Regression often occurs among physically ill people. In the acute stages of illness it can be adaptive, enabling the person to accept the requirements of passively accepting intensive medical and nursing care. If it persists into the stage of recovery, however, regression reduces the patient's ability to take responsibility for himself.

Repression is the exclusion from consciousness of impulses, emotions, or memories that would otherwise cause distress. For example, the memory of a humiliating event may be kept out of awareness.

Denial is a related concept: it is inferred when a person behaves as if unaware of something which he may reasonably be expected to know. For example, a person

Table 6.3.

Mechanisms of defence

More common	Less common
Regression	Projection
Repression	Reaction formation
Denial	Rationalization
Displacement	Sublimation
	Identification

Box 6.1 **Some other mechanisms of defence**

Projection is the attribution to another person of thoughts or feelings similar to one's own, thereby rendering one's own feelings more acceptable. For example, a person who dislikes a colleague may attribute reciprocal feelings of dislike to him. In this way the person can more easily justify his own feelings of dislike for the colleague.

Reaction formation is the unconscious adoption of behaviour opposite to that which would reflect true feelings and intentions. For example, excessively prudish attitudes to sex are sometimes (but not always) a reaction to strong sexual urges that the person cannot accept.

Rationalization is the unconscious provision of a false but acceptable explanation for behaviour which has a less acceptable origin. For example, a husband may leave his wife at home because he does not enjoy her company, but he may tell himself falsely that she is shy and does not enjoy going out.

Sublimation is the unconscious diversion of unacceptable impulses into more acceptable outlets; for example, turning the need to dominate others into the organization of good works for charity.

Identification is the unconscious adoption of the characteristics or activities of another person, often to reduce the pain of separation or loss. For example, a widow may undertake the same voluntary work that her husband used to do.

who has been told that he is dying of cancer may continue to behave as if unaware of the diagnosis.

Displacement is the transfer of emotion from a person, object, or situation with which it is properly associated, to another which causes less distress. For example, after the recent death of his wife, a man may blame his doctor for failure in providing adequate care, instead of blaming himself for putting his work before her needs in the last months of her life.

Some less common mechanisms of defence, involved more often in longer-term problems are shown in Box 6.1.

Classification of reactions to stressful experiences

Reactions to stressful experience can be classified according to the type of stressor into reactions to acute stress, to overwhelming acute stress, and to more gradual events. In each, the reaction may be normal or abnormal. Abnormal reactions to stressful experiences can be classified under three headings (Table 6.4):

(1) *acute stress disorder*, which is an immediate and brief response to sudden intense stressors in a person who does not have another psychiatric disorder at the time. They last from a few hours to at most a few days;

(2) *post-traumatic stress disorder*, which is a prolonged and abnormal response to very intense stressors.

(3) *adjustment disorder*, which is a more gradual and prolonged response to stressful changes in the person's life;

Table 6.4.

Classification of abnormal reactions to stressful experiences

- **Acute stress disorder**
  follows a sudden intense stressor
  lasts at most a few days
  is not an exacerbation of a
  pre-existing psychiatric disorder

- **Post-traumatic stress disorder**
  follows very intense stressors
  is prolonged and has special
  features (see Table 6.6)

- **Adjustment disorder**
  follows life changes
  is prolonged
  does not meet criteria for an
  anxiety, depressive, or other
  disorder

Reactions to acute stressful experiences

Normal reactions

As explained above, the normal response to sudden stressful events is an emotional response coupled with a coping strategy or defence mechanism which serves to limit the intensity of the emotional response. The **emotional response** is anxiety or depression. Anxiety is the normal response to threatening experiences; depression is the normal response to loss. These two responses may occur together because a stressful event may combine elements of both danger and loss; for example a road accident in which a companion is killed. There is poor sleep, restlessness, difficulty in concentration, a feeling of being dazed, and physical symptoms of autonomic arousal especially palpitations and tremor.

The usual **coping strategy** is *avoidance* of the situation, of direct reminders of it, and of talking or thinking about it. The most frequent **defence mechanism** is *denial*, experienced as a feeling that the events have not really happened. As the stressors recede, these processes recede: memories of the event return gradually and can be thought over and talked about with less distress.

Acute stress disorder

This term denotes an abnormal reaction to sudden stressful events. (The term, taken from DSM-IV, is used in preference to the corresponding ICD-10 term 'acute stress reaction' because the former indicates more clearly that the condition is abnormal.)

The emotional response is more severe than in the normal reaction to acute stressors and there may be panic attacks as well as generalized anxiety. Sweating, palpitations, tremor, and other autonomic symptoms of anxiety are common and troublesome.

Coping and defence mechanisms are intense and may sometimes be abnormal. The person avoids talking or thinking about the stressful events, and avoids reminders of them. Denial may be intense: the patient feels as though the events have not really taken place. Abnormal coping responses include 'flight', for example, running away from the scene of a road accident; histrionic or aggressive behaviour; excessive use of alcohol; or deliberate self-harm.

Aetiology

Many kinds of event can provoke an acute stress disorder: for example, involvement in an accident or fire; or a sudden and intense personal misfortune such as the break-up of an intimate relationship; or physical assault or rape. Since the stress response does not become abnormal in everyone exposed to the same events, there is presumably some personal predisposition but it is not known what it is.

Treatment

The treatment of acute stress disorder is summarized in Table 6.5. There are four elements: reducing emotional response; encouraging recall; helping with more effective coping; helping with residual problems. Most acute stress disorders can be managed by the family doctor, physician, or surgeon who is caring for the patient. Few require referral to a specialist.

Reduce the emotional response This is usually achieved when the person is comforted by relatives or friends, and is able to talk to them about the stressful

Table 6.5.

Treatment of acute reactions to stressful experiences

1. Reduce emotion by sympathetic listening and, in severe cases, short-term anxiolytics
2. Encourage recall of, and coming to terms with the events
3. Help with more effective coping
4. Help with residual problems (e.g. loss, or expected disability)

experience. If no close friend or relative is available, or if the anxiety is severe, support may be given by a doctor, nurse, or social worker. In some cases, an anxiolytic drug may be needed for a few days to reduce anxiety, or a hypnotic drug for a few nights to improve severe sleep disturbance.

Encourage recall As anxiety is reduced, associated denial and avoidance usually subside and the person is able to think about and come to terms with the experience. When avoidance and denial persist, the patient should be helped to recall the stressful events by gradual and repeated questioning and encouraging the expression of emotion. Emotional release shortens the acute reaction (some think that it also reduces the incidence of subsequent post-traumatic stress disorder but recent evidence does not confirm this).

Help with more effective coping Some people react maladaptively to crises in personal relationships; for example, by drug overdose, excessive drinking, or histrionic behaviour. Such people need help to improve their coping skills and so deal with future crises more effectively. This management of such patients is discussed further in the section on deliberate self-harm, and the relevant counselling techniques ('crisis intervention') are described on p. 366.

Help with residual problems Sometimes an acutely stressful situation results in lasting adverse circumstances to which the person has to adjust; for example, a serious car accident may lead to permanent disability. Thus the treatment of an acute reaction may need to be followed by help in readjustment (see p. 95).

Reactions to extremely severe stressful events

Normal reactions

The immediate reaction to extremely severe stressful events is severe anxiety, a feeling of numbing, and avoidance of thinking about the events which is interrupted at times by sudden, vivid, and distressing recall of these events ('intrusive thoughts'). The events that provoke this intense reaction include natural disasters such as earthquakes; man-made calamities such as major fires, serious accidents, or the effects of war; and serious physical assault or rape. Most of those involved in such events recover over days or a few weeks but a minority develop an abnormal reaction called 'post-traumatic stress disorder' (PTSD).

Post-traumatic stress disorder

Clinical features

There are three groups of features (see Table 6.6). The first are symptoms of increased arousal: severe anxiety, irritability, insomnia, and poor concentration. Sometimes there are panic attacks or episodes of aggression. The second group reflects persisting defences of avoidance and repression: avoidance of reminders of the events; difficulty in recalling the events at will; detachment, inability to feel emotion ('numbness'), and diminished interest in activities. The third group are intrusions, in which memories of the traumatic events break through the repression as repeated intense imagery ('flashbacks'), or distressing dreams. Anxiety increases further during flashbacks or reminders of the traumatic event. Sometimes there are additional maladaptive coping responses, namely

Table 6.6.

Post-traumatic stress disorder

1. **Increased arousal**
   - Persistent anxiety
   - Irritability
   - Insomnia
   - Poor concentration
2. **Avoidance and repression**
   - Avoidance of reminders of the events
   - Difficulty recalling stressful events at will
   - Detachment
   - Inability to feel emotion ('numbness')
   - Diminished interest in activities
3. **Intrusions**
   - Intense intrusive imagery ('flashbacks')
   - Recurring distressing dreams

persistent histrionic or aggressive behaviour, or excessive use of alcohol or drugs.

Post-traumatic stress disorder may be a the immediate response to the stressor, or may follow an interval of days or occasionally months. Post-traumatic stress disorder usually improves within months, but may persist for years.

Aetiology

The necessary cause is an *exceptionally stressful event* in which the person was involved directly or as a witness. Although PTSD is more common among those most involved in the stressful events, the variation in response is not accounted for solely by the *degree of personal involvement*, so that some form of *personal vulnerability* is involved. Children and old people are particulary vulnerable and so are people with previous psychiatric disorder. Twin studies of Vietnam veterans suggest that, among young adults, part of this vulnerability is genetic. Neurophysiological studies show abnormalities consistent with hyperarousal but do not explain the individual differences in response.

Assessment

Assessment should include: the nature and severity of the stressful event; the nature and duration of the symptoms; previous personality; and any previous psychiatric history. If the traumatic event has included injury to the head (e.g. from an assault or transport accident) neurological examination should be carried out to exclude a subdural haematoma or other forms of cerebral injury.

Treatment

Early treatment If the early response is not severe, most patients need no more than sympathetic support and help with practical problems consequent on the disaster. More intensive counselling is sometimes offered in the hope that talking through the events and emotional release will reduce the frequency of PTSD. The evidence for this is not convincing and it may be better to concentrate the more intensive help on those with severe initial reactions and those that have not resolved in a few weeks. This early care is best carried by the general practitioner or the specialist treating any associated physical injury.

For the most severe disorders, a few doses of an anxiolytic drug may be needed to calm the person, together with a hypnotic drug for a few nights to restore sleep. The person is helped to talk about and reconsider the events and express feelings about them. This may need to be done repeatedly ('working through').

Chronic PTSD is difficult to treat. The same general approach is used: in a series of interviews the patient is encouraged to recall, re-experience, and *work through the emotion* associated with the events. Even with skilled treatment, the response of chronic cases is often limited. *Cognitive-behaviour techniques* have been used to desensitize patients to reminders and images of the stressful events. Several forms of *medication* have been tried. Anxiolytics should be avoided because of the risk of dependence after prolonged usage. SSRIs (specific serotonin reuptake inhibitors) have been claimed to be effective but the evidence is equivocal a the time of writing (see Chapter 4 for ways of seeking new evidence).

Normal and abnormal adjustment reactions

Normal adjustment

These refers to the psychological reactions involved in adapting to new circumstances. Examples of life changes that commonly provoke adjustment disorders are: divorce and separation; a major change of work and abode such as the transition from school to university; the birth of a handicapped child. Bereavement and the onset of a terminal illness involve special kinds of adjustment.

The normal reaction to stressful changes is a brief period of anxiety and depression sometimes with irritability and poor concentration. There may be a brief period of denial but this is soon followed by problem solving.

Adjustment disorder

The response is recorded as abnormal—as an adjustment disorder—if the distress is judged to be:

(1) greater than that which would be expected to the particular stressful events. (This judgement is subjective, and the diagnostic manuals offer no objective criteria.);

(2) or accompanied by impairment of social functioning.
    To diagnose adjustment disorder, it is also necessary that:

(3) the reaction is reasonably close in time to the life change: a period of one month is specified in ICD (but a longer period, three months, is allowed in DSM);

(4) the reaction is not severe enough to meet criteria for diagnosis of an anxiety, depressive, or other psychiatric disorder.

General practitioners see many patients of this kind and physicians see similar cases in relation to the life changes imposed by physical illness. The physician can judge better than a psychiatrist whether the reaction is greater than the normal response to a similar illness.

Treatment

Treatment is designed to assist the natural processes of adjustment by overcoming denial and avoidance, encouraging problem solving, and discouraging maladaptive coping responses. All these changes are easier to make when anxiety has been reduced.

Anxiety reduction Anxiety can usually be reduced by encouraging patients to talk about the problems and express their feelings. Anxiolytic drugs may be needed when anxiety is severe but they should not be prescribed routinely. Occasionally, a hypnotic drug is required for a few nights to restore sleep.

Problem solving Patients with adjustment disorder often feel overwhelmed by a series of life problems and greatly helped by problem-solving treatment. This treatment is described on p. 365 and the essential steps are: (1) the patient is helped to *list the problems* and suggest ways of overcoming them; (2) the advantages and disadvantages of various *solutions* to the problem are *considered*; (3) the patient is helped to *select and implement* a course of *action* that seems most likely to succeed.

If this succeeds, the process is repeated with another problem; if the first attempt fails, the patient tries another approach to the original problem.

Crisis intervention This approach is used when the patient has encountered a sudden crisis such as the breaking up of an intimate relationship. Anxiety is severe and there may be maladaptive coping mechanisms such as deliberate self-harm. The approach (see p. 366) resembles problem solving and the patient is helped to examine the maladaptive coping responses, to recognize their disadvantages, and to consider other ways for dealing with similar problems in the future.

Special forms of normal and abnormal adjustment

Adjustment to serious physical illness

Physically ill people often feel *anxious* and *depressed*, and *sometimes angry*. Most of these reactions are transient, subsiding quickly as the person adjusts to the new situation. As in other adjustment reactions, *denial* protects the patient against overwhelming anxiety in the early stages, but must be given up before the problems can be worked through and a full adjustment achieved. Prolonged denial is particularly unhelpful during physical illness since it prevents the patient from complying fully with treatment. Denial can be reduced by helping the patients discuss their fears and providing information to correct misunderstandings, for example, about the amount of pain that is likely to be felt.

Adjustment to physical illness involves a special set of adaptations, sometimes called **illness behaviour** which include, seeking medical advice, taking medication, asking from relatives and friends, and sometimes giving up activities. These behaviours are adaptive in the early stages of illness, but if they persist when no longer needed they become maladaptive and prolong invalidism. Occasionally, a person who has no physical disease adopts these illness behaviours, seeking medical help, demanding medication, and giving up responsibilities. This is called *abnormal illness behaviour*, though it is not the behaviour itself which is abnormal but the circumstances in which it occurs—that is, without medical reason.

As well as acting as a stressor, physical illness may induce common psychiatric symptoms through *direct physiological effects*; such symptoms include anxiety, depression, fatigue, weakness, weight loss, or abnormal behaviour. These associations are considered in Chapter 11 on psychiatry and medicine (see p. 213). Likewise, some *drugs* used in the treatment of physical illness may affect mood, behaviour, and consciousness (see p. 209).

Treatment

When adjustment to physical illness is slow and incomplete, simple measures are needed which can be provided effectively by the general practitioner or specialist dealing with the physical illness. The nature of the illness and its treatment are explained and the patient's anxieties discussed. The latter may concern the effects of the illness on family, or the threat of loss of job. As anxiety diminishes, so do any maladaptive behaviours such as overdependence or lack of compliance. Effective counselling requires a trusting relationship between patient and physician. To achieve this relationship sufficient time must be set aside and rushed consultations are unlikely to be effective. It is important, however, to ensure that the relationship does not become unduly intense with overdependence on the doctor instead of efforts at self-help.

Some reactions to physical illness develop into depressive or anxiety disorders. In these cases treatment appropriate to these disorders should be given (see pp. 109, 143).

Adjustment to terminal illness

After terminal illness has been diagnosed, many people become anxious, depressed, guilty or angry, and some adopt maladaptive ways of coping. Among patients dying in hospital about half have emotional symptoms. **Anxiety** may be provoked by the possibilities of experiencing severe pain or of becoming disfigured or incontinent, and also by concerns about the family. **Depression** may be provoked by the loss of valued activities and the prospect of separation from loved ones. Depression or anxiety can be induced directly by the physical disease or the medication used to treat it (see also Tables 11.4 and 11.5). **Confusion** is another frequent symptom among dying patients, caused, for example by dehydration, drug side effects, and secondary infection (see p. 189). Other features of adjustment to terminal illness include:

- **Guilt** from the belief that excessive demands are being placed on relatives or friends.
- **Anger** about the unjustness of impending death.

Understandably, among dying patients these emotional reactions are more common in the young than in the elderly, and less common in the religious. The prospect of dying activates defences of denial, dependency, and displacement, which may be followed by acceptance.

Denial is usually the first reaction to the news of fatal illness. It may be experienced as a feeling of disbelief and may lead to an initial period of calm. Denial then diminishes as the patient gradually comes to terms with the situation. It may return with signs of the progress of the disease, and the patient may again behave as if unaware of the nature of his condition.

Dependency is common among terminally ill people and is adaptive at times when the patient needs to comply passively with treatment. Excessive dependency makes other treatment more difficult, and increases the burden on the family.

Displacement of anger may take place so that it is directed to doctors and nurses and to relatives. The latter may find it difficult to tolerate this anger unless they understand its origins and may be less inclined to spend time with the patient, thereby increasing his feelings of isolation.

Acceptance follows denial, dependency, and displacement. The doctor's aim should be to help the patient to reach this acceptance before the final stage of the illness.

Treatment

The first steps in **treatment** are to *control pain* and *reduce confusion*, as these symptoms prevent patients from concentrating on the psychological work needed to

Table 6.7.
The normal grief reaction

Stage I—hours to days
Denial, disbelief
'Numbness'

Stage II—weeks to 6 months
Sadness, weeping, waves of grief
Somatic symptoms of anxiety
Restlessness
Poor sleep
Diminished appetite
Guilt; blame of others
Experience of the presence of the deceased
Illusions; vivid imagery
Hallucinations of the dead person's voice
Preoccupation with memories of deceased
Social withdrawal

Stage III—weeks to months
Symptoms resolve
Social activities resumed
Memories of good times
(symptoms may recur at anniversaries)

reach a satisfactory adjustment. Next, an explanation of the terminal nature of the illness should be offered. Doctors may worry that such an explanation will further increase the patient's distress. While excessive detail given unsympathetically can have this effect, it is seldom difficult to decide how much to say about the disease and the prognosis, provided that patients are allowed to lead the discussion. If patients ask about the prognosis they should be told the truth; evasive answers undermine their trust in those caring for them. However, at the first interview after diagnosis, if patients do not communicate a desire to know the full extent of his problems, it is better to keep this information for a subsequent interview. At an appropriate stage patients should be given an explanation of what can be done to make the remaining time as comfortable as possible. The whole account should be truthful, but the amount disclosed on a single occasion should be judged by patients' reactions and by their questions. If necessary, the doctor should be prepared to return for further discussion when each patient is ready to continue. It is important to bear in mind that most dying patients become aware of their prognosis whether or not they are told directly, because they infer the truth from the behaviour of those who are caring for them. They notice when answers to questions are evasive, and when people avoid talking to them.

The information given to the patient should be known to all the staff and to the relatives; otherwise conflicting advice and opinions may be given. If those involved know what has been said, they feel more at ease in talking to the patient. Otherwise, they draw back from dying patients, isolating them and increasing their difficulty in coming to terms with the situation.

Relatives need as much help as the patient because they too may be anxious and depressed, and may respond with denial, guilt, and anger. These reactions may make it difficult for them to communicate helpfully with the patient. They need information, an explanation of the disease and its treatment, and opportunities to talk about their feelings and to prepare for the impending bereavement.

In many places, terminal care nurses work with the patient and the family, liaising with the family doctor and with the hospital staff caring for the patient. These nurses are skilled in the psychological as well as the physical care of the dying.

Grief: normal and abnormal responses to bereavement
Normal grief

The normal response to bereavement goes through three stages (Table 6.7). The **first stage** lasts from a few hours to several days. Initial denial is manifested as a lack of emotional response ('numbness') often with a feeling of unreality, and incomplete acceptance that the death has taken place.

The **second stage** lasts from a few weeks to six months. There may be extreme sadness, weeping, and often overwhelming waves of grief. Somatic symptoms of anxiety are common. The bereaved person is restless, sleeps poorly, and lacks appetite. Many bereaved people feel guilty that they failed to do enough for the deceased: some project these feelings by blaming doctors or others for failing to provide optimal care for the dead person. Some bereaved people have an intense experience of being in the presence of the dead person, and may experience vivid imagery, illusions, or sometimes hallucinations of that person's voice. The bereaved person is preoccupied with memories of the dead person, and often withdraws from social relationships.

In the **third stage** these symptoms subside, and everyday activities are resumed. The bereaved person gradually comes to terms with the loss, and recalls the good times shared with the deceased in the past. Often, there is a temporary return of symptoms on the anniversary of the death.

Abnormal grief

Grief is said to be abnormal when the symptoms are:

- *more intense* than usual and meet the criteria for a depressive disorder;
- *prolonged* beyond six months;
- *delayed* in onset.

Abnormal grief reactions are more likely in several circumstances:

- after a death that was sudden and unexpected;
- when the bereaved person was very close to, and dependent on, the deceased;
- when the survivor is insecure, or has difficulty in expressing feelings, or has suffered a previous psychiatric disorder;
- when the survivor has to care for dependent children and so cannot show grief easily.

Helping the bereaved

Help for the bereaved follows the general rules that apply to the treatment of other kinds of adjustment reaction. The first step is to listen to the bereaved person talking about the loss and enable him to express feelings of sadness or anger. When the person is seen soon after the loss, it is helpful to explain the normal course of grieving, and to forewarn about the possibility of feeling as if the dead person were present, or experiencing illusions or hallucinations. Without this warning, these experiences may be very alarming.

The bereaved person may need help to move from the early stage of denial of the loss to accepting the reality by viewing the body and by later putting away the dead person's belongings. Practical problems should be discussed, for example, funeral arrangements and possible financial difficulties. A widow may need help in maintaining and caring for young children. As time passes, the bereaved person should be encouraged to resume social contacts; to talk to other people about the loss; to remember happy and fulfilling experiences that were shared with the deceased; and to consider positive activities that the latter would have wanted survivors to undertake.

Similar measures are used when grief is prolonged. When it is abnormally intense, and meets criteria for depressive disorder, antidepressant drug treatment may be required. However, antidepressants do not relieve the distress of normal grief. An anxiolytic or hypnotic drug is helpful in the first few days after bereavement when anxiety is severe or sleep greatly disrupted. This medication should not be continued for more than a few days, and in most cases distress can be reduced by the opportunity to talk and weep.

Support groups are helpful, especially for young widows. The groups enable newly bereaved people to talk with others who have dealt successfully with the emotional and practical aspects of bereavement.

Further reading

Parkes, C. M. (1998). *Bereavement: Studies of Grief in Adult Life* (3rd edn). Pelican, Harmondsworth.
Latest edition of classic description of bereavement reactions.

Joseph, S., Williams, R., and Yule, W. (1997). *Understanding Post-traumatic Stress*. Wiley Chichester.
Comprehensive overview of the syndrome and approaches to treatment.

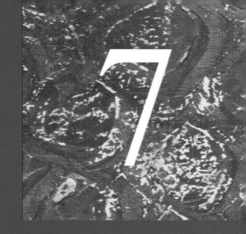

Anxiety and obsessional disorders

- Normal and abnormal anxiety

- Anxiety disorders

- Obsessive-compulsive disorder

Anxiety and obsessional disorders

Anxiety disorders are common in both primary care and general hospital practice. Many patients present with physical rather than psychological symptoms so all doctors should be able to diagnose anxiety disorders, arrange simple treatment, and know when to refer to a specialist. Anxiety disorders are divided into generalized anxiety, phobic, and panic disorders each with a characteristic pattern of symptoms and disabilities, and each requiring somewhat different treatment.

Mixed anxiety/depressive disorders are also common. They are considered with the affective disorders on p. 135, since they are more closely related to them than to the other anxiety disorders.

Benzodiazepine drugs reduce anxiety but their prolonged use may cause dependency and a withdrawal syndrome. The less severe anxiety disorders generally respond to psychological and social measures from non-specialists or treatment with drugs other than benzodiazepines. More severe cases require specialist care with more intensive drug treatment or cognitive-behaviour therapy.

Obsessive-compulsive disorders are less common than anxiety disorders. Severe cases run a chronic course and are difficult to treat, but mild disorders may respond to appropriate advice and medication provided in primary care. Severe disorders require intensive medication, usually with SSRIs (specific serotonin reuptake inhibitors), or behaviour therapy.

Normal and abnormal anxiety

Anxiety is a normal emotion experienced in threatening situations. The mental state of apprehension is accompanied by physiological changes that prepare for defence or escape, including increased heart rate, blood pressure, respiration, and muscle tension. Attention is focused on the threatening situation to the exclusion of other matters. There may be associated changes resulting from increased sympathetic nervous activity, including tremor, polyuria, and diarrhoea. These changes will be familiar to the reader as normal responses to threatening situations.

Anxiety is abnormal when it is out of proportion to the threat and is more prolonged. The clinical features of anxiety disorders are those of normal anxiety; they differ in severity and duration but not in kind. There is, however, an important difference in the focus of attention in normal and pathological anxiety. In normal anxiety, attention is focused on the external threat; in pathological anxiety, attention is focused also on the person's response to the threat, such as increased heart rate, often with worried concerns that the response is abnormal, for example, that rapid heart action signifies heart disease, or that other people will think it abnormal; for example, social phobics' concern that others will think them foolish because their hands are trembling.

Anxiety disorders

Classification

Anxiety disorders are states with marked and persistent mental and physical symptoms of anxiety which are not secondary to another disorder. Anxiety disorders are classified into those with continuous symptoms (**generalized anxiety disorder**) and those with episodic symptoms. The latter are divided into those in which episodes of anxiety occur in particular situations (**phobic anxiety disorders**) and those in which episodes can occur in any situations (**panic disorder**)—see Fig. 7.1. Phobic anxiety disorders are classified further into **simple phobia**, **social phobia**, and **agoraphobia** (these terms are explained later). Some patients have both the episodes of anxiety in the particular situations characteristic of agoraphobia and the random episodes characteristic of panic disorder. In the two systems of classification, these mixed cases are given different names: **panic with agoraphobia** in DSM and **agoraphobia with panic** in ICD.

Prevalence

Anxiety disorders are common and are encountered frequently in general hospital practice. However, many patients do not complain of anxiety but ask for help with one or more of the physical symptoms of anxiety, such as palpitations. The approximate frequency of the various kinds of anxiety disorder is shown in Table 7.1. The figures are approximate and also uncertain because different criteria have been used in the various surveys, particularly in the diagnosis of patients who have both anxiety and depressive symptoms.

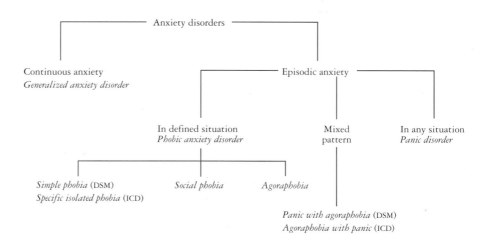

Fig. 7.1 Principles of classification of anxiety disorders.

Table 7.1.

Prevalence of anxiety and obsessive-compulsive disorders in the population*

	Approximate 1-year prevalence per 1000
Generalized anxiety disorder	50
Phobic disorders	
Agoraphobia	30
Social phobia	25
Specific phobia	100
Panic disorder	10
Obsessive-compulsive disorder	15
Mixed anxiety and depression	50

*Published estimates vary considerably; these figures are, however, useful in showing the relative frequency of the various disorders.

Source: OPCS (1995) household survey in the UK and data from the Epidemiological Catchment Area Study in the USA.

Generalized anxiety disorder

Clinical features

The **appearance** of a person with a generalized anxiety disorder is characteristic. The face looks strained and the brow furrowed; the posture is tense and the patient is restless and may tremble. The skin is pale, and there is often sweating especially from the hands, feet, and axillae. Readiness to tears, which may erroneously suggest depression, reflects a generally apprehensive state.

The **psychological symptoms** are listed in Table 7.2 and a few require comment. Patients who concentrate badly sometimes complain of poor memory but true memory impairment does not occur in an anxiety disorder; if it is present a careful search should be made for an organic syndrome. Repetitive *worrying thoughts* are characteristic of generalized anxiety disorder. These thoughts may concern personal illness, fears about the safety of other people, or social anxieties.

The **physical symptoms** of a generalized anxiety disorder result from overactivity in the sympathetic nervous system and from increased tension in skeletal muscles. The list of symptoms is long, but they can be grouped conveniently by the systems of the body as in Table 7.2. A few comments are required about the list: excessive wind results from the swallowing of air; the difficulty in inhaling caused by anxiety contrasts with the expiratory difficulty of asthma; overbreathing causes further physical symptoms as explained below. Among the neurological symptoms, dizziness is not rotational but rather a feeling of unsteadiness. Some patients report blurring of vision although their visual acuity is normal. Headache is typically in the form of constriction or pressure, which is usually bilateral and frontal or occipital. Aching, especially in the back and shoulders, is another common complaint.

Table 7.2.

Symptoms of generalized anxiety disorder

1. Psychological	Fearful anticipation
	Irritability
	Sensitivity to noise
	Restlessness
	Poor concentration
	Worrying thoughts
2. Physical	
• Gastrointestinal	Dry mouth
	Difficulty in swallowing
	Epigastric discomfort
	Excessive wind
	Frequent or loose motions
• Respiratory	Constriction in the chest
	Difficulty inhaling
	Overbreathing
• Cardiovascular	Palpitations
	Discomfort in chest
	Awareness of missed beats
• Genitourinary	Frequent or urgent micturition
	Failure of erection
	Menstrual discomfort
	Amenorrhoea
• Neuromuscular	Tremor
	Prickling sensations
	Tinnitus
	Dizziness
	Headache
	Aching muscles
3. Sleep disturbance	Insomnia
	Night terrors
4. Other symptoms	Depression
	Obsessions
	Depersonalization

It is important to remember that patients may not complain of anxiety but report instead any of these physical symptoms. Conversely, it is important that each of the physical symptoms of anxiety may be caused by physical disease. Both these points are considered further under differential diagnosis (see p. 107).

Sleep is disturbed in a characteristic way. On going to bed patients lie awake worrying; when at last they fall asleep, they wake intermittently. They often report unpleasant dreams; occasionally they experience 'night terrors' in which they wake suddenly feeling intensely fearful, sometimes remembering a nightmare, and sometimes uncertain why they are so frightened. Early waking with inability to go back to sleep again is much less common among patients with a generalized anxiety disorder than among patients with a depressive disorder (see p. 127). Therefore, early waking should always suggest that the anxiety symptoms may be part of a depressive disorder.

Although the **other symptoms** listed in Table 7.2 are not major features of the syndrome, they too may be the symptoms first reported by patients with anxiety disorders.

Hyperventilation is breathing, usually in a rapid and shallow way, that is excessive in that it results in a fall in the concentration of carbon dioxide in the blood. The resultant symptoms are listed in Table 7.3. Paradoxically, overbreathing produces a feeling of breathlessness which causes the patient to breathe even more vigorously. When a patient has unexplained bodily symptoms, the possibility of persistent overbreathing should be considered. The diagnosis should be made on the definite occurrence of this group of symptoms during episodes of anxiety, or on observations of the patient's respiration during a naturally occurring attack. The finding that similar symptoms can be produced by deliberate overbreathing in the clinic does not prove that involuntary hyperventilation is the cause of the physical symptoms experienced at other times.

Some patients with generalized anxiety disorder experience occasional *panic attacks*, that is, sudden episodes of very severe anxiety. However, panic attacks are more characteristic of panic disorder (see p. 117).

Duration of symptoms By convention, *generalized anxiety disorder* is diagnosed only when symptoms of anxiety have been present for several months (in DSM-IV, six months is specified). When symptoms have been present for a shorter time, the formal diagnosis is *adjustment disorder* (see p. 95).

Prevalence

Generalized anxiety disorder occurs in about 50 per 1000 of the population. It is slightly more common among women than men. The disorder is frequent among patients with psychological symptoms in primary care.

Differential diagnosis

Generalized anxiety disorders have to be distinguished from other psychiatric disorders in which anxiety may be prominent and from physical illnesses that produce similar symptoms.

• **Depressive disorder** can usually be distinguished from anxiety disorder by the greater severity of the depressive symptoms relative to the anxiety symptoms and by the order in which the symptoms appeared: anxiety before depression in generalized anxiety disorders. Whenever possible, information on these points should be obtained from a relative or other informant as well as from the patient.

Sometimes the agitation of a severe depressive disorder (see p. 130) may be mistaken for anxiety. These diagnostic errors can be reduced by enquiring routinely about depressive symptoms in patients presenting with anxiety.

• **Schizophrenia.** Patients sometimes complain of anxiety before they reveal other symptoms of schizophrenia, even when questioned directly. Errors in diagnosis can be reduced by asking anxious patients what they think is the cause of

Table 7.3.

Symptoms and signs of hyperventilation

- Rapid shallow breathing
- Dizziness
- Tinnitus
- Headache
- Precordial discomfort
- Weakness
- Faintness
- Numbness and tingling in the hands and feet
- Carpopedal spasm

their symptoms. In reply, schizophrenic patients may reveal unusual ideas (e.g. that their anxiety is due to threatening influences).

- **Presenile** or **senile dementia** may first come to notice when the patient complains of anxiety. When this happens, the clinician may overlook an accompanying memory disorder or ascribe it to poor concentration. For this reason, memory should be assessed appropriately when older patients present with anxiety.

- Withdrawal from **drugs** or **alcohol** or excessive use of **caffeine** can cause anxiety, and the cause may be overlooked because patients wish to hide their drug dependency or alcohol misuse. Reports that anxiety is particularly severe on waking in the morning suggests alcohol dependence (withdrawal symptoms are most likely at this time see p. 266), though anxiety symptoms secondary to depressive disorder may also be worse on waking.

- **Certain physical illnesses** present symptoms similar to those of anxiety disorder. This possibility should be considered in every case, but particularly when no psychological explanation can be found for the anxiety.

  - *Thyrotoxicosis* leads to irritability, restlessness, tremor, and tachycardia. Patients should be examined for an enlarged thyroid, atrial fibrillation, and exophthalmos, and thyroid function tests arranged in appropriate cases.

  - *Phaeochromocytoma* and *hypoglycaemia* should be considered as occasional causes of episodic anxiety

  - *Other physical illness* may cause anxiety through psychological rather than physiological mechanisms (e.g. when the patient fears a fatal outcome). This sequence is particularly likely when the patient has a special reason to fear a serious outcome (e.g. because a relative has died after developing symptoms similar to those of the patient). It is useful to ask anxious patients whether they know anyone who had similar symptoms.

The **opposite diagnostic error** can be made: generalized anxiety disorders with prominent physical symptoms can be mistaken for physical disease. The patient may then be subjected to investigations intended to reassure the patient which actually increase anxiety because their negative results do not explain the symptoms. This error will be less common if the doctor remembers the diversity of anxiety symptoms; palpitations, headache, frequency of micturition, abdominal discomfort, indeed any of those listed in Table 7.2 can be the presenting complaint of a patient with a generalized anxiety disorder.

Aetiology

Predisposing factors Three factors have been proposed: genetic, childhood upbringing, and personality type.

1. **Genetic** causes are important in predisposing to anxiety disorders. The concordance for anxiety disorders of all kinds is greater among monozygotic than among dizygotic twins. However, most studies have not distinguished between the different kinds of anxiety disorder, so the size of the contribution of genetic factors to generalized anxiety disorder is uncertain.

2. **Childhood upbringing** has often been proposed as predisposing to generalized anxiety disorder in adult life. However, despite much speculation, no

specific causes have been identified. Anxiety is a common emotional disorder in childhood but most anxious children grow into healthy adults and not all anxious adults have been anxious children.

3. **Personality**. The anxious personality (see p. 78) is linked with anxiety disorder but other kinds of personality can predispose by making people less able to cope with stressful events.

Precipitating factors Generalized anxiety disorder usually begins in relation to **stressful events**, especially those that are threatening such as problems in relationships, physical illness, and problems in employment.

Maintaining factors Generalized anxiety disorders are often maintained by the **persistence of the stressful** events that provoked them. They are also maintained also by **ways of thinking** that make the symptoms of the disorder stressful: for example, fears that other people will notice that the patient is anxious; or that anxiety will impair performance at work. Such fears can cause a vicious circle which increases and prolongs anxiety.

Prognosis

By convention, the diagnosis of generalized anxiety disorder cannot be made until the symptoms have been present for several months (more than six months is specified in DSM-IV). Without treatment, about 80% still have the disorder three years after the onset. Prognosis is worse when symptoms are severe, and when there is agitation, derealization, conversion symptoms, or suicidal ideas. Brief episodes of depression are frequent among patients with a chronic generalized anxiety disorder and it is often during one of these episodes that further treatment is sought.

Treatment

Patients with generalized anxiety disorder are often treated with benzodiazepines. Although patients improve with this treatment, many relapse when the medication is stopped, and if it is continued for longer than three weeks, dependency may develop. Psychological treatment usually produces improvement similar to that of drug treatment and need take no more time (Table 7.4).

Initial treatment

The first step is to **exclude a depressive disorder**, first, because many patients with chronic anxiety come for treatment during a concomitant depressive disorder and second because depressive disorder can present with anxiety symptoms (see p. 95).

Supportive and social measures General practitioners see many anxious patients before the disorder has been present for the six months needed to make a formal diagnosis of generalized anxiety disorder. At this early stage, when the formal diagnosis is an adjustment disorder, many patients respond to **discussion and reassurance** (see p. 95). Interviews need not be lengthy but patients should feel that they have the doctor's undivided attention and that their problems have been understood sympathetically. A clear **explanation** should be given of the nature of any physical symptoms of anxiety; for example, that palpitations are an exaggeration of a normal reaction to stressful events and not a sign of heart disease.

The patient should be helped to deal with or come to terms with any **social problems** that appear to be maintaining the disorder.

If anxiety is severe, short-term **benzodiazepine** treatment may be prescribed but it should seldom last more than three weeks because of the risk of dependence.

Table 7.4.

Treatment plan for generalized anxiety disorder

Initial treatment
- Exclude concomitant depressive disorder
- Explain nature and cause of symptoms, reassure about specific concerns
- Help in solving or coming to terms with stressful problems
- If anxiety severe, short-term benzodiazepine treatment

Further treatment
Continue the above and consider
- Relaxation training
- Respiratory control if hyperventilating
- Referral for anxiety management training
- Medication if anxiety still severe—see text

Further treatment

Anxiety is prolonged by uncertainty and a **clear plan** of treatment helps to reduce it (see Table 7.4). These measures are important also for patients whose symptoms have lasted for more than six months when first seen by the doctor.

Relaxation training Relaxation training (see p. 369) can reduce anxiety if the patient practises regularly but it is often difficult to persuade patients with generalized anxiety disorder to do this. Relaxation training in a group may improve motivation, and some patients prefer to relax as part of yoga exercises. Some family doctors provide relaxation groups for their patients.

Treatment for hyperventilation

- To *terminate an acute episode*, the patient should rebreathe expired air from a paper bag thereby increasing the alveolar concentration of carbon dioxide. Rebreathing during an episode is also an effective way of demonstrating that certain symptoms are caused by hyperventilation.

- To *prevent further episodes* of hyperventilation, patients should practise slow, controlled breathing, at first under supervision and then at home. A tape recording can be used to help the patient time his breathing appropriately. Such a tape can be made by the doctor or obtained from many departments of clinical psychology.

Anxiety management (see also p. 372) As explained above, patients with generalized anxiety disorders worry about their symptoms in ways that prolong the disorder. These worries include concerns that symptoms are the forerunner of a serious medical condition such as a heart attack, embarrassment that other people notice signs of anxiety, and worries of a more general kind; for example, about the safety of family members. Anxiety management enables patients to control these fearful concerns with distraction and by questioning their logical basis so that more rational ways of thinking can be substituted. Relaxation training is the third component of anxiety management. Anxiety management is usually carried out by a member of a specialist psychiatric team.

Drug treatment *Benzodiazepines* bring symptoms under control quickly, but their use should not be prolonged because the patient may become dependent on them. Generally, their use should be reserved for brief exacerbations of the symptoms (see p. 337). Many benzodiazepines are available; diazepam is commonly prescribed in doses ranging from 5 mg twice daily in mild cases to 10 mg three times daily in severe ones.

Buspirone, a non-benzodiazepine anxiolytic (see p. 338), is less likely than the benzodiazepines to cause dependence and therefore more suitable for prolonged use. Its effects appear more slowly than those of benzodiazepines.

Tricyclic antidepressants and SSRIs have anxiolytic as well as antidepressant effects, and they do not produce dependence. They may be used for long-term control of anxiety disorders, as an alternative to benzodiazepines. Although their long-term effect is anxiolytic, their initial effect may be to increase anxiety and for this reason they are started cautiously and sometimes with a benzodiazepine for a few days. No one preparation is definitely more effective then the rest and the choice depends on the patient's tolerance of side effects and of any contraindications (see pp. 245–6).

Amitriptyline is often used as an inexpensive and well-tried drug. Anticholinergic side effects are seldom troublesome, since the dose required for anxiolytics is less than that required in the treatment of depressive disorder (75–100 mg of amitriptyline) is usually adequate. If side effects are troublesome, or there is a risk of self-harm, an *SSRI* or other drug should be chosen with fewer side effects and less toxicity in overdose than the tricyclics.

Monoamine oxidase inhibitors (MAOIs) have been used to treat chronic anxiety disorders. Because they interact with some drugs and foodstuffs (see p. 350) they are now used infrequently for this purpose and then usually after a specialist opinion. The precautions described on p. 351 and in the manufacturer's literature should be followed carefully.

Beta-adrenergic antagonists are used occasionally to control severe and persistent palpitations unresponsive to other anxiolytic treatment. Care should be taken to observe the contraindications for the use of these drugs and the precautions described in the manufacturer's literature.

Phobic anxiety disorders

The symptoms of phobic anxiety disorder are the same as those of generalized anxiety disorders, but they occur only in particular circumstances. In some phobic disorders these circumstances are few in number and the patient is free from anxiety for most of the time; in other cases many circumstances provoke anxiety. Two other features characterize phobic disorders: **avoidance** of circumstances which provoke anxiety; and **anticipatory anxiety** when there is the prospect of encountering such circumstances. The circumstances which provoke anxiety include *situations,* such as crowded places, *living things,* such as spiders, and *natural phenomena,* such as thunder. For clinical purposes it is usual to recognize three principal groups of phobic disorder: simple phobia, social phobia, and agoraphobia.

In most respects the classification of phobias is the same in ICD-10 and DSM-IV but there is one important difference. In DSM-IV, patients who experience both agoraphobia and non-situational panic are classified as panic disorder with (additional) agoraphobia; in ICD-10 the same cases are classified as agoraphobia with (additional) panic. The reason why panic attacks are given diagnostic priority in DSM-IV is explained on p. 116.

Simple phobia

A person with simple phobia is inappropriately anxious in the presence of a particular object or situation, or when anticipating this encounter and tends to avoid the object or situation. The symptoms experienced are those of any anxiety disorder (see p. 103). The urge to avoid the stimulus is strong, and in most cases there is actual avoidance. Anticipatory anxiety is often severe, for example, a person who fears storms may become extremely anxious even when there are black clouds that might precede a storm.

Simple phobias are sometimes classified further by adding the name of the stimulus; for example, spider phobia. Sometimes terms such as arachnophobia (to denote spider phobia) or acrophobia (to denote phobia of heights) are used, but this is unnecessary. The following varieties of simple phobia are met sufficiently often as clinical problems to require separate comment:

- **Phobias of blood, injection, and injury** These phobias differ from other types of simple phobia in that there is a strong vasovagal response instead of the usual sympathetic reaction. Fainting is common.

- **Phobia of dental treatment** About 5% of adults have specific fears of this kind which can become so severe that all dental treatment is avoided and serious caries develops.

- **Phobia of flying** Anxiety during aeroplane travel is common. A few people have such intense fear that flying is impossible. This fear develops occasionally among pilots, usually following a serious flying accident.

- **Phobia of excretion** Some people with this phobia become anxious when attempting to pass urine in public lavatories. Others have frequent urges to pass urine when away from home, fear being incontinent, and arrange their lives so as never to be far from a lavatory. A few patients have similar symptoms centred around defecation.

- **Phobias of vomiting** People with this phobia fear that they may vomit in a public place, such as a bus or train, or fear that other people may do so.

- Some patients experience repeated fearful thoughts that they may have cancer, venereal disease, or some other serious illness. Such fears are a type of hypochondriacal symptom (see p. 218).

Prevalence Simple phobias are common but very few patients seek medical help. The one-year prevalence is about 100 per 1000 population.

Differential diagnosis A **depressive disorder** should be considered since some patients with longstanding simple phobias seek help when an unrelated depressive disorder makes them less able to tolerate the phobic symptoms. Otherwise the diagnosis is usually straightforward.

Aetiology Most of the simple phobias of adult life began in childhood when simple phobias are extremely common (see p. 405). Why most childhood phobias disappear and a few persist into adult life is not known except that the most severe phobias are more likely to do so. Simple phobias which begin in adult life often develop after a very frightening experience; for example, a phobia of horses following a dangerous encounter with a bolting horse. For a few, no cause can be identified.

Prognosis There has been no systematic study of prognosis. Clinical experience indicates that simple phobias which began in childhood continue for many years, while those starting after a stressful experience in adult life have a better prognosis.

Treatment The exposure form of behaviour therapy (see p. 369) generally gives good results. Such treatment is straightforward but time consuming and most general practitioners arrange treatment from a clinical psychologist.

Social phobia

Social phobia is inappropriate anxiety in situations in which a person is observed and could be criticized by others. There is anticipatory anxiety at the prospect of entering situations, which are avoided wholly or in part. Partial avoidance involves, for example, entering a social group but failing to make conversation, or sitting in an inconspicuous place. The *situations* that provoke anxiety include: restaurants, canteens, and dinner parties; seminars, board meetings, and other places where it is necessary to speak in public; occasions when some action is open to scrutiny; for example, writing, eating, or drinking in front of another person. (Table 7.5.) The *symptoms* of social phobia are the same as those of generalized anxiety disorder (see p. 105), although complaints of *blushing and trembling* are particularly frequent. People with social phobia have specific *concerns about being observed critically* by other people (and realize that this concern is irrational). Some take *alcohol* to relieve anxiety and alcohol abuse is more common among social phobics than among people with other phobias. The condition usually begins with an acute attack of anxiety in some public place. Subsequently, anxiety occurs in similar places with episodes that become gradually more severe and increasing avoidance.

Prevalence The one year prevalence is about 25 per 1000. It is about equally common in men and women. Thus, it is less frequent than simple phobia (see above) but a greater proportion of patients with social phobia seek treatment than do patients with simple phobia.

Table 7.5.

Situations feared and avoided by patients with social phobia

Common theme	Being observed and open to criticism
Examples	Committees, seminars
	Eating or drinking in public
	Social gatherings
	Writing or performing in front of others

Differential diagnosis

• **Generalized anxiety disorder**. Social phobia is distinguished by the pattern of situations in which anxiety occurs.

• **Depressive disorder**. Social phobia is distinguished by the pattern of situations and the absence of the typical pattern of depressive symptoms on mental state examination.

• **Schizophrenia**. Some patients with schizophrenia describe anxiety in and avoid social situations because of persecutory delusions. Diagnosis may be difficult when patients do not reveal the delusions or other symptoms of schizophrenia. Patients with social phobia may have ideas of being watched which at first seem to be delusions but further questioning reveals that the patient knows that they are untrue.

• **Anxious/avoidant personality disorder**, with lifelong shyness and lack of self-confidence, may closely resemble social phobia. The distinction is based on the time of onset, which is earlier in personality disorder; also the onset is sudden in most cases of social phobia but gradual in personality disorder.

• **Social inadequacy** is a primary lack of social skills with secondary anxiety. Diction is hesitant, dull and inaudible, facial expression and gestures are awkward, and the person fails to look appropriately at other people when making conversation. Patients with social phobia possess these basic social skills although they may be prevented from using them by anxiety in the social situation.

Aetiology The cause of social phobia is uncertain. Symptoms begin usually in late adolescence, when many young people are concerned about the impression they are making on other people. It is possible that social phobias begin among people in whom these normal concerns are most pronounced, perhaps after a stressful event leading to an episode of severe anxiety. After the initial episode symptoms seem to be maintained by concerns that other people will respond critically to signs of anxiety.

Prognosis There are no systematic data on the long-term course of social phobia. Clinical experience suggests that the phobias persist for many years, although most improve by mid life.

Treatment **Anxiolytic drugs** provide short-term relief, for example, in dealing with an important social situation. They should not be used regularly because of the risk of dependence (see p. 339). **Monoamine oxidase inhibitors**, such as phenelzine and moclobemide, produce longer-term improvement although some patients relapse when treatment ends. The usual precautions about diet and drug interactions must be taken (see pp. 350–1).

SSRIs: fluoxetine has been reported to be effective in this condition.

Cognitive-behaviour therapy (see p. 367) combines exposure to feared situations with measures to reduce the patients' concerns that others are evaluating them critically. Most patients improve with this treatment which is usually provided by a psychiatrist or clinical psychologist.

Dynamic psychotherapy (see p. 375) is effective in some patients whose social phobia is associated with low self-esteem and longstanding problems in personal relationships.

Agoraphobia

Clinical features Agoraphobic patients are anxious when they are away from home, or in crowds, or in situations they cannot leave easily. Many patients also fear open spaces and social situations. The symptoms resemble those of generalized anxiety disorder (see p. 106), together with a varying combination of *depression and depersonalization*. As in the other phobic disorders, there is *anticipatory anxiety* and *avoidance* of the situations which cause anxiety.

Panic attacks are frequent in agoraphobics, both in response to environmental stimuli and spontaneously. *Anxious thoughts* about fainting and loss of control are common.

Many **situations** provoke anxiety and avoidance (Table 7.6). As explained above, the situations have in common: distance from home, crowding, and confinement. Examples include: buses and trains, shops and supermarkets, and places that cannot be left suddenly without attracting attention, for example, the hairdresser's chair or a seat in the middle of a row at the cinema. Less common situations are open spaces, for example, parks and open country, and social situations, such as a party or a business meeting. As the condition progresses, patients avoid more and more of these situations until in severe cases they may be almost confined in their homes.

The anxiety experienced in these situations may be reduced in several ways. Most patients are less anxious when accompanied by a trusted companion, and some are helped even by the presence of a child, pet dog, or even a reassuring object such as a bottle of tablets (which are not taken).

Anticipatory anxiety may be severe and appear several hours before the person has to enter a feared situation.

Agoraphobia usually begins in the early or mid twenties, with a further period of high onset in the mid thirties. (Contrast the usual onset of simple phobias in childhood and of social phobias in late teenage years.) The *first episode* of agoraphobia often occurs while the person is waiting for public transport, or shopping in a crowded store. Suddenly the person develops an unexplained panic attack, and either goes home or seeks help at a hospital. The person recovers from the first episode, but when they encounter the same or a similar situation again, anxiety returns and another hurried escape is made. This sequence recurs over the next weeks and months with panic attacks in more and more places, and a growing habit of avoidance. It is unusual to discover any immediate cause for the first panic attack, although some patients describe a background of problems at the time (e.g. worry about a sick child).

As the condition progresses, agoraphobic patients may become increasingly *dependent on the spouse or other relatives* for help with activities, such as shopping, that provoke anxiety. The consequent demands on the spouse may lead to arguments, but serious marital problems are not usually common among agoraphobics.

Prevalence The one-year prevalence of agoraphobia is about 30 per 1000, with twice as many women as men.

Differential diagnosis

- **Generalized anxiety disorder** These patients may experience anxiety in public places but it is part of a pattern of anxiety in many other situations, without the pattern of avoidance characteristic of agoraphobia. In doubtful cases it is useful

(see p. 106)

Table 7.6.

Situations feared and avoided by agoraphobics

Common themes	Distance from home
	Crowding
	Confinement
	Open spaces
	Social situations
Examples	Public transport
	Crowded shops
	Empty streets
	School visits
	Cinemas, theatres

to ask whether anxiety was situational or generalized in the early stages of the condition.

• **Social phobia** Many patients with agoraphobia feel anxious in social situations and some social phobics avoid buses and shops when they are crowded. Detailed enquiry into the pattern of avoidance and the symptoms in the early stages of the disorder will usually settle the point.

• **Depressive disorder** These patients may avoid shops and crowds because of low mood but mental state examination will reveal depressive symptoms. Sometimes a recent depressive disorder is superimposed on a longstanding agoraphobic disorder (see treatment, below).

• **Schizophrenia** Occasionally, patients with paranoid delusions avoid going out and meeting people in a way that resembles agoraphobia. If they hide the delusions diagnosis may be difficult but repeated examination of the mental state will eventually reveal the diagnosis.

Aetiology Agoraphobia often begins with a spontaneous panic attack from which anticipatory anxiety and avoidance develop in a way that suggests conditioning. Some investigators consider that agoraphobia is a form of panic disorder; others consider that it is a separate disorder arising from a single unexpected panic attack. Both groups agree that the spread and persistence of the symptoms can be explained by the conditioning of anxiety to an increasing number of situations. They agree also that agoraphobia is **maintained** by avoidance behaviour, which prevents deconditioning, and by apprehensive thoughts, such as fears of fainting or social embarrassment, which cause vicious circles of anxiety. (This difference of opinion is reflected in the systems of classification. The American system, DSM-IV, classifies cases with agoraphobia and panic as a form of panic disorder, the international classification, ICD-10, classifies the same cases as a form of agoraphobia, see p. 111.)

Prognosis When agoraphobia has been present continuously for a year, it is likely to persist for at least five years. Brief episodes of depressive symptoms often occur in the course of chronic agoraphobia.

Treatment (Table 7.7) Since depressive episodes are common in panic disorder and agoraphobia symptoms can occur in depressive disorder, the first step is to exclude a depressive disorder.

Table 7.7.
Management plan for agoraphobia

- Look for associated depressive disorder: treat if present
- Assess severity of the agoraphobia: obtain specialist help for severe cases
- If essential, prescribe anxiolytics until other effects of treatment appear
- Prepare a hierarchy, arrange exposure
- Teach anxiety management
- Prescribe imipramine if spontaneous panic attacks interfere with exposure
- Specialist advice if little improvement

Avoidance is the most important factor maintaining agoraphobia, patients should be strongly encouraged to return to situations they are avoiding, a procedure known as 'exposure'. **Exposure** is described on p. 369. It begins with situations that provoke little anxiety, and proceeds through a graded series of situations that provoke increasing anxiety (a hierarchy). When patients first enter one of these situations they feel anxious, but as they manage their anxiety (see below) the anxiety subsides. It is essential that patients do not leave the situation until anxiety has subsided, otherwise the experience may increase rather than diminish the phobic response when the situation is encountered again.

To help patients remain in the phobic situations for the required time they are taught **anxiety management**, a combination of relaxation and other coping techniques (see p. 372). If this does not control anxiety sufficiently, a benzodiazepine can be given shortly before exposure. However, patients who have taken benzodiazepines during exposure may relapse partially when they are stopped. Also, the aim of treatment should be to encourage self-help rather than reliance on anxiolytics.

Agoraphobic patients who have many spontaneous panic attacks respond less well to exposure treatment. Spontaneous panic attacks can usually be controlled with medication (see p. 119) while exposure continues.

If the patient does not improve with the above treatment specialist advice should be sought to arrange more intensive cognitive-behaviour therapy.

Panic disorder

Clinical features

The symptoms of a panic attack are listed in Table 7.8. Important features of panic attacks are that severe anxiety builds up quickly and there is fear of a catastrophic outcome. The diagnosis of panic disorder is made when the attacks occur unexpectedly (i.e. not in response to a known phobic stimulus), and when they are repeated. As the condition develops, situational panic may be added to the original spontaneous attacks. This progression blurs the distinction between agoraphobia and panic disorder.

Panic disorder patients often seek advice from general practitioners, cardiologists, and other physicians about episodic physical symptoms, such as bouts of palpitations and fears that cardiac or other physical disease might be the cause of the physical symptoms.

Prevalence

The prevalence of panic disorder meeting diagnostic criteria is about 10 per 1000, it is about twice as frequent among women than men. Many other people have panic attacks that are not sufficiently frequent to satisfy formal criteria for panic disorder: they number about 30 per 1000.

Differential diagnosis

Panic attacks occur in many conditions other than panic disorder, notably *generalized anxiety disorder*, *phobic anxiety disorder* (*especially agoraphobia*), *depressive disorders*, and during *withdrawal from alcohol*. Diagnosis is made by searching for symptoms of these other disorders and considering which symptoms developed first; for example, whether depression preceded or followed the onset of panic.

Table 7.8.
Symptoms of a panic attack

- Palpitations
- Dyspnoea
- Chest discomfort
- Sweating
- Trembling
- Dizziness or fainting
- Flushing
- Nausea
- Fears of an impending medical emergency
- Depersonalization

Aetiology

There are three main hypotheses about the causes of panic disorder. The first proposes a biochemical abnormality, the second hyperventilation, and the third a cognitive abnormality.

It seems likely that panic disorder is caused by a combination of the first and third sets of causes; panic disorder develops when a person with poorly regulated autonomic responses to stressful events also fears that the symptoms of autonomic arousal are evidence of a forthcoming medical catastrophe.

Prognosis

Systematic follow-up data have not been reported but clinical observation indicates that some patients with panic disorder recover within weeks. Those cases

Additional information **Aetiology**

The **biochemical hypothesis** is based on three sets of observations. First, certain *chemical agents can induce panic* attacks more readily in patients with panic disorder than in healthy people or patients with other kinds of anxiety disorder. These agents include yohimbine, an alpha-adrenergic antagonist which increases central sympathetic activity, carbon dioxide inhalation, and sodium lactate infusions which act in an unknown way. Second, *certain drugs reduce panic attacks* (e.g. imipramine and SSRIs). Third, panic disorder is *more frequent among relatives* of panic disorder patients than among the general population, a finding consistent with a genetic cause but also with social transmission. So far there have been insufficient twin studies to be sure that the family aggregation is not due to the latter.

It has been proposed that regulation of the adrenergic and possibly also the 5-HT systems are abnormal in panic disorder. While there is no doubt that the nor-adrenergic system is highly active during panic attacks, it has not been shown that this activity is the cause of the disorder rather than the pathway through which another disorder is expressed.

The **hyperventilation hypothesis** proposes that panic attacks are caused by overbreathing. Although some of these patients hyperventilate, measurements of $p\text{CO}_2$ during panic attacks indicates that hyperventilation does not occur in every case. Thus, although hyperventilation increases symptoms in a few cases, is unlikely to be a general cause.

The **cognitive hypothesis** is based on the observation that, compared with other anxious patients, patients with panic disorder have greater fears concerning the physical symptoms of anxiety. They fear, for example, that palpitations will be followed by a heart attack. It is proposed that cognitions cause panic attacks by initiating a vicious circle in which anxiety leads to physical symptoms which activate patients' fears of the significance of these symptoms which leads in turn to greater anxiety. Experimental evidence supports this hypothesis; for example, reducing fearful cognitions reduces panic.

Some patients carry out actions intended to avert the feared catastrophe, for example, breathing deeply or relaxing. Because they believe that these actions have prevented the feared events, for example a heart attack, patients do not find out that the catastrophe never occurs and so they continue to fear it. These so-called *safety behaviours* thereby prolong the panic disorder.

that have persisted for six months or more usually run a prolonged, although often fluctuating course.

Treatment

Early treatment The general practitioner or physician who sees the patient soon after an initial panic attack should attempt to prevent progression to panic disorder by explaining that anxiety produces physical symptoms which may be frightening but are harmless. The physician should also explain that anxiety produces frightening thoughts about dying or losing control and that these cause a vicious circle of anxiety. Patients should be advised about the role of behaviours intended to prevent the feared outcome (see above) and also that they should not avoid situations in which panic attacks have occurred since this will lead to agoraphobia (Table 7.9).

Drug treatment *Benzodiazepines* can be used but it is usually necessary to use high doses to control panic attacks and to continue them for several months with the consequent problems of withdrawal symptoms and dependency when the drug is stopped. In some countries, alprazolam is used for these cases because it has a higher potency than diazepam and is less likely to cause sedation than diazepam in therapeutic doses. Up to 6 mg per day of alprazolam may be needed to suppress panic attacks (equivalent to about 60 mg of diazepam). If used, such high doses should be built up gradually over two to three weeks and withdrawn slowly over about six weeks.

Antidepressant drugs. Some antidepressants have antipanic effects when given in large doses. *Imipramine* is as effective as benzodiazepines in reducing panic attacks and seldom gives rise to withdrawal symptoms and does not cause dependency. However, its effect is slower to appear and causes more side effects (see p. 345). Also, the initial effect of imipramine in panic disorder is increased arousal in the form of apprehension, sleeplessness, and sympathetic activity. For this reason, very small doses should be used at first (see *Additional information*, p. 120). About a third of those who improve with either alprazolam or imipramine, relapse when the drug is stopped after six months, and may need further treatment. *SSRIs* also control the

Table 7.9.
Management plan for panic disorder

Explain
  — the harmless nature of physical symptoms
  — the vicious circle formed by concerns about symptoms and anxiety
  — the effect of safety behaviours and avoidance

Consider medication (see text)
  — if panics severe
  — associated depressive disorder

Arrange cognitive therapy

Additional information **Imipramine for panic disorder**

A starting dose as low as 10 mg per day for 3 days may be needed to avoid overarousal, increased by 10 mg every 3 days until a dose of 50 mg per day has been reached, and then by increments of 25 mg per week to 150 mg per day. If panics persist at this dose the advice of a specialist should be obtained. The specialist may increase the dose cautiously to 175 mg per day or, occasionally, an even higher dose provided that the side effects allow this and the patient is physically fit. Before such high doses are given, appropriate investigations should be carried out if there is any doubt about cardiac, renal, or other functions. If symptoms improve full dosage is continued for up to 6 months; a general practitioner who is asked to continue these high doses should study the manufacturer's literature carefully and watch for side effects.

symptoms of panic disorder and their effect is comparable to that of imipramine. They do not have the anticholinergic or cardiac side effects of imipramine but they have side effects of their own which some patients do not tolerate (see p. 347).

Cognitive therapy This is described on p. 373. It is a specialised treatment provided by a clinical psychologist or psychiatrist. Cognitive therapy is about as effective as drug treatment in the short term and has a lower rate of relapse after treatment. Since it requires specialist skills and is more time consuming than drug treatment, it is often more practical to try medication before cognitive therapy is used.

Obsessive-compulsive disorder

Clinical features

Obsessive-compulsive disorders are characterized by obsessional thinking, compulsive behaviour, and varying degrees of anxiety, depression, and depersonalization (Table 7.10). Obsessional and compulsive symptoms are described on pp. 14–16 but the main features are repeated here.

Obsessional thoughts are words, ideas and beliefs, recognized by the patient as his own. The thoughts intrude forcibly into the patient's mind and the patient attempts to exclude them. It is the combination of this sense of being compelled to think the thoughts and of resistance that characterize obsessional symptoms. Obsessional thoughts may be single words, phrases, or rhymes; they are usually unpleasant or shocking to the patient, obscene or blasphemous.

Obsessional images have the same characteristics of intrusion and resistance but appear as vividly imagined scenes, often of violence or of a kind that disgusts the patient, such as abnormal sexual practices.

Obsessional ruminations are internal debates in which continuous arguments are reviewed endlessly.

Obsessional doubts are thoughts about actions that may have been completed inadequately, such as failing to turn off a gas tap completely; or about actions that

Table 7.10.
Symptoms of obsessional disorder

Obsessions
  – thoughts
  – images
  – ruminations
  – doubts
  – impulse
Rituals
'*Phobias*' (see text)
Slowness
Other symptoms
  – anxiety
  – depression
  – depersonalization

may have harmed other people, for example, the idea that while driving his car past a cyclist the patient might have caused an accident which he did not notice at the time. Doubts may also be related to religious observances, such as the adequacy of confession.

Obsessional impulses are urges to perform acts, usually of a violent kind, for example, leaping in front of a car or striking a child, or of an embarrassing kind, such as shouting blasphemies in church. The urges are resisted strongly, and are not carried out, but the internal struggle may be very distressing.

Obsessional rituals are repeated but senseless activities. They may be mental activities, such as counting repeatedly in a special way or repeating a certain form of words, or behaviours, such as washing the hands twenty or more times a day. Rituals are usually followed by temporary release of distress (although occasionally they increase it). Some rituals have an understandable connection with obsessional thoughts that precede them, for example, repeated hand-washing following thoughts about contamination. Other rituals have no such obvious connection; for example, routines concerned with laying out clothes in a complicated way before dressing may follow obsessional symptoms of an unconnected kind. The ritual may be followed by doubts whether it has been completed in the right way, and the sequence may be repeated over and again. Patients are aware that their rituals are illogical, and usually try to hide them.

Obsessional phobias Obsessional thoughts and compulsive rituals may worsen in certain situations; for example, obsessional thoughts about harming other people often increase in a kitchen or other place where knives are kept. When this happens, patients avoid the situations and this combination of fearful thoughts and avoidance is sometimes called obsessional phobia because it resembles the fear and avoidance of phobic patients (though the latter do not have fears that have the special features of obsessional thoughts).

Obsessional slowness Obsessional thoughts and rituals lead to slow the patient's performance of everyday activities. A minority of obsessional patients are afflicted also by extreme obsessional slowness that is out of proportion to other symptoms. The cause is not known.

Anxiety is an important additional component of obsessive-compulsive disorders. **Depressive symptoms** are often present. In some patients these are an understandable reaction to the obsessional symptoms, but in others there are recurring depressive moods that arise independently of the other symptoms. **Depersonalization** occurs sometimes, adding to the patient's disability.

The **obsessional personality** is described in Chapter 5. Although they share the same name, obsessional personality and obsessive-compulsive disorders do not have a simple one-to-one relationship. Obsessional personality is over-represented among patients who develop obsessive compulsive disorder, but about a third of obsessional patients have other types of personality. Moreover, although people with obsessional personality may develop obsessive-compulsive disorders, they are more likely to develop depressive disorders.

Prevalence

Obsessive-compulsive disorders are much less frequent that anxiety disorders. The one-year prevalence is about 2 per 1000, with men and women affected about equally.

Differential diagnosis

Obsessive-compulsive disorders have to be distinguished from the following disorders in which obsessional symptoms can occur:

• **Anxiety disorders** Obsessional symptoms are less severe than those of anxiety and develop later in the course of the disorder.

• **Depressive disorder** Diagnosis can be difficult because the course of obsessive-compulsive disorder is often punctuated by periods of depression. However, obsessional symptoms appear after depression in depressive disorders. It is important to make the correct diagnosis because depressive disorders with obsessional features usually respond well to antidepressant treatment.

• **Schizophrenia** When obsessional thoughts have a peculiar content, the clinical picture may suggest schizophrenia. Repeated mental state examination will reveal other symptoms of schizophrenia and an informant may describe other behaviours that suggests this diagnosis.

• **Organic cerebral disorders** Although obsessional symptoms may occur in dementia, they are seldom prominent and other features of dementia are present.

Aetiology

Predisposing causes

1. **Genetic** Obsessive-compulsive disorder occurs more frequently among members of the families of obsessive-compulsive patients than among the general population. It is not certain whether this familial pattern indicates genetic causes rather than family environment because the necessary large-scale twin and adoption studies have not been carried out.

2. **Organic factors** Parents with obsessive-compulsive disorder have an increased rate of minor, non-localizing neurological signs but no specific neurological lesion has been identified. Brain imaging has not shown any definite structural abnormality, but functional changes have been reported in the orbitofrontal cortex and caudate nucleus.

3. **Early experience** Obsessional mothers might be expected to transmit a tendency to obsessional symptoms to their children through social learning. However, although children of such mothers are at increased risk for psychiatric problems, more of these problems are non-specific than obsessional.

Precipitating factors

Obsessive-compulsive disorders often begin when there are stressful events but no specific kind of stressful experience has been shown to be important.

Maintaining factors

Although checking behaviour and other rituals reduce anxiety for a short time their long-term effect is to reinforce the obsessional symptoms. Avoidance of cues that provoke symptoms has the same effect. (These findings are made use of in treatment—see below.)

Prognosis

About two-thirds of patients improve within a year; the remaining third run a prolonged and usually fluctuating course with periods of partial or complete remission lasting a few months to several years. Prognosis is worse when the personality is obsessional, the symptoms are severe, and when there are continuing stressful circumstances.

Treatment (Table 7.11)

Severe obsessional disorders are difficult to treat and specialist advice should be obtained. For less severe cases, the following plan should be followed.

General measures Since patients with an obsessive-compulsive disorder often fear that they are developing schizophrenia or another serious mental disorder and will lose control of their actions, it is important to explain that obsessive compulsive disorder does not progress in this way nor are they likely to act on any of the impulses that they are resisting. It is important to explain that great effort should be made to resist the urge to carry out rituals, since these maintain the disorder. With the patient's agreement it is appropriate to talk to one or more family members to explain the same points so that they can help the patient resist the urge to carry out rituals. Obsessive-compulsive symptoms may be provoked by stressful circumstances, especially those causing anger which the person does not express. Alternative ways of dealing with these situations are discussed or, if this proves difficult, strategies for avoiding the situations.

Drug treatment **5-HT uptake blockers** have specific effect on the obsessive-compulsive symptoms. Effective drugs include the tricyclic drug, clomipramine, and the SSRIs, fluvoxamine and fluoxetine. Clomipramine has to be given in high dosage, sometimes beyond the usual maximum of 150 mg per day, proceeding to a dose of as much as 225 mg per day in fit patients who do not experience severe side effects. (Such large doses should generally be prescribed initially by a specialist.) Response to both clomipramine and SSRIs is slow, taking up to six weeks for the full effect; because they do not have anticholinergic and cardiac effects, SSRIs are generally preferred. Treatment should be maintained for up to six months and then reduced cautiously, watching for recurrence, and increased again for a further two to three months if symptoms reappear.

Table 7.11.

Management plan for obsessive-compulsive disorder

- Refer to a specialist if disorder is severe
- Reassure about fears of progression to schizophrenia and loss of control
- Discourage rituals
- Reduce stressors if possible
- Prescribe 5-HT uptake blocker (see text) continuing for 6 months
- Refer for behaviour therapy if no progress or condition initially severe
- Use anxiolytics only for short-term relief and antidepressants if concurrent depressive disorder

Anxiolytic drugs are useful for short-term relief of the distress associated with obsessional symptoms but they should not be prescribed for more than a few weeks.

Tricyclic antidepressants, such as amitriptyline, are needed when there is an associated depressive disorder. Treatment of this disorder usually leads to an improvement in the obsessive-compulsive symptoms

Behaviour therapy The behaviour therapy technique for obsessional disorders is response prevention, which is a vigorous programme to help the patient suppress rituals while they return to any situations they have avoided. (See p. 370 for further information.) About two-thirds of patients with moderately severe rituals improve substantially though far fewer recover completely. When rituals improve, associated obsessional thoughts usually improve as well. A few patients have obsessional thoughts without rituals. A behavioural technique called 'thought stopping' (see p. 370) may be tried in these cases but the results are seldom satisfactory. For these patients, drug treatment is often of more benefit.

Psychosurgery In the past, psychosurgery was occasionally used to treat severe and intractable cases of obsessive compulsive disorder. Several kinds of operative lesion were used, mainly involving the frontal white matter. The immediate results of these procedures was a marked reduction in the obsessional symptoms but the long-term benefits have not been proved. With improvements in behavioural and drug treatments, psychosurgery is no longer in use except in a very few special centres as a last resort for rare cases resistant to all other treatment.

Further reading

Mavassakalian, M. R. and Prien, R. F. (ed.) (1996). *Long-term Treatments of Anxiety Disorders*. American Psychiatric Press, Washington, DC.
A review of the evidence about the effectiveness of both pharmacological and psychological treatments.

Kennerly, H. (1990). *Managing Anxiety: A Training Manual*. Oxford University Press.
A practical guide to the psychological treatment of anxiety disorders.

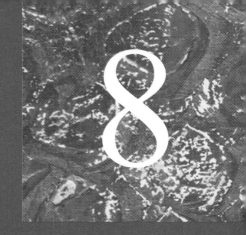

Affective disorders

- Depression

- Mania

- Mixed and alternating affective states

- Classification

- Minor affective disorders

- Differential diagnosis

- Epidemiology of affective disorders

- Aetiology of affective disorders

- Course and prognosis of affective disorders

- Treatment

- Management of depressive disorders

- Management of mania

- Treatment

Affective disorders

The word 'affect' is a synonym for mood, and affective disorders are so named because their main feature is an abnormality of mood, namely depression or elation. These abnormalities are more intense and persistent than normal unhappiness at times of adversity or elation at times of good fortune, and occur as part of syndromes of mood-related symptoms and disturbances of thinking. In addition to the primary mood disorders described in this chapter, both depressed mood and elation (mania) can be secondary to other psychiatric syndromes and also accompany physical illness.

The central features of **depressive disorder** are low mood, pessimistic thinking, lack of enjoyment, reduced energy, slowness and poor concentration, and low self-esteem. Depressive disorder is frequent in general and hospital practice but is often undetected, especially when there are also physical symptoms. Unrecognized depressive disorder is a common cause of distress, and also of slow recovery from physical illness. It is important, therefore, that all doctors should be able to recognize the condition, treat the less severe cases, and identify those requiring specialist care because of suicidal risk or for other reasons.

Depressive disorders are classified as single depressive episodes, mild, moderate or severe, and as recurrent episodes. There are less severe forms of depression known as 'dysthymia'.

The principal treatment of depression is antidepressant medication, but all patients also require psychological and social support. It is essential that medication is prescribed and taken in an adequate dosage for a proper length of time. Failure to show evidence of response within six weeks should lead to reassessment and possible changes in drug treatment. Antidepressant medication should be discontinued with care over a period of months following recovery. Some patients require long-term maintenance medication. Depressive illnesses place a heavy burden on families who require information and support.

The features of **mania** are elevated mood, overactivity, and self-important ideas. Mania is considerably less common than depressive disorder; it occurs as part of bipolar disorder in which there may also be episodes of depression. It is important that mania is recognized in its early stages because in the later stages the patient becomes increasingly unwilling to accept treatment. Prophylactic treatment is available to those with recurrent bipolar illnesses.

Depression

General clinical features

Sadness is a normal emotion commonly experienced by healthy people in response to misfortunes, especially loss, including grief. It is often accompanied by some anxiety, lack of energy, general malaise, and poor sleep.

More severe unhappiness is the central symptom of *primary depressive disorder*—a syndrome of symptoms associated with low mood, depressive thinking, and (in more severe cases) biological symptoms. Depressive symptoms also occur in many other psychiatric disorders, such as schizophrenia and dementia. Together with anxiety, depression is the commonest psychological complaint in patients seen in primary care and many cases are due to depressive psychiatric disorder.

Sometimes the symptoms of depressive disorders are not always immediately obvious because the patient smiles and denies feeling miserable, a condition described as *masked depression*. Diagnosis depends on a careful search for the *whole range of symptoms of depressive disorder* described below, especially lack of pleasure in life, sleep disturbance, diurnal mood variation, and a pessimistic view of the future.

Mild depressive disorder

Mild disorder is frequent and, despite its name, implies an unpleasant and disabling persistent syndrome. The patient's mood, behaviour, and other symptoms are seen by the patient and by others as distinctly different to usual personality and behaviour. As with all depressive disorders, it is a syndrome with a wide range of symptoms.

The patient characteristically complains of low mood, lack of energy and enjoyment, and poor sleep. Other symptoms include anxiety, phobias, and obsessional symptoms. The patient may not be obviously dejected in appearance, or slowed in movement (Table 8.1). Although anxiety may be a symptom in all degrees of depressive disorder, it can be just as severe in the mild as in the severe disorders. There is *sleep disturbance*. The pattern is varied but it is often difficult to fall asleep, and sleep is restless with periods of waking during the night followed usually by sounder sleep a few hours before waking. The 'biological' features of more severe depression (poor appetite, weight loss, and low libido) are uncommon and are described in the next section. Mood may vary during the day; usually it is worse in the evening than in the morning in contrast to the more severe disorder.

Moderately severe depressive disorder

In depressive disorders of moderate severity (Table 8.2), the central features are *low mood, lack of enjoyment, reduced energy,* and *pessimistic thinking*.

Appearance

The patient's **appearance** is often characteristic. **Psychomotor retardation** is frequent, speech movements are slow, there may be **agitation**, that is a state of restlessness, and an inability to relax often accompanied by restless activity. When agitation is severe the patient cannot sit for long and may pace up and down.

Mood

The patient is miserable. The low mood is often experienced as different from ordinary sadness—patients sometimes speak of a black cloud pervading all mental activities. There is **diurnal variation** of mood which is characteristically worse in the morning than in the later part of the day (see biological symptoms, below).

Anxiety and irritability are frequent. Irritability is the tendency to respond with undue annoyance to minor demands and frustrations.

Lack of interest and enjoyment

Lack of interest and enjoyment are frequent and important symptoms, though not always complained of spontaneously. Patients show no enthusiasm for activities and

---

Table 8.1.

Features of mild depressive disorder

- Symptoms are persistent
- Patient's mood and behaviour are seen by others as different to normal character and behaviour
- Depression
- Anxiety symptoms
- Poor sleep
- May be worse in the evenings
- Pessimism, but not suicidal ideation
- Lack of energy or enjoyment

hobbies that they would normally enjoy and describe a loss of zest for living and the pleasure from everyday things. They often withdraw from social encounters.

Reduced energy is characteristic (although when accompanied by physical restlessness it can be overlooked). The patient feels lethargic, finds everything an effort, and leaves tasks unfinished. For example, a normally houseproud woman may leave beds unmade and dirty plates on the table. Understandably, many patients attribute this lack of energy to physical illness and seek help for this rather than for depression.

Poor concentration and complaints of **poor memory** are common. However, if the patient is encouraged to make a special effort, retention and recall can usually be shown to be normal. Sometimes, however, apparent impairment of memory is so severe that the clinical presentation resembles that of dementia. This presentation, which is particularly common in the elderly, is sometimes called **depressive pseudodementia** (see p. 194).

Complaints about **physical symptoms** are common in depressive disorders. They take many forms but complaints of constipation and of aching discomfort in any part of the body are particularly common. Complaints about any pre-existing physical disorders usually increase, and **hypochondriacal** preoccupations are common.

Depressive thinking

Pessimistic thinking ('depressive cognitions') arising from the low mood affects thoughts about the present, future, and the past.

- Concerned with the *present*. Patients see the unhappy side of every event, think that they are failing in everything they do and that other people see them as a failure; they lose confidence and discount any success as a chance happening for which they can take no credit.

- Concerned with the *future*. Patients expect the worst. They may foresee failure in their work, the ruin of their finances, misfortune for their families, and an inevitable deterioration in their physical health. These ideas of **hopelessness** are often accompanied by the thought that life is no longer worth living and that death would come as a welcome release. These gloomy preoccupations may progress to thoughts of, and plans for, **suicide**. *It is important to ask about suicide in every case of depressive illness.* (The assessment of suicidal risk is considered further in Chapter 12.)

- Concerned with the *past*. These thoughts often take the form of unreasonable guilt and **self-blame** about minor matters; for example, patients may feel guilty about some trivial act of dishonesty in the past or about letting someone down. Usually, the patient has not thought about these events for years, but as the depression has developed they have flooded back into their memory accompanied by intense feelings of guilt. Gloomy preoccupations of this kind strongly suggest depressive disorder. Some patients have similar feelings of guilt but do not attach them to any particular event. Other memories are focused on unhappy events; patients remember occasions when they were sad, when they failed, or when their fortunes were at a low ebb. These gloomy memories become more frequent as the depression deepens.

Table 8.2.

The symptoms and signs of moderately severe depressive disorder

Appearance
- Sad appearance
- Psychomotor retardation

Low mood
- Misery and unhappiness
- Diurnal variation—worse in morning
- Anxiety, irritability, agitation

Lack of interest and enjoyment
- Reduced energy
- Poor concentration
- Subjective poor memory

Depressive thinking
- Pessimistic and guilty thoughts
- Ideas of personal failure
- Hopelessness
- Suicidal ideas
- Self-blame
- Hypochondriacal ideas

Biological symptoms
- Early wakening and other sleep disturbance
- Weight loss
- Reduced appetite
- Reduced sexual drive

Other symptoms
- Obsessional symptoms
- Depersonalization, etc.

Biological symptoms

This term is used to denote sleep disturbance, diurnal variation of mood, loss of appetite, loss of weight, constipation, loss of libido and, in women, amenorrhoea. These symptoms are more common in severe depression than in cases of moderate severity (see below).

Sleep disturbance is of several kinds:
- The most characteristic is *early morning waking*, that is waking two or three hours before the patient's usual time. Patients do not fall asleep again, but lie awake feeling unrefreshed and often restless and agitated. They think about the coming day with pessimism, brood about past failures, and ponder gloomily about the more distant future. This combination of early waking with depressive thinking is important in diagnosis.
- *Delay in falling asleep*, and *waking during the night*.
- Some depressed patients *sleep excessively* and wake late although they still report waking unrefreshed.

In depressive disorders, **weight loss** often seems greater than can be explained merely by the patient's **lack of appetite**. Instead of eating too little and losing weight, some patients eat more and gain weight. Sometimes they do this because eating brings them temporary relief from their distressing feelings, in other cases it is a side effect of medication.

Loss of libido is usual.

Other psychiatric symptoms

Many other symptoms may occur as part of a depressive disorder, and occasionally one of these dominates the clinical picture. They include *depersonalization*, *obsessional symptoms*, *phobias*, and *conversion symptoms* such as fugue or loss of function of a limb (Chapter 1).

Severe depressive disorder

As depressive disorders become more severe, all the features described under moderate depressive disorder occur with greater intensity (Table 8.3). There may also be additional symptoms not seen in moderate depressive disorder, namely delusions and hallucinations ('psychotic' symptoms; a disorder with these symptoms is called **psychotic depression**).

The **delusions** of severe depressive disorders are concerned with the same themes as the non-delusional thinking of moderate depressive disorders, namely, *worthlessness*, *guilt*, *ill-health* and, more rarely, *poverty*. Such delusions have been described in Chapter 1, but a few examples may be helpful here. A patient with a *delusion of guilt* may believe that some dishonest act, such as a minor concealment in making a tax return, will be discovered and that he will be punished severely and humiliated. He is likely to believe that such punishment is deserved. A patient with *hypochondriacal delusions* may be convinced that he has cancer or venereal disease. A patient with a *delusion of impoverishment* may wrongly believe that he has lost all his money in a business venture. A patient with *nihilistic delusions* may believe that he has no future, or that some part of him has ceased to exist or function (e.g. that his

Table 8.3.

Symptoms of severe depressive disorder

Delusions of	worthlessness
	guilt
	ill-health
	poverty
	nihilism
	persecution
Hallucinations	auditory
	rarely visual

bowels are wholly blocked). A patient with *persecutory delusions* may believe that other people are discussing him in a derogatory way, or about to take revenge on him. When persecutory delusions are part of a depressive syndrome, typically, the patient accepts the supposed persecution as something he deserves.

Perceptual disturbances may also be found in severe depressive disorders. Sometimes these fall short of hallucinations; a few patients experience true hallucinations, which are usually auditory in the form of voices addressing repetitive words and phrases to the patient. The voices may seem to confirm their ideas of worthlessness (e.g. 'you are evil; you should die'), or to make derisive comments, or urge suicide. A few patients experience visual hallucinations, sometimes in the form of scenes of death and destruction.

Suicidal ideas should be enquired about carefully in any patient with a severe depressive disorder. Rarely, there are **homicidal ideas**. These are particularly important where they relate to young children.

Variants of moderate and severe depressive disorder

The clinical picture of severe depressive disorders is varied and several terms are sometimes used to describe common patterns:

- The term **agitated depression** is applied to depressive disorders in which agitation is particularly severe. Agitated depression occurs more commonly among the middle-aged and elderly than among younger patients.
- The term **retarded depression** is applied to depressive disorders in which psychomotor retardation is prominent. In its most severe form, retarded depression shades into depressive stupor.
- **Depressive stupor** is a rare variant of severe depressive disorder in which retardation is so extreme that the patient is motionless, mute, and refuses to eat and drink. On recovering, patients can recall the events taking place at the time they were in stupor.
- **Atypical depression** A minority of patients have prominent atypical features such as severe anxiety, severe fatigue, increased sleep, and increased appetite.

Seasonal affective disorder (SAD)

Some people repeatedly develop a depressive disorder at the same time of year. In some cases this timing reflects extra demands on the person at a particular time of year; in other cases there is no such extra demand, and it has been suggested that the cause is related to changes in the season, for example, in the length of daylight. Although these affective disorders are characterized mainly by the season at which they occur, they are also said to be characterized by some symptoms that are less common in other affective disorders, for example, hypersomnia and increased appetite with cravings for carbohydrates.

The most common pattern is onset in the autumn or winter, and recovery in the spring or summer. This pattern has led to the suggestion that shortening of daylight is important. Some patients improve after exposure to artificial light given usually in the early morning (see p. 359). It is uncertain for which patients the treatment is effective, or how lasting are its effects.

Mania

Mania, a syndrome which is in some ways the reverse of depression, occurs as part of so-called *bipolar disorder*. This term implies episodes of both mania and depressive disorder but also includes those who, at the time of diagnosis, have only suffered manic illnesses (most patients with mania eventually develop a depressive disorder).

Clinical features

The central features of the syndrome of mania are: *elation or irritability, increased activity,* and *self-important ideas* (Table 8.4).

Most manic patients can exert some **control** over their symptoms for a short time. Many do so when the interviewer is assessing the need for treatment, with the result that the severity of the disorder may be underestimated. For this reason it is important, whenever possible, to interview an informant as well as the patient.

Elevated mood may appear as cheerfulness, undue optimism, and as infectious gaiety. In other cases, it appears as irritability and a tendency to become angry. Mood often varies during the day, although usually not with the regular diurnal rhythm characteristic of severe depressive disorders (see p. 130). Sometimes elation is interrupted by sudden brief episodes of depression.

Appearance often reflects the prevailing mood. Patients often select brightly coloured and ill-assorted clothes. When the condition is severe, they may appear untidy and dishevelled.

Behaviour Patients are *overactive*, often for long periods, leading to physical exhaustion. Manic patients are *distractible*, starting activities and leaving them unfinished as they turn repeatedly to new ones.

Socially inappropriate behaviour includes excessive involvement in pleasurable activities. These may be unrestrained buying sprees or increased sexual energy.

Sleep is often reduced but the patient wakes feeling lively and energetic and may often rise early and engage in noisy activity to the surprise and distress of other people.

Appetite is increased, and food may be eaten greedily with little attention to conventional manners.

Speech is often rapid and copious, reflecting thoughts that occur in quick succession ('pressure of speech'). When severe, the rapid succession of thoughts is difficult to follow; the term **flight of ideas** is used.

Thinking Expansive (grandiose) ideas are common. Patients believe that their ideas are original, their opinions important, and their work is of outstanding quality. Many patients become extravagant, spending more than they can afford, for example, on expensive cars or jewellery. Others make reckless decisions to give up good jobs or embark on plans for risky business ventures.

Table 8.4.

Clinical features of mania

Mood
- Euphoria
- Irritability

Appearance

Behaviour
- Overactivity
- Distractibility
- Socially inappropriate behaviour
- Reduced sleep
- Increased appetite
- Increased libido

Thinking and speech
- Flight of ideas
- Expansive ideas
- Grandiose delusions
- Hallucinations

Impaired insight

In severe cases there may be **grandiose delusions**. For example, the patient may believe that he is a religious prophet or an expert destined to advise statesmen about great issues. At times there are *delusions of persecution*, the patient believing that people are conspiring against him because of his special importance. *Delusions of reference* and *passivity feelings* may occur, and 'first rank' symptoms. The delusions often change in content over days.

Hallucinations also occur in severe cases. They are usually consistent with the mood and fluctuating in content, taking the form of voices speaking to the patient about his special powers or, occasionally, of visions with a religious content.

Insight is invariably impaired. Patients may see no reason why their grandiose plans should be restrained or their extravagant expenditure curtailed. They seldom think themselves ill or in need of treatment.

Clinical patterns

- *Mild mania*—increased physical activity and speech; mood is labile, mainly euphoric but giving way to irritability at times; ideas are expansive, the patient often spending more money than he can afford.

- *Moderate mania*—marked overactivity with pressure and disorganization of speech; the euphoric mood is increasingly interrupted by periods of irritability, hostility, and depression; and grandiose and other preoccupations may become delusional.

- *Severe mania*—frenzied overactivity; thinking is incoherent and delusions become increasingly bizarre; hallucinations are experienced. Very rarely, the patient becomes immobile and mute (manic stupor).

Mixed and alternating affective states

Occasionally, manic and depressive symptoms occur together, as a **mixed affective state**. For example, an overactive and overtalkative patient may have profound depressive thoughts including suicidal ideas. In **alternating affective states** mania and depression follow one another in a sequence of rapid changes. Thus, a manic patient may be intensely depressed for a few hours and then quickly become manic. Occasionally, states of mania and depression follow one another regularly with intervals of a few weeks or months between them. This is sometimes called **rapid cycling**.

Classification

Without more knowledge of the causes of the various kinds of depressive disorders, classification is uncertain. Three broad approaches have been based on:

1. **Aetiology**—the extent to which symptoms are caused by factors within the individual person (*endogenous*) or by external stressors (*reactive*). Both types of cause are present in every case and this is not a useful basis for classification.

2. **Symptoms**—the nature and intensity of depressive symptoms (*neurotic* and *psychotic*). This approach is also unsatisfactory because there appears to be a gradation of severity of the disorder rather than distinct patterns.

Table 8.5.

The classification of affective disorders

ICD-10	DSM-IV
Manic episode	*Manic episode*
Depressive episode	*Major depressive episode*
Mild	
Moderate	
Severe	
Bipolar affective disorder	*Bipolar disorders*
Persistent mood (affective) states	
Cyclothymia	Cyclothymia
Dysthymia	Dysthymia

3. **Course**—apart from classifying depression as a single episode, recurrent or persistent, there is an important distinction between those who only have depressive disorders (*unipolar*) and those who also have manic episodes (*bipolar*). All manic patients are classified as bipolar, even if there has been no episode of depressive disorder. This distinction has a genetic basis and has implications for treatment.

The categories used for classification in ICD-10 and DSM-IV are broadly similar, although the terms are not quite the same (Table 8.5). Depressive episodes can be divided into mild, moderate, or severe, using standard criteria. Within these main diagnostic categories it is possible to specify disorders that have a seasonal pattern and those in which general medical conditions or substance-dependence appear to be aetiological factors.

The classification includes two categories for less severe and more chronic illnesses:

(1) *dysthymia*, with chronic, constant, or fluctuating mild depressive symptoms;

(2) *cyclothymia*, with chronic instability of mood with mild depressive and manic symptoms.

In primary care, the most frequent presentation of mild depressive disorder is a mixture of anxiety and depression; often referred to as *minor affective disorder*. This term does not appear in either ICD-10 or DSM-IV and covers a borderland between adjustment disorder (see p. 95) and the depressive syndromes described below.

Classification and description in everyday practice

For most clinical purposes other than the specialist practice of psychiatry it is more useful to *describe* affective disorders systematically as shown in Table 8.6, than to classify in formal terms.

• The **severity** of the episode is described as mild, moderate, or severe.

• The **type** of episode is described as depressive, manic, or mixed.

• Special features (Table 8.6) are noted.

Table 8.6.

A systematic scheme for the description of affective disorders

The episode	
Severity	mild, moderate, or severe
Type	depressive, manic, mixed
Special features	with neurotic symptoms
	with psychotic symptoms
	with agitation
	with retardation or stupor
The course	unipolar or bipolar
Aetiology	predominantly reactive
	predominantly endogenous

- The **course** of the disorder is characterized as unipolar or bipolar (as explained above, all manic episodes are called bipolar even if there has been no depressive disorder).

- The predominant **aetiology** is recorded. Almost invariably, there are both endogenous and reactive causes.

Minor affective disorders

This term is not included in the standard classifications of disease. It is sometimes applied to conditions in which several emotional symptoms occur together, with none predominating. An alternative term is 'subthreshold disorders'. These conditions are common in general practice. Estimates of prevalence vary from 18 to 79 per 1000 for men, and from 27 to 165 per 1000 for women. Looked at in another way minor affective disorders probably make up about two-thirds of the psychiatric disorders seen in general practice. The most frequent symptoms are:

- Anxiety and worrying thoughts
- Sadness and depressive thoughts
- Irritability
- Poor concentration
- Insomnia
- Fatigue
- Somatic symptoms (see text)
- Excessive concern about bodily function.

Somatic symptoms include abdominal discomfort, indigestion, flatulence, and poor appetite; palpitations, praecordial discomfort, and concerns about heart disease; headache, and pain in the neck, back, and shoulders. All these physical symptoms require a thorough investigation for physical causes because they can occur when a person with physical disease is worried and depressed about his state.

Thorough physical investigation is especially important when the complaint is of difficulty in swallowing or of weight loss, because these symptoms are particularly likely to have a physical cause. For these reasons the diagnosis of minor affective disorder requires a wide range of clinical skills.

Minor affective disorders are not all of the same kind. Some are adjustment reactions (see p. 95); others are mild recurrences of previous anxiety or depressive disorders (not severe enough to meet the diagnostic criteria for anxiety or depressive disorder). It is because the dividing lines between these disorders are arbitrary, and because it is often difficult to determine the exact duration and severity of such disorders, that the term 'minor affective disorder' is useful in clinical practice

Prognosis

About half improve within three months and a further quarter within six months. The rest persist as minor affective disorders, or become more severe so that they are diagnosed as anxiety disorders, depressive disorders, or somatoform syndromes (p. 218).

Differential diagnosis

Depressive disorders

These disorders have to be distinguished from:

• **Normal sadness** As explained on p. 127, the distinction from normal sadness depends on the presence of other symptoms of the syndrome of depressive disorder.

• **Grief** Although depressive disorder resembles **uncomplicated bereavement** in many ways, severe pessimism, suicidal thoughts, profound guilt, and psychotic symptoms are all rare. Severe symptoms persisting more than two months after bereavement suggest a depressive disorder.

• **Anxiety disorder** Mild depressive disorders are sometimes difficult to distinguish from anxiety disorders. Accurate diagnosis depends on assessment of the relative severity of anxiety and depressive symptoms, and on the order in which they appeared. Similar problems arise when there are prominent **phobic** or **obsessional** symptoms. (These points are discussed further in Chapter 7.)

• **Unexplained medical symptoms** It is not uncommon for depressive disorder to present with concern about non-specific and medically unexplained physical symptoms, without a direct complaint of the psychological symptoms. Careful enquiry will elicit these additional symptoms. (See p. 216.)

• **Schizophrenia** The differential diagnosis of depressive disorder from schizophrenia depends on a careful search for the characteristic features of this condition (see Chapter 9). The term **post-psychotic depression** refers to depressive symptoms following treatment of the psychotic symptoms of schizophrenia. Diagnosis may be difficult when a patient has both depressive symptoms and persecutory delusions, but the distinction can usually be made by examining the mental state carefully and establishing whether the delusions followed the depressive symptoms (depressive disorder) or the delusions came first (schizophrenia). Also, in depressive disorder, the supposed persecution is usually accepted as the deserved consequence of the patient's own failings; in schizophrenia it is strongly rejected. Some patients have symptoms of both depressive disorder and of schizophrenia; these **schizoaffective disorders** are discussed in Chapter 9.

• **Dementia** In middle and late life, depressive disorders may be difficult to distinguish from dementia because some patients with depressive disorder complain of considerable difficulty in remembering and some demented patients are depressed. In depressive disorders, difficulty in remembering occurs because poor concentration leads to inadequate registration. The distinction between the two conditions can often be made by careful memory testing; standard psychological tests are required in doubtful cases, but even these may not decide the issue. If memory disorder does not improve with recovery of normal mood, dementia is probable (see also p. 322).

• **Substance abuse** Depressive symptoms are common in substance abuse and some patients with depressive disorder abuse alcohol or non-prescribed drugs to relieve their distress. The sequence of the depressive symptoms and substance abuse should be determined, as well as the presence of the features of depressive disorder other than low mood.

Manic disorders

Manic disorders have to be distinguished from: schizophrenia, organic brain disease involving the frontal lobes (including brain tumour and general paralysis of the insane), and states of excitement induced by amphetamines and related drugs.

• **Schizophrenia** The diagnosis from schizophrenia can be most difficult. In manic disorders, auditory hallucinations and delusions can occur, including some delusions that are characteristic of schizophrenia such as delusions of reference. In mania these symptoms usually change quickly in content, and seldom outlast the overactivity. When there is a more or less equal mixture of features of the two syndromes, the term 'schizoaffective' (or 'schizomanic') is used. These conditions are discussed further in Chapter 9.

• **Dementia** should always be considered, especially in middle-aged or older patients with expansive behaviour and no past history of affective disorder. In the absence of gross mood disorder, extreme social disinhibition (e.g. urinating in public) strongly suggests frontal lobe pathology. In such cases appropriate neurological investigation is essential.

• **Abuse of stimulant drugs** The distinction between mania and excited behaviour due to abuse of amphetamines depends on the history together with examination of the urine for drugs before treatment with psychotropic drugs is started. Drug-induced states usually subside quickly once the patient is in hospital and free from the drugs (see Chapter 13).

Epidemiology of affective disorders

Major depressive disorders are frequent with a prevalence in Western countries of 20–30 per 1000 for men and 40–90 per 1000 for women. The lifetime risk is

70–120 per 1000 for men and 200–250 per 1000 for women. It is not certain why consistently higher figures are reported for women.

Bipolar disorder is much less common. The prevalence is between 1 and 6 per 1000 and the lifetime risk is rather less than 10 per 1000. First degree relatives have a 120 per 1000 lifetime risk of the same disorder and another 120 per 1000 have a lifetime risk of recurrent depressive disorder. An additional 12% have dysthymic or other mood disorders.

A primary care doctor responsible for 2000 patients of all ages may expect to see 20 to 30 patients a year *presenting* with major depression and 1 to 4 with manic illness.

Aetiology of affective disorders

In broad terms, affective disorders are caused by an interaction between: (1) stressful events; and (2) constitutional factors resulting from genetic endowment and childhood experience. These aetiological factors act through biochemical and psychological processes, which have been partly identified by research. More is known about the aetiology of depressive than of manic disorders, and correspondingly more space is given to depressive disorders in this account. Also, since it illustrates the multifactorial approach to aetiology in psychiatry, it is described at length.

Precipitating factors

- Genetic
- Personality
- Predisposing environmental factors
- Precipitating environmental factors
- Physical causes

Genetic causes

These have been studied mainly in moderate to severe cases of affective disorder, rather than in milder cases. Parents, siblings, and children of severely depressed patients have a higher morbid risk for affective disorder (10–15%), than the general population (1–2%). *Twin studies* indicate that these high rates among families are due to genetic factors. Thus the concordance of bipolar disorder is the same (about 70%) among monozygotic twins reared together and monozygotic twins reared apart, and higher than the concordance between dizygotic twins (23%).

Studies of *adopted children* confirm the importance of genetic causes of depressive disorder. Thus the risk of a depressive disorder is

- *higher in a child* who was (i) born to a parent with a history of serious depressive disorder, but (ii) reared by adoptive parents with no such history;
- *lower in a child* who was (i) born to parents with no history of serious depressive disorder, and (ii) reared by adoptive parents with no such history.

Looked at in another way, the biological parents of adoptees with a bipolar disorder have a higher rate of affective disorder than do the biological parents of adoptees without bipolar disorder.

Bipolar disorders are more frequent in the families of bipolar probands than in the families of unipolar probands. However, unipolar cases are frequent in the families of bipolar as well as unipolar probands. Thus unipolar cases may be of more than one genetic type.

It is uncertain whether the *mode of inheritance* is dominant or recessive, or even whether it is sex-linked or not. Attempts to link the inheritance of the disorder to a particular region of the genome have not be successful at the time of writing, although a major research effort is being undertaken.

The same kinds of study indicate that genetic factors are less important in the less severe depressive disorders.

Personality

It has been suggested that genetic factors might predispose to affective disorder through an effect on personality, or alternatively that variations in personality reflect the same genetic factors that cause illness. **Cyclothymic personality** (see p. 85) with its repeated mood swings is related to bipolar disorder but the relationship is not one-to-one; not all cyclothymic personalities develop a bipolar disorder, and not all bipolar disorders occur in people with cyclothymic personality.

Unipolar disorders are not associated with a single personality type although in an individual case it is often apparent that personality has played a part by sensitizing the patient to events that another personality would not find stressful.

Predisposing environmental factors

Clinical experience indicates that depressive disorders often begin after prolonged adversity, such as difficulties in marriage or at work. These adverse circumstances (*chronic difficulties*) seem to prepare the ground for a final acute stressor, which precipitates the disorder. For example, there is evidence that having the care of several young children, poor economic circumstances, and unsupportive marriage increase vulnerability to depression.

There is also evidence that certain factors *protect* against the action of stressors and that the person is more vulnerable if they are removed. Thus, some women appear to be more vulnerable to depressive disorder when they have nobody with whom they can confide.

Precipitating environmental factors

Everyday clinical experience indicates that depressive disorders often follow stressful **life events**. This association is not necessarily causal: instead it might be coincidental or non-specific (that is present but to no greater extent than in other kinds of disorder). Further difficulties in interpretation are that the events may have been perceived as stressful only after the depressive disorder began and that events can be consequences of the early, but unrecognized, stages of the illness (e.g. losing a job because of deteriorating performance) rather than causes (e.g. losing a job when a whole factory closes).

Using such methods it has been shown that there is an excess of life events *independent* of the illness in the week preceding a depressive disorder, but this association is *non-specific* since life events also occur in excess in the weeks before the onset of schizophrenia, and before acts of deliberate self-harm. The findings do not mean that the association is unimportant: in fact, the risk of developing a depressive disorder is increased about sixfold in the six months after experiencing moderately severe life events (the corresponding figure for schizophrenia is about threefold).

Simply counting events disregards the possibility that *particular kinds of event* are more likely to cause depressive disorder. Since bereavement and other kinds of loss provoke ordinary feelings of sadness, it is natural to suggest that loss events might provoke depressive disorder. Research confirms that loss events have this effect.

Life events also provoke mania but less often than depressive disorder. Surprisingly, mania can follow an event that would be expected to produce a depressive response (e.g. a bereavement) as well as an event that would be expected to produce elation (e.g. success and excitement).

Physical conditions as predisposing or precipitating factors

Most physical conditions are non-specific stressors but a few appear to precipitate depressive disorder by direct biological mechanisms. They include influenza, childbirth (see p. 234), and Parkinson's disease (see p. 215).

A number of psychoactive substances, brain injury, some neurological endocrine disorders, and several other physical illnesses can produce secondary manic illnesses. In addition, in some people with a family history of bipolar disorder, antidepressant medication can precipitate a manic episode.

Mediating processes

Two kinds of complementary mediating processes have been studied: psychological and biochemical.

Psychological mediating processes

Depressed patients think in a gloomy, self-deprecating way that worsens and prolongs the initial change of mood. Their abnormal thinking can be divided into three components: (1) they *remember unhappy* events more easily than happy ones; (2) they have intrusive gloomy thoughts ('negative thoughts'), for example, 'I am a failure as a mother'; (3) they have *unrealistic beliefs*, for example, 'I cannot be happy unless I am liked by everyone I know'. Repeated negative thoughts deepen the depressive mood, while unrealistic beliefs convert everyday experiences into stressful problems.

Depressed patients also think in illogical ways ('*cognitive distortions*') such as drawing a general conclusion from a single event; for example 'I have failed in this relationship, so I will never be loved by anyone'. These illogical ways of thinking allow the intrusive gloomy thoughts and the unrealistic expectations to persist despite evidence to the contrary. These ways of thinking may also explain why some disorders persist after the original causes have passed, since they set up a vicious circle in which depressive thinking generates low mood, which then perpetuates the depressive thinking. It is not known whether these modes of thought precede the depressive disorder and play a part in its onset.

Biochemical mediating processes

Since it is not possible to examine directly the biochemistry of the living human brain, biochemical theories of depression rest on indirect information. There is increasing evidence of biochemical abnormalities, at least in the more severe depressive disorders, but their nature is uncertain. Also, it is not known whether there is a single abnormality present in every patient with depressive disorder, or different abnormalities leading to the same clinical picture.

The strongest evidence is for an abnormality of **5-HT (serotonin) function**. There are three main strands of evidence:

(1) *concentrations of the main 5-HT metabolite (5-HIAA) are reduced* in the cerebrospinal fluid (CSF) of patients with severe depressive disorders. This is very indirect evidence since concentrations of 5-HT in the brain could be very different from those in CSF;

(2) *5-HT concentrations are reduced* in the brains of depressed patients who have died by suicide. This reduction could, however, be caused by drugs used to commit suicide or by post-mortem changes;

(3) *neuroendocrine functions that involve 5-HT transmission are reduced* in depressed patients. However, the findings of an abnormality in neurones controlling endocrine function is not necessarily evidence for the same abnormality in neurones controlling mood.

If low 5-HT function is important in causing depressive disorder, then increasing this function should be therapeutic. All antidepressant drugs increase 5-HT function but until recently most have also had effects on other neurotransmitter systems. Recently, drugs have been developed that have specific 5-HT effects (the SSRIs, see Chapter 16) and these have antidepressant effects. The action of transmitter systems in the brain, however, is through checks and balances; hence it cannot be argued that, because increasing 5-HT function improves depressive disorder, reduced 5-HT function causes the disorder. The point becomes more obvious when parkinsonism is considered: in this disorder, anticholinergic drugs have therapeutic effects but the abnormality is a loss of dopaminergic function. Recently, the picture has become more complex with the discovery that there are several kinds of 5-HT receptor, each with different functions. It seems possible that antidepressant drugs exert their effects mainly on 5-HT_2 receptor function.

Noradrenergic function also seems to be reduced in depressive disorders. Most antidepressant drugs affect this transmitter system; they affect both pre- and post-synaptic noradrenergic neurones in a complicated way, but the overall action is a brief initial increase of function followed by a decrease. It seems unlikely, therefore, that the beneficial effect of antidepressant drugs can be due to a direct effect on noradrenergic receptors since, as just mentioned, noradrenergic function appears to be decreased in depressive disorders.

Endocrine abnormalities

A causal role for endocrine abnormalities is suggested by the association of mood disorder with Cushing's syndrome, Addison's disease, and hyperparathyroidism (Cushing's syndrome is sometimes associated with elation rather than depression of mood). It has also been suggested that depressive disorders occurring after childbirth or at the menopause are related to endocrine changes at these times but there is no strong evidence for this.

Among endocrine causes, interest has centred on **cortisol**. In about half of patients with depressive disorder plasma cortisol is increased, although the patients do not show evidence of hypercortisolism possibly because the number of cortisol receptor sites is reduced. However, this increase in cortisol is not specific to depressive disorder; it occurs also in mania and schizophrenia. The change does not seem to be just a reaction to the stress of being ill, for it involves a change in the diurnal pattern of secretion of cortisol (being high in the afternoon and early evening after which time it normally decreases), a change not seen after exposure to stressors. Moreover, the normal suppression of cortisol secretion, induced by giving the synthetic corticoid, dexmethasone, at midnight of the preceding day, is not observed in depressive disorder. However, this abnormal response to dexmethasone is observed also in mania, chronic schizophrenia, and dementia, indicating that the changes in cortisol function in depressive disorder may be caused by the mental disorder and not be a cause of it.

Even though the cortisone changes in depressive disorder are not those seen in response to acute stress, it has been suggested that cortisone may be involved in the aetiology of depressive disorders arising after a *prolonged* life stress. It is suggested that such stress leads to prolonged elevation of cortisol production and thereby to abnormal brain 5-HT function and thereby to depression. Direct evidence is lacking.

Conclusion

The most important **predisposing** causes for depressive disorder and mania are genetic, although the precise mode of inheritance is unknown. Adverse social circumstances also predispose to depression. While there is good evidence relating to recent chronic difficulties, it is less clear to what extent and in what way childhood experiences are important.

Depressive disorder is **precipitated** by stressful life events (especially loss), and by certain kinds of physical illness. People who lack confiding relationships seem to be more vulnerable than others to stressful circumstances. An accumulation of long-term problems may increase vulnerability to acute stressors.

Depressive disorders are **maintained** by continuing stressors and constitutional factors. There is evidence that 5-HT function is decreased in depressive disorder and psychological processes may do the same.

Course and prognosis of affective disorders

Unipolar depressive disorders may **start** at any time from adolescence to late life, the average age of onset being in the late twenties (some probably start in childhood). With treatment, each episode lasts two to three months on average; untreated illnesses last six months or more with a significant minority lasting for years. Except among the elderly (see p. 321), most patients eventually recover from the episode, although recurrences are common. At least half of those who have a single episode followed by complete recovery will eventually have another episode.

Bipolar disorders These disorders usually begin in the first half of life, 90% starting before the age of 50. They run a recurring **course** with recovery between episodes of illness. Each episode generally lasts several months—on average about three. Most patients experience depressive as well as manic episodes, but a few have only manic episodes.

Suicide is substantially more frequent among patients with affective disorder than among the general population. Among patients with severe depressive disorder about 1 in 10 eventually commit suicide.

Treatment

Depressive disorder

This section is concerned with the effectiveness of various forms of treatment for depressive syndromes. (More details of treatment with drugs and electroconvulsive therapy is given in Chapter 16, which should be consulted when reading this account.) Advice on the selection of treatments and the day-to-day care of patients is given in the section on management (see p. 150).

Drug treatment

There are three main groups of antidepressant drugs (see pp. 344–53): tricyclics, specific serotonin reuptake inhibitors (SSRIs), and monoamine oxidase inhibitors (MAOIs).

Tricyclic antidepressants A wide range of tricyclic antidepressant drugs has been tested in clinical trials. Imipramine and amitriptyline (see p. 345) were the first to be introduced and are still the standards against which others are judged. These drugs are effective in mild as well as in severe depressive disorders. They are probably the first choice in severe disorders as they are as effective as electroconvulsive therapy (ECT) but take two weeks before their therapeutic effect begins, while ECT has a more rapid action.

The side effects and hazards of the tricyclic antidepressants are described on p. 345. The anticholinergic side effects most often cause patients to stop taking these drugs. The main hazards are in patients who have heart disease, glaucoma, prostatic hypertrophy, or epilepsy.

Specific serotonin reuptake inhibitors (SSRIs) More recently, drugs with specific 5-HT uptake blocking effects have been developed (see p. 347). They appear to be as effective as tricyclic drugs in mild and moderate depression, and do not have anticholinergic side effects (but they do have other side effects, see p. 347). They are safer in overdose. They are also particularly useful for patients in whom tricyclic antidepressants are contraindicated because of their anticholinergic and cardiovascular side effects and when sedation is undesirable.

Monoamine oxidase inhibitors (MAOIs) These drugs are generally less effective than tricyclics for severe depressive disorders, and no more effective for the mild disorders. However, some patients who do not respond to tricyclic antidepressants do respond to MAOIs. These drugs reach their maximum effect slowly, and up to six weeks may be needed. MAOIs potentiate the effects of naturally occurring pressor amines including tyramine, found in some common foods (see p. 350) and of synthetic amines used as decongestants and vasoconstrictors (see p. 350) and these interactions can cause dangerous increases in blood pressure (see p. 349). Although these reactions can be avoided by careful choice of diet and by avoiding prescription of synthetic amines, it is better not to use MAOIs as the first treatment, but to reserve them for patients who have not improved with adequate dosage of a tricyclic drug.

The so-called *reversible type MAOI*, moclobemide, is less likely to have harmful interactions than the conventional MAOI drugs.

Other antidepressants There are many other antidepressants (see also Chapter 16). Some are useful in treating patients resistant to standard drug therapy. They are not discussed here because specialist psychiatric advice should generally be sought before prescribing them.

Combined drug regimes

When lithium is combined with an antidepressant the combination is effective in some patients who have not responded to the antidepressant alone. Combined treatment should be initiated by a specialist and used cautiously, especially when lithium is given with a MAOI.

Combinations of tricyclics and MAOIs and tricyclics and a SSRI are effective in some patients unresponsive to either drug given separately. Combinations can cause hazardous side effects so they should be initiated by a specialist, although other doctors may continue the combined medication after its safety and effectiveness have been established.

Electroconvulsive therapy (ECT)

ECT was the first effective physical treatment of severe depressive disorder; it retains an important clinical role in selected cases. As noted above, the antidepressant action of ECT is quicker than that of tricyclics: it starts earlier and is significantly greater after four weeks of treatment. After three months, however, the results of the two treatments are similar. The procedure for ECT and its side effects are described on p. 358.

ECT has been compared with placebo ECT (i.e. the whole procedure except for the passage of current to induce a seizure) and shown to be more effective—on average about 70% improvement versus 40%. The 40% improvement rate with placebo ECT is a reminder that even among the most severe depressive disorders some improve with good medical and nursing care and with the passage of time.

ECT is most effective for severe depressive disorders, especially those with marked weight loss, early morning wakening, retardation, and delusions. It is much less effective when there is evidence of poor premorbid adjustment, hypochondriacal, and histrionic features, and a fluctuating course—features that also predict a poor response to imipramine. In clinical trials, delusions and retardation were the best predictors of improvement with ECT as against improvement during placebo treatment.

Psychological treatment

All depressed patients and their families need *supportive care* to sustain them until improvement takes place. The least severe illnesses can usually be treated by psychological and social methods or support and problem solving alone; more severe illnesses require drug treatment or intensive cognitive therapy.

Although depressed patients often express guilt and regrets about experiences in their recent or remote past, these feelings generally resolve as mood improves and there is no evidence that dynamic psychotherapy speeds this process; indeed, it is better not to dwell on past events in the early stages of treatment for this may only increase the patient's guilty introspection.

Persistent interpersonal problems maintain depression and *problem solving* can resolve the difficulties and may reduce the risk of relapse.

Cognitive therapy (see p. 367) has been used to treat depressive disorders. When these disorders are up to of moderate severity, cognitive therapy has been reported to produce results similar to those of antidepressant drugs and also to prevent relapse as well as maintenance medication. In practice, cognitive therapy is seldom used for these purposes, because antidepressant drug treatment is simple, generally effective, and less time consuming. Cognitive therapy is sometimes used for recurrent or chronic depressive disorders in which depressive thinking seems to make the patient more vulnerable to life events, or to perpetuate the disorder. However, this use has not been thoroughly evaluated by clinical trials.

Treatment for mania
Antipsychotic drugs
Antipsychotic drugs, such as chlorpromazine and haloperidol, have proven value in the treatment of acute mania. **Lithium carbonate** (p. 353) is also effective but takes longer, usually a week or more, to produce its effects and is therefore not the usual first choice for acutely disturbed patients. **Carbamazepine** and **sodium valproate** are widely used alternatives to lithium (see p. 357).

ECT
Clinical experience indicates that ECT has a therapeutic effect in mania as well as in depressive disorder. To produce a sustained effect, this treatment has to be given more frequently in mania than in depressive disorder (usually three times as against twice a week). ECT is not a first-line treatment; its use is mainly in the uncommon cases when antipsychotic drugs are ineffective and the patient is so seriously disturbed that to spend time trying further medication or awaiting natural recovery is not justified (see p. 358).

Continuation therapy

This refers to prevention of *relapse* (i.e. return of symptoms after initial improvement during a single episode of illness). *Recurrence* means the start of a new episode of illness after recovery from the first.

For **unipolar depressive disorders**, the relapse rate is reduced by *antidepressant treatment for six months* after recovery from the acute illness. Longer treatment prevents later recurrence. *Lithium carbonate* also reduces recurrence, though it may be less effective than tricyclic antidepressants.

For **bipolar depressive disorders**, continuation treatment with *lithium carbonate* is effective in preventing relapse into mania, and is as effective as antidepressant drugs in preventing relapse into depressive disorder (lithium carbonate is discussed on p. 353). For patients who do not respond to lithium carbonate, *carbamazepine* (p. 357) or *sodium valproate* may be used, although the evidence for their preventative effects is less strong than for lithium. Relapse into mania may be induced by the continued use of antidepressant medication to prevent the depression that is the other feature of bipolar disorder.

Social and psychological factors also contribute to relapse in unipolar and bipolar disorders. Marital disharmony seems to be important, particularly in the form of repeated criticism of the patient by the spouse. Although there is no definite proof that attention to these factors is helpful, it is reasonable to try to reduce social stresses in patients who relapse despite adequate drug treatment.

Maintenance therapy

Patients with a history of relapse relatively soon after successful treatment of depression or on the ending of continuation therapy require *antidepressant drug* maintenance therapy in a dosage high enough to achieve the best possible mood. *Lithium* is used in recurrent bipolar disorder (see p. 353).

It has been proposed that *cognitive therapy* (see p. 367) reduces the relapse rate after a moderately severe depressive disorder but the effect is no greater than that of drug maintenance. The treatment is sometimes tried for patients who have **repeated** episodes of depression in response to maintenance medication and apparently related depressive forms of thinking.

Management of depressive disorders

Assessment

In the **assessment** of a patient complaining of depression (Table 8.7) the steps are to:

(1)   decide whether the diagnosis is depressive disorder;

(2)   judge the severity of the disorder and the effect of the disorder on the patient's life, including the risk of suicide, risk to others (e.g. driving a pub-

Table 8.7.

Assessment of depressive disorder*

Diagnosis	history
	mental state
	relevant physical examination
	relevant physical investigation
	informants' accounts
Severity	biological symptoms
	psychotic symptoms
	suicide risk, risk to others
	effect on social functioning
Aetiology	psychological
	social
	physical illness
	drug therapy
	constitutional
Social consequences	patient's everyday life
	partner and family
	dangers at work
Social resources	family support
	housing
	work

*The assessment of mania is similar, see text.

lic service vehicle or caring for children); key questions relate to low mood, pessimism, lack of pleasure in life, and depressive delusions.

(3) identify any primary condition causing secondary depression: medical illness, prescribed medication (see p. 209), substance abuse and other psychiatric disorder;

(4) assess the role of psychological and social predisposing and precipitating factors;

(5) assess the patient's social support and other resources;

(6) understand the effect of the disorder on other people.

Diagnosis depends on thorough history taking and examination of the physical and mental state. Differential diagnosis has been discussed earlier in this chapter (p. 136). Particular care should be taken not to overlook a depressive disorder in a patient who complains of the physical symptoms of depression such as fatigue or poor sleep rather than depressed mood ('masked depression'). It is equally important not to diagnose a depressive disorder simply on the grounds of prominent depressive symptoms; the latter could be part of another disorder, for example, an organic psychiatric syndrome caused by cerebral neoplasm (see p. 199). It should be remembered that certain drugs can induce depression (see p. 209).

The **severity** of the disorder is judged from the symptoms and behaviour. Whenever possible, an informant should be interviewed as well as the patient. Greater severity is indicated by 'biological' symptoms, and considerable severity by the presence of 'psychotic' symptoms, i.e. hallucinations and delusions). The risk of **suicide** must be judged in every case (the methods of assessment are described in Chapter 12). It is also important to assess how far the depressive disorder has reduced the patient's capacity to work or to engage in family life and social activities. In this assessment, the duration and course of the condition should be taken into account as well as the severity of the present symptoms. The length of history not only affects prognosis, it also gives an indication of the patient's capacity to tolerate further distress. A long continued disorder, even if not severe, can bring the patient to the point of desperation.

Aetiology is assessed next. First, the identification of known medical and psychiatric causes and second, precipitating, predisposing, maintaining, and pathoplastic factors. The importance of both external and internal causes should be evaluated in every case.

Precipitating causes may be psychological and social (the 'life events' discussed earlier in the chapter) or they may be physical illness or its treatment. In assessing such causes enquiries should be made into the patient's work, finances, family life, social activities, general living conditions, and physical health. Problems in these areas may be recent and acute, or may take the form of chronic background difficulties such as prolonged marital tension, problems with children, and financial hardship.

Social consequences The impact on the patient's everyday life should be considered by asking about ability to work, effects on leisure interests, and particularly consequences for family life. Such information is not only an indication of the severity of the disorder, but may bring up issues that require advice and discussion with the patient and family.

Consideration should be given to the **effect of the disorder on other people** in the household, especially young children. A severely depressed mother may neglect her children. Depressive disorder in either parent is associated with the development of emotional disorder in the children. It is important to consider whether the patient could *endanger other people* by remaining at work (e.g. as a bus driver). Danger may also arise when there are depressive delusions that could lead to action. Severely depressed mothers may sometimes kill their children because of the belief that they are doomed to suffer if they remain alive. Severely depressed patients occasionally kill their spouses.

The patient's **social resources** are considered next. Enquiries should cover family, friends, and work. Supportive families and friends can help patients through periods of depressive disorder by providing company, encouraging them when confidence is lost, and guiding them into suitable activities. For some patients, work is a valuable social resource, providing distraction and comradeship. For others it is a source of stress. A careful assessment is needed in each case.

Treatment

Further management has these stages:

- an **acute phase** to achieve recovery;
- **continuation** therapy to preserve the improvement;
- a **maintenance phase** to protect the vulnerable patients from further episodes. (See also Fig. 8.1.)

Mild depressive disorders

Mild depressive disorders may not require treatment with antidepressant drugs, especially when they are clearly reactions to stressful life events that have resolved. Patients should be encouraged to talk about their feelings and to discuss their problems. If provoking factors can be altered, patients should be encouraged to change them; if these factors cannot be altered, patients should be helped to come to terms with their situation. Such help is particularly important after bereavement or other kinds of loss (see p. 98).

Among patients with mild depressive disorders, a history of several weeks poor sleep is common. A hypnotic drug may be given for a few days to restore sleep, but such treatment should not be prolonged. If the depressive symptoms do not respond quickly to social and psychological measures and if sleep problems persist, antidepressants should be prescribed to be taken at night.

Moderately severe and severe depression
Is psychiatric referral appropriate?

Moderately severe depression may be treated by non-specialists. However, it is essential to consider whether psychiatric referral is required (Table 8.8) and, if so, whether there is an indication for hospital in-patient or out-patient care. It is also necessary to consider a number of other questions about advice to the patient and the nature of the treatment.

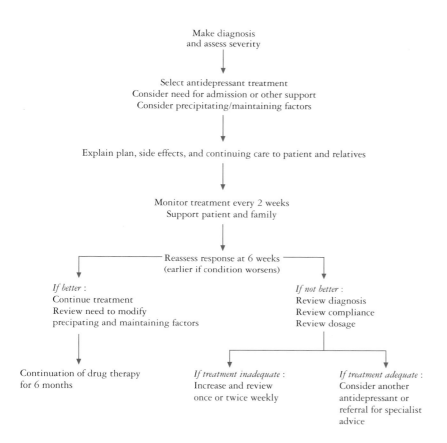

Make diagnosis
and assess severity

Select antidepressant treatment
Consider need for admission or other support
Consider precipitating/maintaining factors

Explain plan, side effects, and continuing care to patient and relatives

Monitor treatment every 2 weeks
Support patient and family

Reassess response at 6 weeks
(earlier if condition worsens)

If better :
Continue treatment
Review need to modify
precipitating and maintaining factors

If not better :
Review diagnosis
Review compliance
Review dosage

Continuation of drug therapy
for 6 months

If treatment inadequate :
Increase and review
once or twice weekly

If treatment adequate :
Consider another
antidepressant or
referral for specialist
advice

Fig. 8.1 Treatment of depressive illness.

When is hospital care needed?

In deciding the need for in-patient or day-patient care, consideration is given not only to severity and risk but also to the availability of social support. A patient living alone may need hospital care for a disorder that could be treated at home if there were a supportive family member who could be present day and night.

Should the patient remain at work?

When the disorder is mild, work can be a valuable distraction from depressive thoughts, and can provide companionship. When the disorder is more severe, retardation, poor concentration, and lack of drive are likely to impair perform-ance, and this failure may add to feelings of hopelessness. Sometimes, poor per-formance at work may endanger other people, and when the potential for such danger is great (as in the case of driving a heavy goods vehicle) the patient should not work even if the risk of failure is small.

Is antidepressant drug treatment required?

This treatment is indicated for most patients with a depressive disorder of at least moderate severity, and particularly those with 'biological' symptoms. A history of

Table 8.8.

Referral for specialist advice

- in all severe and some moderately severe cases, especially when there is a substantial risk of suicide or harm to the welfare or life of another person (particularly dependent children)
- when the diagnosis is in doubt
- when a patient has failed to respond to antidepressant treatment
- when day- or in-patient care is required
- when cognitive-behaviour treatment (CBT) may be required

previous response to medication and severe symptoms both suggest a likely good response to treatment.

Which drug is appropriate?

No single antidepressant is clearly more effective than another and selection for a particular patient depends the history of previous response to medication, side effects, any concurrent medical illnesses or medication, toxicity in overdose, and cost. Doctors should become familiar with the use of one or two drugs from each group. Tricyclic drugs are usually considered to be the first choice for severe depression, but with more serious illnesses the choice between a tricyclic and an SSRI depends consideration of their side effects, any contraindications (e.g. heart disease contraindicates tricyclics), and concern about safety and overdosage.

Tricyclic drugs are effective in all types of depression. Amitriptyline is an example of a more sedative drug, while imipramine is also well proven but less sedative. Lofepramine has somewhat fewer side effects and is safer in overdosage. Tricyclic drugs are contraindicated in patients with cardiovascular disease, glaucoma, or prostatic problems.

The **SSRIs** (fluoxetine, sertraline, paroxetine, etc.) are generally as effective as tricyclics but it is uncertain whether this extends to the most severe depressive disorder. They have different side effects and are generally well tolerated. They have an advantage in patients with a history of overdoses, those who are unable to tolerate the side effects of tricyclics, and those with medical illnesses for which tricyclics are contraindicated.

What information do the patient and family need?

It is essential to make sure that the drugs are taken in the full prescribed dose. A depressed patient's adherence to antidepressant treatment can be improved by informing the patient and the family about the medication, its potential side effects, the importance of continuing a full dosage for an adequate period of time, and the likelihood of success. It is important to explain that, although side effects will appear quickly, the therapeutic effect is likely to be delayed for two to three weeks. Patients should be warned about the effects of taking alcohol because of its sedative effects. They should be advised about driving, particularly that they should not drive while experiencing sedative or any other side effects that might impair their performance.

Continuing the treatment

During the initial weeks of treatment, patients should be seen and supported; those with severe disorders may need to be seen every two or three days; others usually weekly.

Suitable activity should be considered for every patient. Depressed patients give up activities and withdraw from other people. In this way, they become deprived of social stimulation and rewarding experiences, and their original feelings of depression increase. It is important to make sure that patients are occupied adequately, but also that they are not pushed into activities in which they may fail because of slowness or poor concentration. Hence, the range of activity appropriate for a depressed patient is narrow and changes as the illness runs its course. If the patient is treated at home, it is important to discuss with relatives how much the patient should do each day.

Relatives should be **helped to accept** the disorder as an illness, to avoid criticizing the patient, and to encourage appropriate activity.

Psychological treatment. All depressed patients require support, encouragement, and repeated explanation that they are suffering from illness not moral failure. When the depressive disorder appears to have been precipitated by life problems, discussion and problem-solving counselling may be required. However, when the depressive disorder is severe, discussion of problems may increase hopelessness. The more depressed the patient, the more the doctor and others should take over problems in the early days of treatment. When mood improves, the problems can be reconsidered.

Lack of response to treatment within 6 weeks

Around 30% of those with a depressive disorder do not respond within about six weeks to a combination of antidepressant drugs, graded activity, and psychological treatment. In these cases the *treatment plan should be reviewed* (Table 8.9).

- *Is the diagnosis correct?* The diagnosis should be reviewed carefully and a check made for stressful life events or continuing difficulties that may have been overlooked (Table 8.9).

- *Is the patient taking the full prescribed dose of medicine?* Check again that the patient has been taking the medication in the full amount. If not, the reasons should be sought. Some patients are convinced that no treatment can help, others are unable to tolerate drug side effects.

- *Should the dose be increased?* If the preceding enquiries reveal nothing, the dose of antidepressant may be increased if it is not already maximal.

- *Would it be sensible to change the medication?* If the patient cannot tolerate full dosage, or there has been no response to adequate dosage, an antidepressant drug from another group may be tried.

Table 8.9.

Lack of response to antidepressant treatment

- Review diagnosis
- Check compliance with present treatment
- Review psychological and social causes
- Increase dose to maximum
- Consider change to antidepressant of a different group*
- Obtain specialist opinion concerning need for hospital admission and further treatment*
- Combined drug treatment*
- Consider ECT*

*These steps usually require a specialist opinion (see text).

- *Supportive interviews* should be continued and the patient reassured that depressive disorders almost invariably eventually recover. Meanwhile, provided that the patient is not too depressed, any problems contributing to the depressed state should be discussed further. In resistant cases it is particularly important to *watch carefully for developing suicidal intentions.*
- *Is a specialist opinion required?* If serious depression persists, specialist advice should be obtained concerning the need for day care or admission to hospital, combined antidepressant drugs treatment or, in the most severe cases, ECT.

Combined treatment

Some patients who have failed to respond to one antidepressant drug, respond to a combination of drugs. Combined treatment is usually started by a psychiatrist although other doctors may be asked to continue it. Several combinations are used (see p. 351):

- Lithium may be added to a tricyclic or MAOI. The addition of lithium to a 5-HT uptake blocker may produce neurotoxic side effects in a few cases.
- MAOI added to a tricyclic drug: the reverse procedure of adding a tricyclic drug to MAOI should not be used because it is more likely to cause serious toxic effects. Specialist advice should be sought.

ECT

ECT has an important place in the treatment of a small number of patients with depressive disorders that do not respond to drugs. The decision will be made by a psychiatrist, who may recommend ECT when there is a need for rapid improvement; for example, depressed patients who refuse to drink enough to maintain an adequate output of urine or those with a high risk of suicide.

Preventing recurrence

- *Maintenance antidepressant therapy* is indicated for patients with histories of relapse or recurrence following successful treatment of depression.
- *Lithium prophylaxis.* If the patient has had manic as well as depressive disorders in the past, and if recurrences have been frequent, lithium prophylaxis should be considered, balancing advantages against risks (see p. 353).
- *Social and psychological measures.* If the depressive disorder was related to stressors such as overwork or complicated social relationships, the patient should be helped to change to his lifestyle in the hope that this will reduce recurrence.

Management of mania

Assessment

The assessment of a manic patient is difficult, and the help of a *specialist will usually be required*. In the assessment of mania, the steps are those already outlined for depressive disorders. They are: (1) decide the diagnosis; (2) assess the severity of the disorder; (3) form an opinion about the causes; (4) assess the patient's social resources; and (4) judge the effect on other people.

Recovery

As patients recover, they should be encouraged gradually to resume responsibility for their own affairs.

After recovery from a depressive disorder the patient should be followed up for several months either by the family doctor or by a psychiatrist. At this stage it is often valuable to discuss possible precipitants of the illness with the patient and also in joint interviews with close relatives. This discussion is particularly important when there have been repeated depressive disorders provoked by life events.

If recovery appears to have been brought about by an antidepressant drug, the latter should usually be continued at the full therapeutic dose for about six months.

Maintenance therapy Antidepressants should be continued for longer when there have been recurring depressive disorders and a careful watch should be kept for signs of relapse. With the patient's consent, relatives should be warned about the possibility of relapse and asked to report any signs of returning illness.

Diagnosis depends on a careful history and examination. Whenever possible, the history should be taken from relatives as well as from the patient because the patient seldom recognizes the full extent of the abnormal behaviour. Differential diagnosis has been discussed earlier in this chapter; it is important to remember that mildly disinhibited behaviour can result from intoxication with drugs or alcohol or, rarely, from frontal lobe lesion causes (e.g. by a cerebral neoplasm).

Severity is judged next. For this purpose it is essential to interview another informant. Manic patients are able to exert a degree of self-control during an interview with a doctor, and then behave in a more disinhibited and grandiose way immediately afterwards (see p. 132). At an early stage of the disorder it is easy to be misled by patients in this way and to miss the opportunity to persuade them to enter hospital before causing difficulties for themselves, for example, through ill-judged decisions at work or unaffordable extravagance.

Usually, the **causes** of a manic disorder are largely endogenous; some cases follow physical illness, treatment by drugs (especially steroids), or operations. It is important to identify any life events that may have provoked the onset and also to identify maintaining factors.

The patient's **resources** and the **effects of the illness** on other people should be assessed along the lines already described for depressive disorders. Even for the most supportive family, it is extremely difficult to care for a manic patient at home for more than a few days unless the disorder is exceptionally mild. The patient's responsibilities in the care of dependent children or at work should always be considered carefully.

Treatment

In most cases, the general practitioner will be involved in only the first stages of treatment since admission to hospital is nearly always advisable to protect patients from the consequences of their own behaviour. If the disorder is not too severe, patients usually agree to enter hospital after some persuasion. When the disorder is more severe, compulsory admission is likely to be needed.

The *immediate treatment* is with an antipsychotic drug. Haloperidol is a suitable choice, chlorpromazine a more sedating alternative. The first dose should be large enough to bring the abnormal behaviour under rapid control. At this stage it is important that the patient is not left under-treated, overactive, and irritable. In emergencies, the first dose may need to be given by intramuscular injection (see p. 226 for further advice about the use of antipsychotic drugs in urgent cases).

In hospital, the subsequent dosage should be adjusted frequently in relation to fluctuations in the condition. The doctor, psychiatrist, and nurses should reassess the patient's condition frequently until symptoms have been brought under control. During this early phase, it is important to avoid angry confrontations which often arise because the patient makes unreasonable demands that cannot be met. It is usually possible to avoid an argument by taking advantage of the manic patient's easy distractibility; instead of refusing demands, it is better to delay until the patient's attention turns to another topic.

When the patient is well enough to co-operate, tests of renal and thyroid function are carried out so that results are available if lithium treatment should be required later. Practices vary about the use of lithium. Some psychiatrists continue to use haloperidol or chlorpromazine throughout the manic episode, and reserve lithium for prophylactic treatment. Others start lithium as soon as the acute symptoms are under control, although taking precautions not to introduce it when the dose of haloperidol is high (because occasional serious interactions have been reported, see p. 342). The use of lithium rather than haloperidol at an early stage can have the advantage that the patient is more alert; it may also have the advantage of making a depressive disorder less likely to follow.

ECT is used occasionally for the uncommon manic patient who does not respond to drugs given in such high doses that intolerable side effects are produced. In such cases, ECT may be followed by a reduction in symptoms sufficient to allow treatment to continue with drugs.

Progress is judged not only by the mental state and general behaviour, but also by the pattern of sleep and by the regaining of any weight lost during the illness. As progress continues, antipsychotic drug treatment is reduced gradually. It is important, however, not to discontinue the drug too soon, otherwise relapse may occur.

A careful watch should be kept for the appearance of depressive symptoms because transient but profound depressive mood change and depressive ideas are common among manic patients. Also, the clinical picture may change rapidly from mania to a sustained depressive disorder. In either case, suicidal ideas may appear. A sustained change to a depressive syndrome may require antidepressant drug treatment, which should be used cautiously to avoid a return to mania.

Following recovery, regular follow-up is necessary to monitor mood (relapse into mania or the onset of depression). Patients should be helped to deal with or to come to terms with any precipitating causes of the episode, and with the consequences of any ill-judged actions during the acute illness.

The monitoring of prophylactic lithium includes review of mental stage, measurement of plasma lithium concentration, and tests of thyroid and renal function at regular intervals. These arrangements, which are started by specialists but may be continued by general practitioners, are summarized on p. 356.

Further reading

Checkley, S. (ed.) (1998). *The Management of Depression*. Blackwell, Oxford.
Includes chapters on both drug therapy and psychological treatment of depressive disorders.

Paykel, E. (ed.) (1992). *Handbook of Affective Disorders*. Churchill Livingstone, Edinburgh.
Comprehensive textbook including aetiology, classification, treatment and prognosis. Covers depressive disorders and bipolar affective disorders.

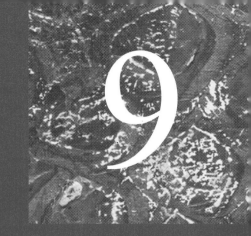

9

Schizophrenia and related disorders

- Epidemiology

- Aetiology

- Diagnosis and clinical features

- Treatment

- Assessment and management

- Delusional syndromes

- Appendix: ICD-10 criteria for schizophrenia

Schizophrenia and related disorders

Schizophrenia and related disorders are characterized by psychotic symptoms such as delusions and hallucinations. There is a spectrum of severity. In *schizophrenia*, the patient suffers from psychotic symptoms and functional impairment. In *delusional disorders*, the patient experiences delusions, but there is no evidence of hallucinations or any of the other symptoms characteristic of schizophrenia.

Schizophrenia is a particularly disabling illness because of its course which, although variable, is frequently chronic and relapsing. The care of patients with schizophrenia places a considerable burden on all carers, from the patient's family through to the health and social services. Schizophrenia makes up a good deal of the work of the specialist mental health services.

Although general practitioners may have only a few patients with chronic schizophrenia on their lists, the severity of their problems and the needs of their families will make these patients important.

This chapter aims to provide sufficient information for the reader to be able to recognize the basic symptoms of schizophirenia and related disorders and to be aware of the main approaches to treatment. The chapter focuses on schizophrenia.

Epidemiology

Incidence

The annual incidence of schizophrenia is between 0.1 and 0.2 per 1000 of the population. In men, schizophrenia usually begins between the ages of 15 and 35. In women, the mean age of onset of the disorder is later (Fig. 9.1). Although the incidence of schizophrenia is similar world-wide, it may be higher in certain ethnic groups (e.g. Afro-Caribbean immigrants in the UK).

Prevalence

The **point prevalence** of schizophrenia is about 4 per 1000 (much higher than the incidence because the disorder is chronic). The **lifetime risk** of developing schizophrenia is about 10 per 1000. The prevalence of schizophrenia is higher in socioeconomically deprived areas: in people who are homeless, the prevalence is 100 per 1000.

The general practitioner with an average list of 2000 may expect to have about 8 patients with schizophrenia. An inner city doctor, with a large homeless population, may have considerably more cases (50–100). Although the numbers are usually small, the needs of these patients for medical care are great.

Aetiology

The aetiology of schizophrenia is uncertain, although there is evidence for several risk factors (Table 9.1). There is strong evidence for genetic causes, and good

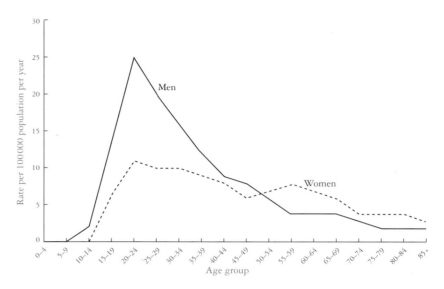

Fig. 9.1 Age- and sex-specific incidence rates for schizophrenia in men and women. Source: Information and statistics Division, NHS in Scotland, 1993.

Table 9.1.
Risk factors for schizophrenia

	Risk factors	Relative risk of developing schizophrenia
Predisposing		
Genetic	Monozygotic twin of a schizophrenic patient	40
	Dizygotic twin of a schizophrenic patient	15
	Child of a schizophrenic patient	10–15
	Sibling of a a schizophrenic patient	10–15
Environmental	Abnormalities of pregnancy and delivery	2
	Maternal influenza (2nd trimester)	2
	Fetal malnutrition	2
	Winter birth	1.1
Precipitating	Chronic cannabis consumption	2

reason to believe that stressful life events may provoke the disorder. Structural changes have been found in the brains of some schizophrenic patients, particularly in the temporal lobes, but it is not yet certain how they are caused. These and some other aetiological factors will be discussed briefly; a longer account can be found in *The Oxford Textbook of Psychiatry*.

Genetic factors

There is strong evidence for the heritability of schizophrenia from three sources:

(1) **Family studies** have shown that schizophrenia is more common in the relatives of schizophrenic patients that in the general population (where the lifetime risk is approximately 1%). The risk is 10–15% in the siblings of schizophrenics; among the children of one schizophrenic parent, 10–15%; and among the children of two schizophrenic parents, about 40%.

(2) **Twin studies** indicate that a major part of this familial loading is likely to be due to genetic rather than to environmental factors. Among monozygotic twins, the concordance rate (the frequency of schizophrenia in the sibling of the affected twin) is consistently higher (about 40%) than among dizygotic twins (about 10–15%).

(3) **Adoption studies** confirm the importance of genetic factors: among children who have been separated from a schizophrenic parent at birth and brought up by non-schizophrenic adoptive parents, the likelihood of developing schizophrenia is no less than that among children brought up by their own schizophrenic parent.

Although twin studies point to genetic factors, they also indicate that environmental factors are important because, even among identical twins, half the siblings do not develop schizophrenia (see below).

Specific genes and the mode of inheritance

No specific genes have been yet been identified for schizophrenia. It remains unknown whether schizophrenia is:

• monogenic (i.e. caused by a single gene);

• polygenic (i.e. caused by the cumulative effect of several genes); or

• heterogeneous (i.e. schizophrenia could be not one disorder but several, each caused by a different gene or genes).

With advances in molecular genetics, it is hoped that the gene(s) for schizophrenia will be identified in the next decade.

Environmental factors

These can predispose to the development of schizophrenia, precipitate the onset, provoke relapse after initial recovery, and maintain the disorder in persisting cases.

Predisposing factors Some factors putatively implicated in the development of schizophrenia are summarized in Table 9.1. The role of most of the environmental factors remains controversial. Abnormalities of pregnancy and labour associated with increased risk of schizophrenia include premature rupure of membranes, low birth weight, and birth events which are linked to infection and hypoxia. There is also an association with low **social class** and this is probably both cause and effect: social deprivation increases exposure to several risk factors and it is likely that people who develop schizophrenia tend to become increasingly socially deprived.

Precipitating factors of schizophrenia include stressful life events occurring shortly before the onset of the disorder.

Maintaining factors include strongly expressed feelings, especially in the form of critical comments, among family members ('high emotional expression'). High expressed emotion may lead to increased relapse rates and can be modified by family therapy.

Finally, it has been suggested that inconsistent forms of **child rearing** predispose to schizophrenia, but such ideas are not supported by evidence. Such speculations have caused unjustified guilt in some parents.

Pathophysiology

The response of some schizophrenic symptoms to antipsychotic drugs suggests that they may have a biochemical basis. The potency of the antipsychotic drugs depends on their ability to block dopaminergic neurotransmission. A schizophrenia-like disorder can be induced by amphetamine, a drug that increases dopamine functions. It is therefore possible that the pathophysiology of schizophrenia involves a disorder of dopaminergic function. However, there is currently little direct evidence that abnormal dopaminergic transmission is the cause of schizophrenia. In any case, the effect of antipsychotic drugs is not specific to schizophrenia; they reduce hallucinations and delusions in delirium, dementia, and severe depressive disorder.

Schizophrenia as a disorder of brain development

It is currently thought that schizophrenia is a *neurodevelopmental disorder* caused by one or more genes—possibly interacting with environmental factors. This idea is based on several pieces of evidence:

1. Evidence of brain abnormalities, particularly in the temporal lobes, has been consistently found in studies performing computerized tomography (CT) and magnetic resonance imaging (MRI) scans of patients with schizophrenia. These abnormalities do not appear to progress during the course of the disorder.

2. Patients with schizophrenia are more likely to have dermatoglyphic abnormalities (sometimes associated with central nervous system developmental disorder) and separate 'soft' neurological signs than controls.

3. Post-mortem studies have not found gliosis in the brains of schizophrenic patients. This means that it is likely that the brain abnormalities occurred early in life.

4. Subjects who subsequently develop schizophrenia are more likely than controls to have developmental problems during childhood.

Taken together, this evidence suggest a pathological process which takes place early in life and results in abnormal neurodevelopment that is sometimes observable during childhood. This theory does not explain why the age of onset of schizophrenia is usually so much later or why the illness is often episodic.

Diagnosis and clinical features

Clinical features of schizophrenia

The clinical presentations and the outcome are varied and schizophrenia can be a confusing illness to gain understanding of. It is best to start by considering simplified descriptions of two common presentations: (1) the acute syndrome; and (2) the chronic syndrome. It is then easier to understand the core features as well as the diversity of schizophrenia.

The acute syndrome (positive symptoms) (Table 9.2)

The main clinical features of the acute syndrome can be illustrated by a short *case study* (p. 164) of a patient, which illustrates the following common features of acute schizophrenia.

Common features

- Hallucinations
- Persecutory ideas
- Social withdrawal
- Impaired performance at work
- The false idea of being referred to (a delusion of reference, see p. 12).

The term **positive syndrome** is sometimes used to refer to these features. It refers to the appearance of hallucinations and delusions in contrast to the loss of function in the chronic syndrome—the negative syndrome.

Table 9.2.

The acute syndrome (positive symptoms)

Appearance and behaviour	– preoccupied, withdrawn, inactive
	– restless, noisy, inconsistent
Mood	– mood change
	– blunting
	– incongruity
Disorders of thinking	– vagueness
	– formal thought disorder
	– disorders of the stream of thought
Hallucinations	– auditory
	– visual
	– tactile, olfactory, gustatory
Delusions	– primary
	– secondary (especially persecutory)
Orientation	– normal
Attention	– impaired
Memory	– normal
Insight	– impaired

> ## *Case study: acute schizophrenia*
>
> A previously healthy 20-year-old male student had been behaving in an increasingly odd way. At times he appeared angry and told his friends that he was being followed by the police and secret services; at other times he was seen to be laughing to himself for no apparent reason. For several months he had spent more time on his own, apparently preoccupied with his own thoughts, and his academic work had deteriorated. When seen by the family doctor he was restless and appeared frightened. He said that he had heard voices commenting on his actions and abusing him. He also said that the police had conspired with his university teachers to harm his brain with poisonous gases and take away his thoughts, and that the police had arranged for items referring to him to be inserted into television programmes.

Appearance and behaviour Many patients with acute schizophrenia appear entirely normal. Some appear awkward in their social behaviour, preoccupied and withdrawn, or otherwise odd. Others smile or laugh without obvious reason, or appear perplexed by what is happening to them. Some are restless and noisy, and a few show sudden and unexpected changes in behaviour. Others retire from company, spending much time alone in their rooms, perhaps lying immobile on the bed apparently deep in thought.

Mood Abnormalities of mood are common. There are three main kinds:

1. *Mood change* such as depression, anxiety, irritability, or euphoria. Depressive symptoms in the acute syndrome may develop in one or more of three ways:
   - as an integral part of the disorder—caused by the same processes that cause the other symptoms such as the delusions and hallucinations;
   - as a response to insight into the nature of the illness and the problems to be faced;
   - as side effects of antipsychotic medication.

2. A reduction in the normal variations of mood, which is called *blunting* (or flattening) of affect. A patient with this disorder may seem indifferent to others because of unchanging mood.

3. Emotion not in keeping with the situation, a condition known as *incongruity* of affect. A patient may, for example, laugh when told about the death of his mother.

Speech and form of thought Speech may be difficult to follow. In the early stages, a patient's talk may be vague so that it is difficult to grasp the meaning. Later there may be more definite abnormalities (*formal thought disorder*). These abnormalities are of several kinds. Some patients have difficulty in dealing with abstract ideas (a phenomenon called *concrete thinking*) while others become preoccupied with vague pseudoscientific or mystical ideas. There is a lack of connection between the ideas expressed by the patient (*loosening of associations*). The links between ideas may be illogical, or they may wander from the original theme. In its most extreme form, loosening of association leads to totally incoherent thought and speech (*word salad*).

There may be **disorders of the stream of thought**, such as pressure of thought, poverty of thought, and thought blocking (all of which are described on p. 9).

Perception **Auditory hallucinations** are among the most frequent symptoms of schizophrenia. They may be experienced as simple noises or complex sounds of voices or music. Voices may utter single words, brief phrases, or whole conversations. The voices may seem to give commands to the patient. A voice may speak the patient's thoughts aloud, either as he thinks them or immediately afterwards. Sometimes, two or more voices may seem to discuss the patient in the third person. Other voices may comment on his actions. As explained later, these last three symptoms have particular diagnostic value (see p. 168).

In schizophrenia, **visual hallucinations** are less frequent than auditory, and seldom occur without other kinds of hallucination. A few patients experience **tactile**, **olfactory**, **gustatory**, and **somatic** hallucinations, which are often interpreted in a delusional way; for example, hallucinatory sensations in the lower abdomen may be attributed to unwanted sexual interference by a persecutor.

Abnormalities of the content of thought **Delusions** occur commonly in schizophrenia. *Primary delusions* (see p. 11) occur occasionally and when present are important because they occur seldom in other disorders and are therefore of value in diagnosis. Most delusions are *secondary*, that is, they arise from a previous mental change. Delusions may be preceded by so-called *delusional mood* (see p. 11), which is seldom found in conditions other than schizophrenia, or by hallucinations. Several kinds of delusion occur. *Persecutory delusions* are common, but not specific to schizophrenia. Less common but of greater diagnostic value are: *delusions of reference* (false beliefs that objects, events, or people have a special personal significance, see p. 12); *delusions of control* (the feeling of being controlled by an outside agency, see p. 13); and *delusions about the possession of thought* (the idea that thoughts are being inserted into or withdrawn from the person's mind, or 'broadcast' to other people, see pp. 13–14).

Cognitive function In acute schizophrenia **orientation** is normal. **Attention** and **concentration** are commonly impaired, and there may be consequent apparent difficulties in remembering, although **memory** itself is not impaired. Delusional memory (i.e. delusional meaning given to past events), occurs in a few patients.

Insight **Insight** is usually impaired. Most patients do not accept that their experiences result from illness, often ascribing them instead to the malevolent actions of other people. This lack of insight is often accompanied by unwillingness to accept treatment.

The combination of disturbed behaviour, hallucinations, and delusions is often referred to as **positive symptoms**. Schizophrenic patients do not necessarily experience all these symptoms. The clinical picture is variable, as explained later in this chapter (see p. 167).

The chronic syndrome (negative symptoms) (Table 9.3)

In contrast to the 'positive' symptoms of the acute syndrome, the **chronic syndrome** is characterized by 'negative' symptoms of:

- Underactivity
- Lack of drive

Table 9.3.

The chronic syndrome (negative symptoms)

Lack of drive and activity	
Social withdrawal	
Abnormalities of behaviour	
Abnormalities of movement	— stupor and excitement
	— abnormal movements
	— abnormal tonus
Speech	— reduced in amount
	— evidence of thought disorder
Mood disorder	— blunting
	— incongruity
	— depression
Hallucinations	— especially auditory
Delusions	— systematized
	— encapsulated
Orientation	— age disorientation
Attention	— Normal
Memory	— Normal
Insight	— Variable

- Social withdrawal
- Emotional apathy
- Thought disorder.

The syndrome can be illustrated by a brief *case study* of a typical patient. This description illustrates several of the features of what is sometimes called a 'schizophrenic defect state'.

Case study: the chronic syndrome

A middle-aged man lives in a group home for psychiatric patients and attends a sheltered workshop. In both places he withdraws from company. He is usually dishevelled and unshaven, and cares for himself only when encouraged to do so by others. His social behaviour is odd and awkward. His speech is slow, and its content vague and incoherent. When questioned, he says that he is the victim of persecution by extraterrestrial beings who beam rays at him. He seldom mentions these ideas spontaneously and he shows few signs of emotion about them or about any other aspects of his life. For several years this clinical picture has changed little except for brief periods of acute symptoms which are usually related to upsets in the ordered life of the group home.

Impairment of volition The most striking feature is diminished **volition**, that, is a lack of drive and initiative. Left to himself, the patient may be inactive for long periods, or may engage in aimless and repeated activity.

Impairment of daily living skills Social behaviour often deteriorates. Patients neglect personal hygiene and their appearance. They may withdraw from social encounters. Some behave in ways that break social conventions, for example talking intimately to strangers, shouting obscenities in public, or behaving in a sexually uninhibited manner. Some patients hoard objects, so that their surroundings become cluttered and dirty.

Movement disorders A variety of disturbances of movement occur which are often called **catatonic**. They will be described only briefly here (they are detailed in *The Oxford Textbook of Psychiatry*). **Stupor** and **excitement** are the most striking catatonic symptoms. A patient in stupor is immobile, mute, and unresponsive, although fully conscious. Stupor may change (sometimes quickly) to a state of uncontrolled motor activity and excitement.

Patients with chronic schizophrenia sometimes make repeated odd and awkward movements. Repeated movements that do not appear to be goal-directed are called **stereotypies**; repeated movements of this kind that do appear to be goal-directed are called **mannerisms**. Occasionally, patients have a disorder of muscle tone which can be detected by placing the patient in an awkward posture; when the sign is present, the patient maintains this posture without apparent distress for much longer than a healthy person could without severe discomfort (*waxy flexibility*). When catatonic symptoms are prominent the illness is referred to as *catatonic schizophrenia*.

Speech and form of thought **Speech** is often abnormal, reflecting **thought disorder** of the same kinds as those found in the acute syndrome (see above).

Affect and perception **Affect** is generally blunted; and when emotion is shown, it may be incongruous. **Hallucinations** are common, and any of the forms occurring in the acute syndrome may occur in the chronic syndrome.

Thought content In chronic schizophrenia **delusions** are common and often systematized. They may be held with little emotion. For example, patients may be convinced that they are being persecuted but show neither fear nor anger. Delusions may also be 'encapsulated' from the rest of the patient's beliefs. Thus, a patient may be convinced that his private sexual fantasies and practices are widely discussed by strangers; but his remaining beliefs are not influenced by this conviction, nor is his work or social life affected.

Cognitive function **Orientation** is normal. **Attention** and **concentration** are often impaired. **Memory** is not generally abnormal except that some patients have difficulty in giving their age correctly.

Insight **Insight** is often impaired; the patient does not recognize that his symptoms are due to illness and is seldom fully convinced of the need for treatment.

Factors modifying the clinical features

In schizophrenia several factors can interact with the disease process to modify the clinical picture.

Age of onset The symptoms of adolescents and young adults often include thought disorder, mood disturbance, and disrupted behaviour. With increasing age, paranoid symptomatology is more common, and disrupted behaviour is less frequent.

Sex The course of the illness is generally more severe in males.

Social background may affect the content of delusions and hallucinations. For example, delusions with a religious content are more common among patients from a religious background. Recent technological innovations are often used to explain symptoms. For example, a patient thought that his auditory hallucinations were due to nanotechnology.

The amount of **social stimulation** has a considerable effect on the type of symptoms. *Understimulation* increases 'negative' symptoms such as poverty of speech, social withdrawal, apathy, and lack of drive, and also catatonic symptoms. *Overstimulation* induces 'positive' symptoms such as hallucinations, delusions, and restlessness. Modern treatment is designed to avoid understimulation; as a result 'negative' features including catatonia are less frequent than in the past. This policy can, however, result in a degree of overstimulation leading to more positive symptoms.

High emotional expression by people with whom the patient is living is one form of social stimulation that increases symptoms. Overt expressions of criticism seem to be particularly important. The more time the patient spends in the company of highly critical people, the more likely he is to relapse. This is a reason why some patients are less disturbed when living in a hostel than with their family.

Diagnosis

The diagnosis of schizophrenia is based entirely on the clinical presentation (history and examination). The only diagnostic tests used are those needed to exclude other disorders when there is clinical suspicion. Because the diagnosis is based on clinical findings, it is made more reliable when **diagnostic criteria** are used to specify patterns of symptoms which must be present to make the diagnosis. The currently most widely used diagnostic criteria are those in the International Classification of Diseases (ICD-10) (see Appendix) and the Diagnostic and Statistical Manual of the American Psychiatric Association (DSM-IV). Currrent diagnostic criteria for schizophrenia include:

1. Individual symptoms that have been found to be highly specific for schizophrenia and therefore have a high **positive predictive value**. These are called **Schneider's 'first rank' symptoms** after the clinician who first described them (Table 9.4 and described more fully in Chapter 1). They occur in about 70% of patients who meet the full diagnostic criteria for schizophrenia.

2. Symptoms that are more frequent but less discriminating than first rank symptoms (e.g. prominent hallucinations, loosening of association, and flat or inappropriate affect).

3. Impaired social and occupational functioning.

4. A minimum duration (6 months in DSM-IV but, unfortunately, a different period—1 month—in ICD-10).

Table 9.4.

Schneider's 'first rank' symptoms of schizophrenia*

- Hearing thoughts spoken aloud
- 'Third person' hallucinations
- Hallucinations in the form of a commentary
- Somatic hallucinations
- Thought withdrawal or insertion
- Thought broadcasting
- Delusional perception
- Feelings or actions experienced as made or influenced by external agents

* The terms used in this list are explained in Chapter 1.

5. The exclusion of: (a) organic mental disorder; (b) major depression; (c) mania, or; (d) the prolongation of autistic disorder (which is a mental disorder of childhood—see p. 416).

Classification of psychotic disorders which do not meet the diagnostic criteria for schizophrenia

Both ICD-10 and DSM-IV provide categories for disorders that resemble schizophrenia but fail to meet the diagnostic criteria for schizophrenia in one of the following three ways:

1. **Duration too short** Cases lasting for less than 1 month are called **acute psychotic disorders** in both classifications. DSM-IV has an extra category for cases lasting less than the 6 months required in this classification for the diagnosis of schizophrenia. These cases are called **schizophreniform**. (Since ICD-10 requires a duration of only 1 month, it does not require this extra category.)

2. **Prominent affective symptoms** These cases are called **schizoaffective** in both classifications (see p. 170).

3. **Delusions without other symptoms of schizophrenia** These are called **delusional disorders** (in ICD-10 the term is persistent delusional disorder). Delusional disorder is described later in the chapter.

Differential diagnosis

Schizophrenia needs to be distinguished from four other types of disorder.

1. Organic syndromes In **younger patients** the most relevant organic diagnoses are:

- *drug-induced states* especially that induced by *amphetamines* (see pp. 285–6);
- *temporal lobe epilepsy* should be considered when the condition is brief and there is evidence of clouding of consciousness. (In a few patients, chronic temporal lobe epilepsy gives rise to a persistent state resembling schizophrenia more closely.)

In **older patients**, the organic brain diseases which should be excluded include:

- *Delirium* can be mistaken for an acute episode of schizophrenia, especially when there are prominent hallucinations and delusions; the cardinal feature of this disorder is clouding of consciousness (see pp. 187–8).

- *Dementia* can resemble schizophrenia, particularly when there are prominent persecutory delusions; the finding of memory disorder suggests dementia.

- Some other *diffuse brain diseases* can present a schizophrenia-like picture without any neurological signs or gross memory impairment; for example, *general paralysis of the insane*, a form of neurosyphilis.

To exclude organic disorders, history taking and mental state examination should focus on cognitive impairment (including disorientation and memory deficit) which is characteristic of organic disorder but not of schizophrenia; and a thorough physical examination should be carried out including a neurological examination.

2. Affective disorder The distinction between **affective disorder** and schizophrenia depends on:

(1) the degree and persistence of mood disorder (greater in affective disorder);

(2) the congruence of any hallucinations or delusions to the prevailing mood (close in affective disorder);

(3) the nature of the symptoms in any previous episodes (if previously affective, then current affective disorder is more likely).

Sometimes, affective and schizophrenic symptoms are so equally balanced that it is not possible to decide whether the primary disorder is affective or schizophrenic. As explained above these cases are diagnosed as **schizoaffective** disorder (see below).

3. Personality disorders Differential diagnosis from **personality disorder** may be difficult, especially when there have been insidious changes of behaviour in a young person who does not describe hallucinations or delusions. As well as interviewing relatives it may be necessary to make prolonged observations for first rank and other features of schizophrenia before a definite diagnosis can be reached.

4. Schizoaffective disorder Some patients have at the same time definite schizophrenic symptoms and definitive affective (depressive or manic) symptoms of equal prominence. These disorders are classified separately because it is uncertain whether they are a subtype of schizophrenia, or of affective disorder. Schizoaffective disorders usually require both antipsychotic and antidepressant drug treatment. When they recover, affective and schizophrenic symptoms improve together, and most patients lose all their symptoms although many have further episodes. Some of these subsequent episodes are schizoaffective, but others have a more typical schizophrenic or a more typical affective form.

Course and prognosis

The *course* of schizophrenia is variable:

- Acute illness with complete recovery   20%
- Recurrent acute illness   20%
- Chronic illness starting acutely   20%
- Chronic illness starting insidiously   20%
- Suicide   10–15%

Patients with recurrent acute episodes often do not recover to the previous level after each relapse and so gradually deteriorate. The risk of *suicide* is high among young patients in the early stage of the disorder when insight is still present into the likely effect of the illness on the patient's hopes and plans.

The best *outcome* is in disorders of acute onset following stress. Other predictors of outcome, some related to the illness, some to the ill person, are listed in Table 9.5. Although of some value, these predictors cannot be used to make a definite prediction for an individual patient. For this reason, advice to patients and relatives should be given cautiously, especially at the first episode of illness. The factors listed in Table 9.5 are those operating before or at the onset of schizophrenia. Factors acting after the onset are discussed next.

Life events

As noted above, stressful life events can precipitate relapses, and patients exposed to many life events generally have a less favourable course. In general, as explained

Table 9.5.

Factors predicting poor outcome in schizophrenia

Features of the illness
Insidious onset
Long first episode
Previous psychiatric history
Negative symptoms
Younger age at onset

Features of the patient
Male
Single, separated, widowed, divorced
Poor psychosexual adjustment
Abnormal previous personality
Poor employment record
Social isolation
Poor compliance

above, an overstimulating environment increases positive symptoms, while an understimulating one increases negative symptoms. Prognosis depends in part on how far a balance can be achieved between these extremes.

Family life

In general, after discharge from hospital, schizophrenics returning to their families have a worse prognosis than those entering hostels. As explained above, relapse is especially likely in families where relatives make many critical comments, express hostility, and show signs of emotional over-involvement. In such families the risk of relapse is greater if patients spend much time in contact with their close relatives (35 hours a week has been suggested as a cut-off point). Reducing this contact by arranging day care appears to improve prognosis and so may family therapy.

Cultural background

There is some evidence that the outcome of schizophrenia is more benign in less developed countries, in which fewer demands are made on schizophrenics and there is greater family support, as part of a traditional rural way of life.

Treatment

In this section, we describe the specific interventions which have been shown to be effective in the management of schizophrenia. Management of specific situations is dealt with in the next section. Specific treatments are needed for:

1. The acute psychotic symptoms

2. Drug-resistant symptoms

3. Prevention of relapse

4. Associated depressive symptoms

5. Psychosocial care and rehabilitation

1. Treatment of acute psychotic symptoms

Antipsychotic drug therapy

The most effective treatment for acute psychotic symptoms is antipsychotic drug therapy (see p. 340–4). Antipsychotic drugs have an immediate sedative effect, followed by an effect on psychotic symptoms (especially hallucinations and delusions) which may take up to three weeks to develop fully.

There are many antipsychotic drugs which differ more in side-effect profiles than in effectiveness. Equivalent doses of these drugs are shown in Table 9.6. These equivalents should only be used as a rough guide, and the manufacturer's instructions should be followed.

Antipsychotic drugs should be started at a low dose and increased gradually. For an acutely ill patient effective treatment usually begins at a dose of chlorpromazine 100 mg three times a day or an equivalent dose of another drug: depending on side effects, the dose can be increased if there is no response, but not above 900 mg of chlorpromazine a day. Prescribers should follow the manufacturer's literature or a work of reference.

Table 9.6.

Commonly used antipsychotic drugs with normal daily dose range

Conventional		'Atypical'	
Haloperidol	(2–30 mg)	Risperidone	(4–16 mg)
Chlorpromazine	(100–600 mg)	Olanzapine	(5–20 mg)
Trifluoperazine	(5–30 mg)	Sertindole	(12–20 mg)
Sulpiride	(400–800 mg)	Clozapine	(100–900 mg)*

* Sometimes effective in schizophrenia resistant to other antipsychotics.

Extrapyramidal side effects occur frequently when antipsychotic drugs are prescribed in full doses. *Anticholinergic medication* can be used to prevent the development of extrapyramidal symptoms including acute dystonic reactions, akathisia, or parkinsonism. However, the aim of treatment should be to adjust the dose of the antipsychotic to avoid the side effects.

Electroconvulsive therapy (ECT)

ECT is not used regularly in the treatment of schizophrenia but there are two important indications:

(1) when there are severe depressive symptoms accompanying schizophrenia; and

(2) in the rare cases of catatonic stupor.

ECT is often rapidly effective in both these conditions. ECT may be effective also in acute episodes of schizophrenia, even without severe depression or stupor, but it is seldom used because drug treatment is simpler and equally beneficial. The main exception is a post-partum psychosis, when a rapid response is particularly important (see p. 235).

2. Drug-resistant symptoms

In about 70% of acute episodes symptoms respond to antipsychotic drug treatment. Drug-resistant symptoms can be treated in two ways:

1. *Alternative drug therapy*. Clozapine has been shown to be effective in some patients where symptoms are resistant to treatment with conventional antipsychotics (see p. 340).

2. *Psychological treatments*. There is some evidence suggesting that cognitive therapy may reduce preoccupation with drug-resistant hallucinations and delusions.

3. Prevention of relapse

Two kinds of intervention are effective in reducing relapse: **drug therapy** and **family therapy**.

Drug therapy

Continuation therapy reduces the risk of relapse. Since compliance with medication is often poor and intramuscular depot injections are often used instead of oral medication. There are two main problems. First, 20% of patients remain well without drugs and long-term conventional antipsychotic medication leads to persistent tardive dyskinesia in 15% of subjects after four years of treatment. Therefore, if all patients receive continuation treatment, some will be exposed unnecessarily to the risk of developing side effects. Unfortunately, it is not possible to predict which patients will benefit from continuing drug treatment. The clinician and patient therefore need to work together to judge the benefit of continuation treatment by reducing the drugs cautiously when the patient has been free from symptoms for several months. Patients taking long-term continuation therapy should be assessed every six months for signs of tardive dyskinesia (see pp. 342–3).

Although anticholinergic drugs reduce parkinsonian side effects, they may increase the likelihood of dyskinesia. They should not be prescribed routinely but only if there are extrapyramidal side effects that cannot be avoided by adjusting the dose of antipsychotic drug.

Family therapy

Family psychoeducation aimed to reduce emotional involvement and criticism has been shown to reduce the rate of relapse in schizophrenic patients living with their families (see p. 171).

4. Treatment of associated depressive symptoms

Depressive symptoms in schizophrenia have several causes (see p. 164).

Antidepressants

When depressive symptoms are severe, antidepressant medication can be given, although it is probably less effective in this situation than in depressive disorder. Antidepressants are also indicated in schizoaffective disorder.

Lithium

Lithium is beneficial for schizoaffective disorders, especially when there is a mixture of schizophrenic and manic symptoms (see pp. 353–7).

4. Psychosocial care and rehabilitation

The main aim of psychosocial care and rehabilitation is to reduce the long-term disability experienced by many patients with schizophrenia. In practice, psychosocial care is usually tailored to the individual patient needs. Skill is required to arrange a care plan which is optimally stimulating but not too stressful. The approach is a general one including supportive care from community nurses and others. Specific methods that may be included in this programme are:

Social skills training

Social skills training use a behavioural approach to help patients to improve interpersonal, self-care, and coping skills needed in normal life.

Employment training

This includes a range of activities from help in developing the skills necessary to obtain and hold down a job, to the provision of sheltered employment or other occupational activities.

Assessment and management

Unlike most patients with depressive disorders, who are treated in primary care, the majority of schizophrenic patients are treated mainly by the specialist psychiatric services. However, the first evidence of schizophrenia is usually detected by general practitioners and assessment and referral should be made as soon as possible. There is evidence that a delay in starting treatment is associated with poorer outcome.

Assessment of non-urgent cases

Sometimes the patient asks for help with the symptoms of schizophrenia but more often relatives or other people draw attention to problem behaviours that could be caused by schizophrenia. For example, a general practitioner may be asked to help a young person who is becoming increasingly withdrawn and showing odd behaviour, or an elderly woman who is reclusive and suspicious. In these situations, family doctors are in a good position to make an initial assessment because they will often know the family and the patient's background. The doctor should try to:

- Obtain a good description of the patient's symptoms and behaviour. When possible this should be supplemented by information from an informant.

- Assess the patient's level of functional impairment. For example, is the patient still working?

- Make an assessment of the degree of risk the patient poses to himself and others (pp. 244–7).

- Clearly inform the patient of the results of the assessment and try to persuade the patient to accept referral to the specialist mental health services.

- When the patient will not accept referral, the presentation should be discussed with a psychiatrist. Treatment can then sometimes be commenced, although it is advisable to maintain contact with a psychiatrist in case the situation deteriorates.

Assessment and management of acutely disturbed patients

Sometimes the family doctor's first encounter with a schizophrenic patient is during an episode of disturbed behaviour. This may occur when the patient is in the early stages of the disorder, or during a relapse of the established condition. If the patient has been or seems likely to become aggressive, special care should be taken. It is unwise to be alone with such a patient until an assessment of dangerousness has been made. On the other hand, the doctor is sometimes called to see a patient who is being restrained by several people. An attempt should then be made to calm the patient and, if possible, remove the physical restraint while ensuring that helpers remain close at hand during the assessment.

Table 9.7.

Assessment and management of acutely disturbed patients

1. Make a provisional diagnosis
   - acute organic disorder
   - alcohol or drug intoxication or withdrawal
   - personality disorder
   - schizophrenia
   - mania
2. Appropriate examination and blood and urine specimen (if patient permits)
3. Antipsychotic drug treatment if needed
4. Decide the need for admission to hospital (may require Mental Health Act powers)

Since not all overactive, aggressive, or otherwise disturbed behaviour is due to schizophrenia the doctor's first task when confronted with this problem is to **make a provisional diagnosis**. The main task is to exclude any acute organic disorder or non-psychotic disorder (such as personality disorder). At this stage the diagnosis between *schizophrenia* and *mania* may be difficult to make but the distinction does not affect the immediate management (Table 9.7).

If the cause of the behaviour disturbance appears to be a psychotic disorder, it is usually appropriate to call for a psychiatric opinion immediately in order to admit the patient to hospital. If the patient refuses and his (or other people's) health or safety appears to be at risk, compulsory powers for admission to hospital may be required (see pp. 451–4). Less severe disturbance may be managed at home if there is sufficient social support or if intensive community nursing is available.

Hospital management of an acute episode of schizophrenia

Following admission to hospital, acute behavioural disturbance sometimes subsides with the change of environment. When this happens and if the diagnosis is uncertain it may be desirable to arrange a few days without further drug treatment to allow the diagnosis to be clarified (Table 9.8).

When the diagnosis is sufficiently clear, antipsychotic medication is started. The antipsychotic effect may take two to three weeks to begin, but antipsychotics also have a calming effect which may reduce the need for a separate sedative.

If the patient is very excited or abnormally aggressive, drug treatment may be needed for immediate behavioural control. A sedative drug such as lorazepam (see pp. 337–8) is usually used for behavioural control. It is best to avoid administering large doses of antipsychotic drugs simply for behavioural control, as side effects may be unpleasant and discourage patients from continuing, even with smaller maintenance doses.

Table 9.8.

Hospital management of an acute episode of schizophrenia

Antipsychotic medication

Appropriate activities

Counselling for patient and family

Good response and good prognosis
- continue medication for 6 months gradual return to work and social activities
- regular review and counselling

Incomplete response and or poor prognosis
- long-term medication (consider depot)
- counselling and support for family (reduce 'expressed emotion')
- assess needs for sheltered work or housing

Choice of antipsychotic drug (see also pp. 340–4)

There are many antipsychotic drugs (see Table 9.6) which are divided into two groups: the *conventional* and '*atypical*' antipsychotics. The conventional antipsychotics include chlorpromazine and haloperidol. They have been available for many years and are effective but cause troublesome extrapyramidal side effects (EPS). The second group, the 'atypical' antipsychotics, cause fewer EPS. The atypicals include risperidone, olanzapine, and clozapine. Clozapine is currently the only drug which has been shown to be effective in illnesses which do not respond to adequate courses of conventional antipsychotics. The main problem with clozapine is that it causes agranulocytosis in <1% of cases which, rarely, may be fatal. The main side effects of antipsychotics are shown in Table 9.9.

The usual initial choice of drug is a conventional antipsychotic. Within this group the drugs have different side-effect profiles and these usually determine which drug is used. For example, chlorpromazine is suitable when sedation is desirable, and trifluoperazine is appropriate when sedation is not required. If the patient cannot tolerate a conventional antipsychotic drug, an 'atypical' drug should be used. If the patient fails to respond to at least two trials of adequate doses of first-line antipsychotic given for an adequate duration, clozapine should be considered.

The effects of antipsychotics

Following commencement of an antipsychotic, symptoms of excitement, irritability, and insomnia usually improve within a few days. Hallucinations and delusions may take longer to improve, often changing gradually over several weeks. If there is no improvement, a check should be made that the patient is taking the prescribed drugs. If not, the reason should be determined and an attempt made to ensure compliance. If the patient is taking the prescribed dose, this should be increased cautiously unless it is already at the top of the recommended range.

Table 9.9.

Side effects of antipsychotic drugs

Conventional antipsychotics
Sedation 70–80%
Anticholinergic and antiadrenergic effects (including dry mouth, constipation, blurred vision, urinary retention, tachycardia) 10–50%
Extrapyramidal side effects (parkinsonism, dystonia, akathisia, neuroleptic malignant syndrome) 60%
Tardive dyskinesia: 4% per year of antipsychotic medication
Endocrine effects: galactorrhoea and oligomenorrhoea
Weight gain
Sexual dysfunction
Allergy

'Atypical' antipsychotic (clozapine)
Sedation
Weight gain
Hypersalivation
Tachycardia
Orthostatic hypotension
Seizures 3%
Agranulocytosis <1%

Other 'atypical' antipsychotics (e.g. risperidone, olanzapine)
Sedation
Orthostatic hypotension
Sexual dysfunction
Weight gain

Other aspects of hospital treatment

Appropriate activities should be arranged. The patient should not be left unoccupied to become absorbed in his symptoms, nor overstimulated since this prolongs the acute symptoms. Nurses and occupational therapists should work together to arrange a suitable programme.

As well as drug treatment, psychological support and education about the illness and treatment are needed to help the patient accept the limitations imposed by the effects of the illness on his day-to-day life, and on his hopes for the future. With the patient's permission, similar counselling should be offered to the family.

Preventing relapse in patients who recover fully from an acute episode

If the symptoms are well controlled on discharge from hospital, the dual aims of management are to continue to control symptoms with antipsychotic drugs, while making arrangements for daily living that protect the patient from too many stressors, and enable him to return as far as possible to his previous life. Even if the patient is free from symptoms, it is usual to continue antipsychotic medication for six or more months, at a rather lower dose than that required to bring acute symptoms under control. For patients living with their families, family therapy aimed at reducing the number of critical comments, and improving the family's knowledge of the disorder can reduce the relapse rate.

Long-term treatment of patients who do not fully recover from an acute episode

The general aims of treatment are similar to those for patients who recover in hospital, but more attention has to be give to the social aspects of care.

The main approach to management is based on a systematic assessment of the patient's medical and social needs. Patients with schizophrenia who do not fully recover may have multiple social needs (e.g. housing and occupation), which are best met by a multidisciplinary team (see pp. 388–90). A *care plan* should be developed in which the problems are listed with the interventions proposed.

In caring for patients with chronic schizophrenia an experienced community psychiatric nurse (CPN) is often one of the key professionals. The roles of the CPN include:

- Acting as key worker responsible for co-ordinating the care plan.
- Monitoring the mental state.
- Administering depot neuroleptic medication.
- Monitoring compliance with medication and presence of side effects.
- Arranging or carrying out specific behavioural and psychological interventions.
- Education and support of patient and relatives.
- Liaison with other care workers.

Management of schizophrenia in primary care

In general, acute psychotic episodes should be dealt with by the specialist services because successful outcome often needs admission to hospital and/or multidisciplinary team work.

After the acute episode, general practitioners provide the majority of care for up to 25% of schizophrenic patients. As well as requiring care for their psychiatric disorder, schizophrenic patients often have significant physical illness. There is evidence that less notice is taken of the physical problems of schizophrenics than of other patients. Also, drug regimens initiated by psychiatrists tend to be continued without regular reviews by the general practitioner.

To improve the care of schizophrenic patients in the community:

1. Hospital catchment areas should be based on primary care practices rather than administrative boundaries.

2. Psychiatrist and general practitioners should work closely together.

3. Responsibilities of the specialist and primary care teams should be defined clearly.

4. Clear and consistent advice should be provided to patients and carers about diagnosis, treatment, and prognosis.

5. The training of general practitioners and psychiatrists in the care of these patients should be linked.

Management of violent schizophrenic patients

Overactivity and disturbances of behaviour are common in schizophrenia. Violence to others, although often feared by lay persons, is uncommon, and homicide is rare. Nevertheless, the risk of violence should be assessed in all cases: it is greater when there are delusions of control, persecutory delusions, or auditory hallucinations.

Threats of violence should be taken seriously, especially if there is a history of such behaviour in the past, whether or not the patient was ill at the time. The danger usually resolves as acute symptoms are brought under control, but a few patients pose a continuing threat and require regular close supervision.

Treatment for a potentially violent patient is the same as for any other schizophrenic patient, although a compulsory order is more likely to be needed. While medication is often needed to bring disturbed behaviour under immediate control, much can be done by providing a calm, reassuring, and consistent environment in which provocation is avoided. A hospital with a special area with an adequate number of experienced staff is usually able to rely less on the use of large doses of medication.

Delusional syndromes

Delusional disorder

Delusional disorder is a chronic and unshakeable delusional system, developing insidiously in a person in middle or late life. The delusional system is encapsulated, and other mental functions are normal. The patient can often work and maintain a reasonable social life. Disorders conforming strictly to this definition are rare; most eventually turn out to be an early stage of schizophrenia.

Specific delusional syndromes

The remaining delusional syndromes can be divided into two groups: those with special kinds of symptoms, and those occurring in particular situations. Of the first group, only pathological jealousy is described, and of the second group, only induced psychoses are described (the other conditions are described in *The Oxford Textbook of Psychiatry*).

Pathological jealousy

In pathological (or morbid) jealousy, the essential feature is an abnormal belief that the sexual partner is unfaithful. The condition is called 'pathological' because the belief, which may be an overvalued idea or a delusion, is held on inadequate grounds and is unaffected by rational argument. Jealousy is not classified as pathological because of strong feelings of jealousy or a violent response to a lover's infidelity; the condition is classified as pathological when the jealousy is based on unsound reasoning. Various other terms have been given to the syndrome, including sexual jealousy, erotic jealousy, morbid jealousy, psychotic jealousy, and the Othello syndrome.

Clinical features Pathological jealousy is more common in men than women. The main feature is an abnormal belief in the partner's infidelity. This belief may be accompanied by other abnormal beliefs, for example, that the partner is plotting against the patient. The mood is variable and includes misery, apprehension, irritability, and anger.

Commonly, there is intensive seeking for evidence of the partner's infidelity; for example, by searching in diaries and correspondence, and by examining bed linen and underwear for signs of sexual secretions. The patient may follow the spouse about, or engage a private detective. Typically, the jealous person cross-questions the spouse incessantly. This may lead to violent quarrelling and paroxysms of rage in the patient, and sometimes to a dangerous assault or murder. The partner may become worn out and even make a false confession in an attempt at pacification.

Aetiology Pathological jealousy may be secondary to other psychiatric disorders, including *schizophrenia*, *depressive disorder*, *alcoholism*, and *organic disorder*. Pathological jealousy can also arise from a *personality disorder*, in which the person has a pervasive sense of his own inadequacy, and a vulnerability to anything that might increase this sense of inadequacy, such as loss of status. In the face of such threats, the person may project blame on to the partner, in the form of jealous accusations.

Prognosis The prognosis is difficult to predict but generally poor, depending on the prognosis of any underlying psychiatric disorder, and of the patient's personality.

Assessment Because of the risk of violence, the assessment of a patient with pathological jealousy should be particularly thorough, and specialist psychiatric advice is necessary. The spouse should be seen alone to allow a much more detailed account of the patient's morbid beliefs and actions than may be elicited from the patient. In general practice, the spouse may be the first person to seek help. The doctor should try to find out tactfully:

- the **strength of** the jealous person's **belief** in the partner's infidelity;
- **amount of resentment**, and whether vengeful action has been contemplated;
- **provoking factors** for outbursts of resentment, accusation, or cross-questioning;
- the **partner's response** to such outbursts from the patient. An angry response may inflame the problem.
- the **patient's response** to the partner's behaviour;
- whether there has been any **violence** and if so, how it was inflicted; and whether there was any **injury**.
- **Further points** about assessment of risk are listed on p. 40.

In addition to these specific enquiries, the doctor should take a **marital and sexual history** from both partners. It is also important to seek any evidence of an underlying psychiatric disorder (see Aetiology, above) as this will have important implications for treatment.

Treatment The treatment of pathological jealousy is usually difficult, because the jealous person is usually uncooperative. Specialist advice is usually needed. If there is a primary disorder (see above), it should be treated. If no primary disorder is identified, an antipsychotic drug, such as trifluoperazine or chlorpromazine, given in the dosage used for schizophrenia, may reduce the intensity of the jealous beliefs and the emotional disturbance.

Open discussion of the problem may help by reducing emotional tension. The partner should be encouraged to behave in ways that least provoke the patient's jealousy, avoiding argument and aggressive responses to the patient's questions.

If there is no response to such treatment, or if the risk of violence is high from the beginning, in-patient care may be necessary for the jealous patient. The doctor should warn the spouse if there is a risk of serious violence. If treatment fails, it may be necessary to advise temporary or lasting separation to protect the spouse.

Induced psychosis (folie à deux)

An induced psychosis is a paranoid delusional system that develops in a healthy person who is in a close relationship with another person, usually a relative, who has an established, similar delusional system. The delusions are nearly always persecutory.

Induced psychosis is more frequent in women than in men. Before the induced psychosis appears, the person with the fixed delusional state has usually been dominant in the relationship, while the other person (who later develops the induced psychosis) has often been dependent and suggestible. Generally, the two have lived together for a long time in close intimacy, often cut off from the outside world. Once established, the condition persists until the two people are separated, when it usually improves gradually. This occurs sometimes without treatment but more often antipsychotic medication is required.

Further reading

McKenna, P. J. (1997). *Schizophrenia and Related Syndromes*. Psychology Press, Hove, UK. *A readable and comprehensive account of aetiology, diagnosis, treatment and prognosis.*

Appendix: ICD-10 criteria for schizophrenia

(a) thought echo, thought insertion or withdrawal, and thought broadcasting;

(b) delusions of control, influence or passivity, clearly referred to body or limb movements or specific thoughts, actions or sensations; delusional perception;

(c) hallucinatory voices giving a running commentary on the patient's behaviour, or discussing the patient among themselves, or other types of hallucinatory voices coming from some part of the body;

(d) persistent delusions of other kinds that are culturally inappropriate and completely impossible, such as religious or political identity, or super-human powers and abilities (e.g. being able to control the weather, or being in communication with aliens from another world);

(e) persistent hallucinations in any modality, when accompanied either by fleeting or half-formed delusions without clear affective content, or by persistent overvalued ideas, or when occurring every day for weeks or months on end;

(f) breaks or interpolations in the train of thought, resulting in incoherence or irrelevant speech, or neologisms;

(g) catatonic behaviour, such as excitement, posturing, or waxy flexibility, negativism, mutism, and stupor;

(h) 'negative' symptoms such as marked apathy, paucity of speech, and blunting or incongruity of emotional responses, usually resulting in social withdrawal and lowering of social performance; it must be clear that these are not due to depression or neuroleptic medication;

(i) a significant and consistent change in the overall quality of some aspects of personal behaviour, manifest as loss of interest, aimlessness, idleness, a self-absorbed attitude, and social withdrawal.

Diagnosic guidelines The normal requirement for the diagnosis of schizo-phrenia is that a minimum of one very clear-cut symptom (and usually two or more if less clear-cut) belonging to any one of the two groups listed as (a)–(d) above, or symptoms from at least two of the groups referred to as (e)–(h), should have been clearly present for most of the time *during a period of 1 month or more*. Conditions meeting such symptomatic requirements but of duration less than 1 month (whether treated or not) should be diagnosed in the first instance as acute schizophrenia-like psychotic disorder and reclas-sified as schizophrenia if the symptoms persist for longer periods.

Viewed retrospectively, it may be clear that a prodromal phase in which symptoms and behaviour, such as loss of interest in work, social activities, and personal appearnace and hygiene, together with generalized anxiety and mild degrees of depression and preoccupation, preceded the onset of psy-chotic symptoms by weeks or even months. Because of the difficulty in timing onset, the 1-month duration criterion applies only to the specific symptoms listed above and not to any prodromal non-psychotic phase.

The diagnosis of schizophrenia should not be made in the presence of extensive depressive or manic symptoms, unless it is clear that schizophrenic symptoms antedated the affective disturbance. If both schizophrenic and affective symptoms develop together and are evenly balanced, the diagnosis of schizoaffective disorder should be made, even if the schizophrenic symptoms by themselves would not have justified the diagnosis of schizophrenia. Schizophrenia should not be diagnosed in the presence of overt brain disease or during states of drug intoxication or withdrawal. Similar disorders developing in the presence of epilepsy or other brain disease should be diagnosed as organic delusional (schizophrenia-like) disorder and those induced by drugs as psychotic disorder due to psychoactive substance use.

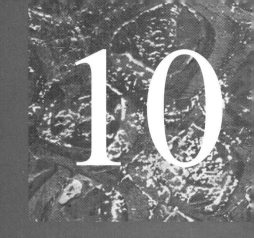

Delirium, dementia, and other cognitive disorders

- Delirium

- Dementia

- Assessment and diagnosis of possible delirium and dementia

- Specific organic psychiatric syndromes

- Neurological syndromes

- Epilepsy

Delirium, dementia, and other cognitive disorders

This chapter deals with organic psychiatric disorders; that is, psychiatric disorders resulting from brain dysfunction caused by organic pathology inside or outside the brain. It should be read in conjunction with the Chapter 11 on psychiatry and medicine and Chapter 15 on psychiatry of the elderly. The former describes the general principles of the psychological impact of major physical disorders of all types; the latter includes sections on the commonest causes of dementia and of their management in old age.

Four types of clinical problem are described in this chapter:

1. Acute generalized impairment, **delirium**, in which the most important feature is impairment of consciousness. The disturbance of brain function is generalized, and the primary cause is often outside the brain, for example, anoxia due to respiratory failure.

2. Chronic generalized impairment, **dementia**, in which the main clinical feature is generalized intellectual impairment. There are also changes in mood and behaviour. The brain dysfunction is generalized, and the primary cause within the brain, for example, a degenerative condition such as Alzheimer's disease.

3. **Specific syndromes**, which include disorders with predominant impairment of memory only (amnesic syndrome), or thinking, or mood, or personality change. We also describe a number of neurological disorders which frequently result in organic psychological complications.

4. The chapter concludes with a review of the psychiatric features of **epilepsy**.

Table 10.1 lists the main categories of psychiatric disorder associated with organic brain disease. The following sections, describing these syndromes and also the psychiatric consequences of a number of neurological conditions, should be read in conjunction with Chapter 11 which describes the general principles of the assessment and management of psychological problems in medical patients.

Delirium

Delirium is characterized by impairment of consciousness. It is a common accompaniment of physical illness, occurring in about 5–15% of patients in general medical or surgical wards, and about 20–30% of patients in surgical intensive care units. It is especially common in the elderly (see Chapter 15). Most patients recover quickly, and only a few need specific treatment. Terms such as **confusional state** and **acute organic syndrome** are outdated and best avoided.

Table 10.1.

Classification of organic mental states

Global syndromes
Delirium
Dementia

Specific syndromes
Amnesic syndrome
Organic mood disorder
Organic delusional state
Organic personality disorder

Clinical features (Table 10.2)

Impairment of consciousness is the most important symptom and is recognized by disorientation (uncertainty about the time, place, and the identity of other people) and poor concentration. The features *fluctuate in intensity* and are often *worse in the evening*.

Behaviour, may be either overactive, with noisiness and irritability, or underactive. Sleep is often disturbed.

Thinking is slow and muddled but the content is often complex. Ideas of reference and delusions are usually transient and poorly elaborated.

Mood may be anxious, perplexed irritable, or depressed and is often labile.

Perception may be distorted with misinterpretations, illusions, mainly visual, and visual hallucinations. Tactile and auditory hallucinations occur but are less frequent.

Disturbance of **memory** affects registration, retention, and recall; and new learning.

Insight is impaired. On recovery there is usually amnesia.

Features of delirium vary between patients, partly reflecting personality. There are two main patterns of presentation: in the first, the patient is restless and oversensitive to stimuli, and may have hallucinations and delusions; in the second, the patient is inactive and lethargic.

Aetiology

There are many causes of delirium the most important of which are listed in Table 10.3. It is more frequent among children and the elderly, among people with previous brain damage of any kind, and in conditions of low sensory input (such as isolation, and low levels of illumination).

Management

Treatment is directed both to identifying and dealing with the underlying physical cause and with measures to treat patients' anxiety, distress, and behavioural problems (Fig. 10.1).

- Patients need *reassurance and reorientation* to reduce anxiety and disorientation; these should be repeated frequently.

- *Relatives should receive a clear explanation* of the nature of the disorder to relieve their own anxiety and to help them reassure and reorientate the patient.

- In a hospital ward, there should be a *predictable consistent routine*. There are advantages in nursing the patient in a quiet side room. At night there should be enough light to enable the patient to know easily where he is but not so much that sleep is disturbed. Relatives and friends should be encouraged to stay or to visit frequently.

- It is important to *give as few drugs as possible* since these may worsen the delirium.

- Small doses of a benzodiazepine or other hypnotic are useful *to promote sleep at night*. Benzodiazepines should be avoided during daytime as their sedative effects may increase disorientation.

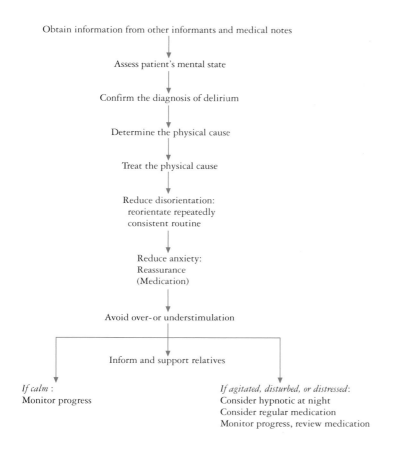

Obtain information from other informants and medical notes

↓

Assess patient's mental state

↓

Confirm the diagnosis of delirium

↓

Determine the physical cause

↓

Treat the physical cause

↓

Reduce disorientation:
reorientate repeatedly
consistent routine

↓

Reduce anxiety:
Reassurance
(Medication)

↓

Avoid over- or understimulation

↓

Inform and support relatives

If calm :
Monitor progress

If agitated, disturbed, or distressed:
Consider hypnotic at night
Consider regular medication
Monitor progress, review medication

Fig. 10.1 Treatment of delirium.

Table 10.3.
Some causes of delirium

- Drug intoxication
- Alcohol withdrawal
- Metabolic failure
  cardiac
  respiratory
  renal
  hepatic
  hypoglycaemia
- Fever
  systemic infection
- Neurological causes
  encephalitis
  space occupying lesions
  raised intracranial pressure
  following an epileptic
  seizure

- When patients are particularly distressed and behaviourally disturbed, carefully monitored antipsychotic medication can be valuable. Following an initial dose sufficient to treat the acute situation, a regular oral dose may be given, adequate to calm the patient without causing excessive drowsiness. Haloperidol is suitable; the effective daily dose usually varies between 10 and 60 mg. If necessary, the first dose of 2–5 mg can be given intramuscularly (see the *case study*).

Case study: delirium

As a general hospital duty doctor you are called in the middle of the night to see a 69-year-old man who has become disturbed and distressed three days after major abdominal surgery. The nursing staff, who have not known the patient before, say the patient has been attempting to pull out his drip, has been shouting incoherently, and seems frightened. He has accused them of being gaolers in a prison. You look at the case notes which contain routine medical information but find that in the nursing notes the patient has been intermittently rather drowsy and that, during the day, his relatives reported that he seemed confused.

You find it difficult to interview the patient who seems unable to concentrate on your questions and makes disconnected comments about being in prison and having been attacked by people who want to kill him. He is unable to say where he is or to tell you the date. He is bewildered and fearful. You diagnose delirium. You notice that he has a pyrexia and the nurses tell you that he appears to be developing a wound infection. Consider physical treatment if required; initiate if required.

You arrange for the patient be moved to a quiet, well-lit side room. You explain to the patient that he is safe in hospital and that you will be able to help him feel better. One of the nurses takes responsibility for looking after the patient and for repeatedly reassuring him that all is well.

Despite reassurance, the patient remains very agitated. Your prescribe 3 mg of haloperidol which the patient is willing to take as syrup. You also prescribe 3 mg of haloperidol to be taken three times a day as a regular regime.

In the morning you review the patient who is calmer. You discuss a consistent, reassuring regime with the day nursing staff, explain to the relatives what has happened and encourage them to spend time with the patient explaining and reassuring what is going on.

You also discuss the response of the patient and your treatment with the responsible medical team so that they are able to continue with a consistent long-term plan.

During the next few days the medical team review the patient's mental state. There is marked improvement in orientation, mood, and behaviour and, over a period of three days, enabling step-by-step reduction and then stopping of the regular medication.

Dementia

Dementia is a generalized impairment of intellect, memory, and personality, without impairment of consciousness. It is an acquired disorder, as distinct from mental retardation in which impairments are present from birth (see Chapter 20). Although most cases of dementia are irreversible, a small but important group are remediable. Dementia before the age of 65 is said to be presenile. Dementias of the elderly are described more fully in Chapter 15.

Clinical features

Dementia usually presents with impairment of memory. Other features include changes in behaviour, mood disorder, delusions, and hallucinations (Table 10.4). Although dementia generally develops gradually, it may come to notice after an acute deterioration caused by either a change in social circumstances or an intercurrent illness. There may also be uncharacteristic aggressive behaviour or sexual disinhibition. In a middle-aged or elderly person any social lapse that is out of character should always suggest dementia. The clinical picture depends in part on the patient's premorbid *personality*; for example, neurotic and paranoid traits may become exaggerated. People who are socially isolated or deaf are less able to compensate for failing intellectual abilities. On the other hand, a person with good social skills may maintain a social facade despite severe intellectual deterioration (Table 10.4).

Disorders of **cognitive function** are central. *Forgetfulness* usually appears early and is prominent; difficulty in new learning is generally a conspicuous sign. *Memory loss* is more obvious for recent than for remote events. Patients often make excuses to hide these memory defects, and some confabulate. In some cases there are specific deficits of aphasia, agnosia, or apraxia. *Attention and concentration* are also impaired. *Disorientation* for time, and at a later stage for place and person, are almost invariable once dementia is well established (but in contrast to delirium are not usually prominent in the early stage).

Behaviour may be disorganized, restless, or inappropriate. Typically there is loss of initiative and reduction of interests. Some patients become restless and wander about by day and sometimes at night. When patients are taxed beyond their restricted abilities, there may be a sudden change to tears or anger (a *'catastrophic reaction'*). As dementia worsens patients care for themselves less well and may become disinhibited, neglecting social conventions. Behaviour becomes aimless. Eventually, the patient may become incontinent of urine and faeces.

In the early stages, **changes of mood** include anxiety, irritability, and depression. As dementia progresses emotions and responses to events become generally blunted, though there may be sudden changes of mood without apparent cause, or the catastrophic reactions noted above.

Thinking slows and becomes impoverished in content. There may be difficulty in abstract thinking, reduced flexibility, and perseveration. Judgement is impaired. False ideas, often of a persecutory kind, gain ground easily and may progress to *delusions*. In the later stages, thinking becomes grossly fragmented and incoherent. Disturbed thinking is reflected in the patient's **speech**, in which syntactical errors and nominal dysphasia are common. Eventually, the patient may utter only meaningless noises or even become mute.

Perceptual disturbances (illusions and hallucinations) may develop as the condition progresses. Hallucinations are often visual.

Insight is usually lacking into the degree and nature of the disorder.

Aetiology

Dementia has many causes, of which the most important are listed in Table 10.5. Among elderly patients degenerative disorders (notably Alzheimer's disease) and vascular causes predominate. Although these and many other causes are irreversible, when assessing a patient, the clinician needs to keep in mind the whole range of causes, so as not to miss any that might be partly or wholly treatable, such as an operable cerebral neoplasm, chronic subdural haematoma, or normal pressure hydrocephalus. Table 10.6 summarizes the 'primary dementias' (i.e. the diffuse diseases of the brain that can cause dementia). The first three are described in Chapter 15.

Table 10.4.
Clinical features of dementia

Cognition
- poor memory
- impaired attention
- aphasia, agnosia, apraxia
- disorientated

Behaviour
- odd and disorganized
- restless; wandering
- self-neglect
- disinhibition

Mood
- anxiety
- depression

Thinking
- slow, impoverished
- delusions

Perception
- illusions
- hallucinations

Insight
- impaired

Table 10.5.

Some causes of dementia

- **Degenerative**
  degenerative neurological disorders causing dementia (see Table 10.6)
  (e.g. multiple sclerosis)
- **Normal pressure hydrocephalus**
- **Intracranial**
  tumour
- **Space-occupying lesion**
  chronic subdural haematoma
- **Traumatic**
  severe head injury
- **Infections**
  postencephalitis, HIV
- **Vascular**
  multi-infarct dementia
- **Toxic**
  alcohol
- **Anoxia**
  cardiac arrest
  carbon monoxide poisoning
- **Vitamin lack**
  B_{12}
  folic acid
  thiamine
- **Metabolic**
  diabetes
- **Endocrine**
  hypothyroidism

Assessment and diagnosis of possible delirium and dementia

Assessment

Any suspicion of a dementia should lead to detailed questioning about intellectual function and neurological symptoms. It is important to interview other informants, since patients are often unaware of the extent of the change in themselves. Also, the details of the mode of onset and progression of symptoms may be provided more accurately by an informant. In doubtful cases, standardized procedures for assessing cognitive state may be of value, but in interpreting the results it is essential to take account of previous education and achievement. The Mini Mental State Examination (see p. 326) is used widely in assessment; it combines standard questions with tests of spatial ability.

Table 10.6.
Degenerative neurological diseases causing dementia

Alzheimer's disease	See Chapter 15
Vascular dementia	See Chapter 15
Lewy body dementia	See Chapter 15
Pick's disease	A rare degenerative disorder. Autosomal dominant. Compared with Alzheimer's disease, the atrophy is more marked in the frontal and less marked in the temporal lobes. Clinical differentiation is difficult.
Huntington's chorea	A rare degenerative disorder. Autosomal dominant. The pathological changes affect mainly the frontal lobes and caudate nucleus. There are choreiform movements of the face, hands and shoulders, dysarthria and abnormal gait. Dementia usually follows these neurological signs but may precede them. Occasionally there are persecutory delusions. A predictive test using a polymorphic DNA marker is available for members of affected families.
Creutzfeld–Jacob disease	A rare rapidly progressive prion disorder which causes dementia and a variety of neurological signs.

Special investigations

The aim should be to perform the minimum of investigations to reveal the cause of the disorder, whether acute or chronic. For *delirium* a common basic routine is: full blood count and ESR (erythrocyte sedimentation rate); blood biochemical screen; urinary sugar and protein; and in selected cases skull X-ray or computerized tomography (CT).

For *dementia* **computerized tomography** is valuable in the diagnosis of both focal and diffuse cerebral pathology. It should be requested if there is any suspicion of organic brain disease in patients up to late middle age, or if there is any suggestion of a focal brain lesion in the elderly.

Psychological testing Specific tests of memory, learning, and other aspects of cognitive function are sometimes used by specialists to identify and quantify patients with localized brain lesions. A commonly used basic test is the **Wechsler Adult Intelligence Scale** (WAIS), which is a well-standardized test providing a profile of verbal and non-verbal abilities. It should be given by a trained tester. Organic impairment is suggested by a discrepancy between performance IQ (as an estimate of current capacity) and verbal IQ (as an estimate of previous capacity).

Aspects of differential diagnosis

Organic or functional?

It is sometimes difficult to distinguish between functional and organic psychiatric disorder, especially when an organic disorder presents with disturbances of behaviour and thinking in the absence of obvious neurological symptoms or signs. In **affective disorder** and **schizophrenia** there may be an impression of impairment of cognitive functions.

Pseudodementia A common diagnostic problem is presented by so-called depressive pseudodementia. In this syndrome, a depressed patient's complains of poor memory and appears intellectually impaired because poor concentration leads to inadequate registration and depressive mood leads to slowness and self-neglect. Characteristic features are:

- A history from another informant that the depressed mood preceded the memory problems.

- Memory testing shows that the poor performance improves when interest is aroused.

- The patient is retarded and unwilling to co-operate in the interview; by contrast, patients with dementia are usually willing to reply to questions but make mistakes.

Conversely, *an organic disorder can present with mood disorder or behaviour change* that suggests a functional disorder. The points in favour of an organic cause are:

- Cognitive disorder preceding mood or other disorder
- Cognitive defects in specific areas of intellectual function
- Neurological signs
- Symptoms not typical of non-organic disorder, such as visual hallucinations.

It is important to consider a possible organic cause in every case of acute psychological or behavioural disturbance especially when there are atypical features. The diagnoses of functional disorder is partly by exclusion of organic causes but also on the finding of positive evidence of psychological aetiology since organic causes may be undetectable in the early stages of disease.

Delirium or dementia?

Delirium is an acute reversible condition, dementia is a chronic disorder. As shown in Table 10.7, delirium is characterized by an acute onset, fluctuating course, impaired consciousness, and disorganized thinking. Also, perceptual disturbance is more frequent and alertness more often impaired in delirium. Especially in the elderly, the two syndromes may occur together; when this happens the underlying dementia may be overlooked or the delirium may not be detected or treated. Sometimes a longstanding dementia becomes apparent only after successful treatment of a more recent delirium.

Stupor

Stupor is a rare condition in which the patient is immobile and unresponsive but has a normal level of consciousness. Stupor can occur in severe affective disorders (see p. 131) and schizophrenia (see p. 167). Lesions of the brainstem or mesen-

Table 10.7.

Delirium vs. dementia

Delirium	Dementia
Acute onset	Insidious onset
Fluctuating course	Stable or progressive*
Impaired consciousness	Normal consciousness
Thinking disorganized	Thinking impoverished
Perceptual disturbance common	Perceptual disturbance uncommon
Alertness usually impaired	Normally alert

*Except multi-infarct dementia.

cephalon can cause a similar clinical picture, although in these cases there may be some impairment of consciousness. Neurological examination and a CT scan help in diagnosis of these neurological causes. Even more rarely the cause is renal or hepatic failure or hypoglycaemia.

The management of dementia

A minority of patients have a treatable cause (see Table 10.5). For the remainder, treatment aims to reduce disability and provide support. Whenever possible, care is outside hospital, either with relatives or in residential accommodation. Management begins with an assessment of the degree of disability and the social circumstances of the patient. The aims of treatment are to:

- maintain remaining ability as far as possible;
- relieve distressing symptoms;
- arrange for the practical requirements of the patient; and
- support the family.

The management of dementia is described more fully in Chapter 15 on the elderly.

Specific organic psychiatric syndromes

Brain pathology may give rise to several specific psychiatric syndromes as well as the generalized disorders described above. Sometimes these syndromes are associated with focal neurological signs, but the psychiatric syndrome may be the only abnormality.

The amnesic syndrome

The amnesic syndrome (otherwise known as the *amnestic syndrome*) is characterized by a prominent disorder of recent memory, in the absence of the generalized intellectual impairment observed in dementia or the impaired consciousness seen in delirium. The condition usually results from lesions in the posterior hypothalamus and nearby midline structures, but occasionally from bilateral hippocampal lesions. It is often described as **Korsakov** syndrome after the Russian neurologist who first described the clinical features, or as the **Wernicke–Korsakov** syndrome because the amnesic syndrome may accompany an acute neurological syndrome described by Wernicke (Wernicke's encephalopathy) characterized by impairment of consciousness, memory defect, disorientation, ataxia, and opthalmoplegia.

Alcohol abuse is the most frequent cause, and seems to act by causing a *deficiency of thiamine*. Other causes include *carbon monoxide poisoning, vascular lesions, encephalitis*, and *tumours of the third ventricle*.

Clinical features (see Table 10.8) The central feature of the amnesic syndrome is a profound *impairment of recent memory*. The patient can recall events immediately after they have occurred, but cannot do so even a few minutes afterwards. Thus, on the standard clinical test of remembering an address, immediate recall is good but grossly impaired 10 minutes later. One consequence of the profound disorder of memory is an associated *disorientation in time*. Gaps in memory are often filled by *confabulation*. The patient may give a vivid and detailed account of recent activities which, on checking, turn out to be inaccurate. It is as though he cannot distinguish between true memories and the products of his imagination or recollection of events from times other than those he is trying to recall. Such a patient is often suggestible; in response to a few cues from the interviewer, he may give an elaborate account of taking part in events that never happened.

Other cognitive functions, including remote memory, are relatively well preserved. Unlike the patient with dementia, the patient with an amnesic syndrome seems alert and able to reason or hold an ordinary conversation, so that the interviewer may at first be unaware of the extent of the memory disorder.

Treatment For cases that may be due to *thiamine* deficiency, this vitamin should be prescribed in the hope of limiting further damage. Otherwise, there is no specific treatment and the *general measures* are those described above for dementia.

Course and prognosis The course is chronic. Prognosis is better when the condition is due to thiamine deficiency, provided that thiamine treatment was started promptly. If the cause continues to act (e.g. excessive drinking that persists), the amnesia may worsen.

Organic personality disorder

Brain damage may result in **personality change** and this may be severe enough to be classified as *personality disorder*. An example is the distinctive syndrome associated with *frontal lobe damage* in which the patient's behaviour is disinhibited, overfamiliar, and tactless. The patient may be overtalkative, make inappropriate jokes, and engage in pranks. He may make errors of judgement and commit sexual indiscretions, and disregard the feelings of others. The **mood** is generally fatuous euphoria. **Concentration** and **attention** may be reduced. Measures of formal intelligence are generally unimpaired, but special testing may show deficits in abstract reasoning. **Insight** is impaired.

Organic mood disorders

Some neurological diseases (e.g. multiple sclerosis), are direct causes of mood disturbance, which may be depression, mania, or anxiety. Some endocrine disorders, for example Cushing's disease, can have the same effect (see p. 215). It is difficult

---

Table 10.8.
Clinical features of amnesic syndrome

- Recent memory severely impaired
- Remote memory spared
- Disorientation in time
- Confabulation
- Other cognitive functions preserved

to distinguish such disorders from emotional disorders that are a normal psychological response to physical illness, or from chance associations between mood disorder and physical disease.

Organic delusional disorder

Occasionally, brain pathology, particularly that associated with temporal lobe epilepsy, causes a delusional disorder resembling schizophrenia.

Neurological syndromes

Normal pressure hydrocephalus

In this variety of hydrocephalus there is no block within the ventricular system. Instead, there is an obstruction in the subarachnoid space such that cerebrospinal fluid can escape from the ventricles but is prevented from flowing over the surface of the hemispheres. There is marked hydrocephalus generally with a normal, or even low, ventricular pressure, although episodes of raised pressure occur sometimes.

The characteristic features are progressive memory impairment, slowness, marked unsteadiness of gait, and in the later stages, urinary incontinence. The condition is more common in the elderly but may occur in middle life. Often, no cause for the obstruction can be discovered although there may be a history of subarachnoid haemorrhage, head injury, or meningitis. Treatment is a shunt operation to improve the circulation of cerebrospinal fluid. This procedure arrests the condition and sometimes the dementia improves. It is important to differentiate this treatable condition from the primary dementias, as well as from depressive disorder with mental slowness.

Head injury

Major head injury has obvious neuropsychiatric consequences such as dementia or personality change. Some more minor head injuries cause less obvious cognitive impairments which may significantly impair functioning and behaviour for many months after the injury. Patients returning to demanding occupations or activities or who complain of difficulties following head injury require full neurological review.

Repeated minor blows to the head, such as occur in boxing, can lead to progressive deterioration in intellectual function. Since the clinical changes are insidious, it is important to obtain information from other informants about how current intellectual function compares with previous function and achievements. Specialist psychological assessment can be helpful.

Acute psychological effects

- **Impairment of consciousness** occurs after all but the mildest closed head injuries.

- After severe head injury there is often a prolonged phase of **delirium** often lasting for days or weeks.

Lasting cognitive impairment

When head injuries are followed by post-traumatic amnesia of more than 24 hours, they are likely to be followed by persisting cognitive impairment. Improvement usually takes place slowly over months or even years.

The impairment is usually global but, after a localized injury, there may be only focal cognitive deficits affecting specific aspects of intellectual function.

Personality change is often the most serious long-term complication after severe head injury, particularly after damage to the frontal lobe. There may be irritability, loss of spontaneity and drive, some coarsening of behaviour, and occasionally reduced control of aggressive impulses. These changes often cause serious difficulties for the patient and his family.

Emotional symptoms may follow any kind of injury. Depression is frequent in those with severe physical disability. There may also be a combination of anxiety, depression, and irritability, with headache, dizziness, fatigue, poor concentration, and insomnia, whatever the injury severity. This *post-concussional syndrome* is probably due to an *interaction* of minor brain damage and anxiety and depression.

Assessment and treatment

A plan for long-term treatment should be made as early as possible after head injury. Three aspects of the problem should be assessed:

(1) neurological signs and the degree of physical disability;

(2) any neuropsychiatric problems and their likely future course;

(3) social circumstances, social support, the possibility of return to work, and the effect of the injury on the patient's responsibilities in the family.

Specialist rehabilitation should include not only physiotherapy and graded increase in physical activity, but work with the patient and family to try and minimize disabilities in everyday life and to find ways of dealing with specific cognitive deficits such as impaired memory.

Cerebrovascular disease

Among people who survive a cerebrovascular accident, about half return to a fully independent life. The rest may have psychological as well as physical problems. The psychological changes are often the more significant, preventing a return to a normal life when the physical disability has ceased to be a serious obstacle.

Cognitive defects Stroke can cause dementia as well as specific deficits of higher cortical function such as dysphasia and dyspraxia, which may handicap the patient to a degree that is underestimated by doctors. If the stroke is repeated the dementia may progress. (The separate condition of *vascular dementia* is described on p. 317.)

Personality change Irritability, apathy, or lability of mood may occur after a cerebrovascular accident. Difficulties in coping with everyday problems is common and failure may result in a 'catastrophic reaction'. Such changes are probably due more to associated widespread arteriosclerotic vascular disease than to a single stroke, and they may continue to worsen even though the focal signs of the stroke are improving.

Depressed mood is common after a stroke. It is partly a psychological reaction to the handicap caused by the stroke but may, in part, be a direct consequence of any localized brain damage. It may contribute to the apparent intellectual impairment and is often an important obstacle to rehabilitation.

Lability of mood is frequent and may be a significant clinical problem.

Even though biological factors may contribute to aetiology, depressed mood should be treated with antidepressant medication. Lability of mood is also frequently helped by antidepressant treatment. Practical help is frequently required by both patient and carers.

Cerebral tumours

Many cerebral tumours cause psychological symptoms at some stage, and in a significant minority these symptoms are the first to appear. Fast growing tumours are more likely to cause an delirium, especially if there is raised intracranial pressure; slow growing tumours are more likely to present with dementia or, occasionally, depressive symptoms.

Transient global amnesia

This syndrome is an occasional but important cause of episodes of unusual behaviour which may present as emergencies to general practitioners and casualty officers. Doctors who are not familiar with the syndrome may misdiagnose it as a dissociative disorder (see p. 223).

It occurs in middle or late life. There are abrupt episodes, lasting several hours, of global loss of recent memory. The patient apparently remains alert and responsive but usually appears bewildered by his inability to understand his experience. There is complete recovery, except for amnesia for the episode. The cause is unknown and there is no specific treatment.

Multiple sclerosis

Psychological symptoms occur early in the disorder, and may rarely be the presenting feature. In the established disease, *depression and elation* may occur, and is sometimes severe enough to require psychiatric treatment.

Occasionally, a *rapidly progressive dementia* occurs early in the disease. In most cases, however, intellectual deterioration occurs later, is less severe, and progresses slowly. In the late stages of the disease *dementia* is common.

Epilepsy

People with epilepsy suffer from the misconceptions and prejudices of other people about epilepsy as well as from the condition itself. Such problems arise in school and later, at work, and also within the family. In caring for people with epilepsy the general practitioner should try to reduce these misunderstandings, and to support the patient and the family. Restriction of the driving of motor vehicles by epileptic individuals further limits their activities.

There are several ways in which epilepsy predisposes to psychiatric disturbance (Table 10.9).

Psychiatric disorder associated with the cause of epilepsy When epilepsy is a consequence of brain damage, this damage may also cause intellectual impairment or personality problems.

Table 10.9.

Associations between epilepsy and psychological problems of epileptic individuals

1. Effects of stigma and social restrictions
2. Psychiatric disorder due to the cause of epilepsy
3. Behavioural disturbance associated with the seizure
   - *Before*: tension, irritability, depression
   - *During*: complex partial seizures
   - *After*: (rarely), automatism
4. Disorders between seizures
   Cognitive impairment
   Personality disorder
   Paranoid disorder
   Sexual dysfunction
   Increased self-harm and suicide

Behavioural disturbance associated with the seizure

Before a seizure there may be a period of increasing tension, irritability, and depression lasting for hours or sometimes a few days.

During seizures of the complex partial type there may be automatic behaviour of a complicated kind. Occasionally, such seizures are prolonged for days as 'complex partial status' in which there may be an abnormal mental state, abnormal behaviour, or social withdrawal.

After the seizure there may occasionally be a prolonged period of abnormal behaviour and impaired awareness: 'automatism'.

Psychiatric disorder occurring between seizures

Cognitive dysfunction The drugs used to treat epilepsy may cause impaired attention. In some patients, there is persistent abnormal electrical activity in the brain between seizures, and this activity can be associated with poor attention and memory. (For both reasons, learning problems are more common in children with epilepsy than in non-epileptic children, see p. 436.)

Personality Most people with epilepsy are of normal personality. When personality disorder does occur, it is not of any single kind. The causes are multiple: social limitations imposed on the epileptic person during childhood and adolescence, self-consciousness, and reactions of other people. In cases in which brain damage has caused the epilepsy, the former may contribute to the personality disorder.

Psychosis Affective disorder may be more common in people with epilepsy than in the general population.

Sexual dysfunction. This problem is more common in epileptics than in non-epileptics. The causes include problems difficult relationships, and the effect of antiepileptic medication. There may be neurophysiological causes in some cases since sexual problems are more common with temporal lobe damage than with other kinds of epilepsy.

Suicide, deliberate self-harm. Among people with epilepsy suicide is four times more frequent, and deliberate self-harm six times more frequent, than in the general population.

Further reading

Lishman, W. A. (1998). *Organic Psychiatry: The Psychological Consequences of Cerebral Disorders* (3rd edn). Blackwell, Oxford.
A comprehensive work of reference, invaluable for the detailed study of specific conditions.

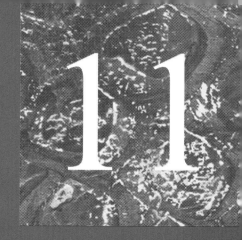

11

Psychiatry and medicine

Psychiatry and medicine

Physical symptoms and psychiatric disorder occur commonly together in patients who consult general practitioners and in those referred to specialists working in all branches of medicine and surgery. In *primary care*, psychiatric disorder often presents with physical complaints; psychological symptoms are a frequent consequence of acute or chronic organic illness. In *hospital out-patients and in-patients*, at least a quarter of patients with physical complaints can be diagnosed as suffering from psychiatric disorder.

There are five important reasons for the association:

1. Chance association: physical and psychiatric disorders are both common.

2. Psychological factors as causes of physical disorder.

3. Psychiatric complications of physical illness and its treatment (e.g. heart disease can provoke anxiety and depression). (Delirium, dementia and focal syndromes have been described in Chapter 10.)

4. Some psychiatric disorders can cause physical symptoms (e.g. palpitations in an anxiety disorder).

5. Physical complications of psychiatric disorder (e.g. deliberate self-harm, eating disorders).

An understanding of the psychological aspects of general medical care is important because:

• A psychiatric disorder may respond to treatment.

• It may be possible to reduce adverse psychologically determined effects on disability and everyday life.

• Untreated psychological problems are often associated with excessive and inappropriate use of medical resources and poor compliance with medical advice.

The first part of this chapter is mainly concerned with psychiatric consequences of physical illness and the role of psychological factors as causes of physical symptoms.

Later parts of the chapter describe a number of clinical problems of special psychiatric importance. These include eating disorders, psychiatric aspects of obstetrics and gynaecology, and sleep disorders.

General principles

Epidemiology

In primary care, unexplained physical symptoms are among the commonest reasons for seeking treatment and are often due to psychiatric disorder. In addition, psychological and social factors are important in the management of many patients with serious acute or chronic physical illness.

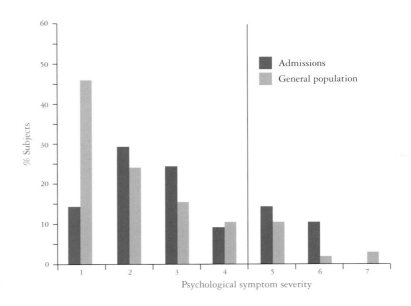

Fig. 11.1 Frequency of psychological symptoms in women admissions to a general hospital as compared with a general population. Scores of 5 and above to the right of vertical line indicate psychiatric disorder (Oxford data provided by R. A. Mayou).

In hospital practice, psychological problems are especially frequent in accident and emergency departments, gynaecological and medical out-patient clinics, medical and geriatric wards, and units treating liver disease. About a quarter of patients in medical wards (Fig. 11.1) have a psychiatric disorder of some kind. *Affective disorders* are common in younger women, *organic mental disorders* in the elderly, and *drinking problems* in younger men. In out-patient clinics about 15% of patients with a definite medical diagnosis have an associated psychiatric disorder, and about 40% of those with no medical diagnosis have a psychiatric disorder.

Associations between psychiatric and physical disorder (Table 11.1)

Psychiatric and physical disorders occurring together by chance Psychiatric and physical disorders are both common and often occur together by chance. They often then interact. For example, a depressive disorder provoked by business failure might make a patient less compliant with treatment or rehabilitation for a coincidental physical condition. Conversely, physical illness may exacerbate psychiatric symptoms; for example, a virus infection could delay recovery from a depressive disorder.

Psychological factors as causes of physical illness It used to be thought that certain diseases—called *psychosomatic*—were caused mainly by psychological factors; asthma and ulcerative colitis are two examples. Research has not supported

Table 11.1.

Associations between physical and psychiatric disorder

- Psychiatric and physical disorder occurring together by chance
- Psychological factors as causes of physical illness
- Psychiatric consequences of physical illness:
  - organic disorders (Chapter 10)
  - functional disorders (especially depression and anxiety)
- Psychological causes of physical symptoms
- Psychiatric disorders with physical complications:
  - deliberate self-harm (Chapter 12)
  - alcohol and other substance abuse (Chapter 13)
  - eating disorders

this idea but there are four ways in which psychological factors may contribute to the aetiology, presentation, and outcome of physical illness:

1. They may lead to **unhealthy habits** such as overeating, smoking, and excessive use of alcohol.

2. They may result in **hormonal, immunological,** or **neurophysiological changes** which contribute to onset or affect late course of the pathological process. It has been suggested that increased mortality among patients depressed after myocardial infarction is caused in this way.

3. Psychological factors can determine **whether a person seeks help** from a doctor about an illness; for example, a person may seek help for backache when he feels depressed, but would have tolerated the pain had he remained in a normal mood.

4. Psychological factors may **affect compliance** with treatment and in this way influence outcome; for example, a depressed patient may neglect the treatment of diabetes.

Psychiatric consequences of physical illness Most people are remarkably resilient when physically ill. It is usual to feel distress during the acute stages of serious illness or drug treatment, but this distress is usually short-lived. A minority develop a more extreme response in the form of an organic or functional psychiatric disorder.

Psychological causes of physical symptoms Psychological and psychiatric factors are an important cause of non-specific physical symptoms for which no organic cause can be found. These *medically unexplained symptoms* are usually transient but, in an important minority of patients, they persist and are often difficult to treat. Such symptoms are described later in this chapter (p. 216).

Psychiatric disorders with physical complications Some common psychiatric disorders cause behaviours that lead to physical illness. Deliberate self-harm and eating disorders are examples.

Table 11.2.

Common psychiatric disorders in the physically ill

More common	Adjustment disorder
	Depressive disorder
	Anxiety disorders
	Delirium
Less common	Somatoform disorders
	Dementia
	Panic
	Phobic disorder
	Anxiety disorder
	Post-traumatic stress disorder
	Mania
	Schizophrenia and delusional disorder

Psychological complications of physical illness

As explained above, most people are resilient when ill and carry on without undue distress. Even so, all physical illness has some psychological impact which in about a quarter of cases may have substantial affect on outcome by leading to:

- Disturbances of mental state, which may be severe enough to be classified as psychiatric disorder.
- Impaired quality of everyday life.
- Unnecessarily poor physical outcome.
- Adverse effects on family and others.
- Inappropriate or excessive consultation.
- Poor compliance with treatment.

The usual reaction to **acute illness** is anxiety which may be followed by depression. In up to a quarter of patients these reactions reach the diagnostic threshold for an anxiety or depressive disorder. Delirium is frequent in those who are severely ill (delirium is discussed in Chapter 10). After the diagnosis of a severe illness, such as myocardial infarction or cancer, complete or partial *denial* of the diagnosis and its meaning may occur. If denial is prolonged it can lead to poor compliance with treatment.

In disabling **chronic illness**, anxiety and depressive disorders are up to twice as common as in the general population and there is also an increase in anxiety and depression below the threshold for diagnosis of a disorder.

Although adjustment disorder and anxiety and depression are the commonest psychological consequences of physical illness, other psychiatric disorders may be precipitated by physical illness (see Table 11.2).

Major medical and surgical treatments are also important causes of psychological symptoms.

Drug treatment. Many drugs have side effects including depression, delirium, psychotic symptoms and elation (the list, which is long, is given for reference in *Additional information*). These symptoms diminish when the drug is stopped or reduced but it is sometimes difficult to do this (e.g. to reduce large doses of steroids). In such a case it may be necessary to prescribe psychotropic medication to treat depression or other psychiatric symptoms.

Chemotherapy of cancer, particularly the long and repeated courses of unpleasant treatment required for certain blood disorders, may cause very great distress. Not infrequently, patients receiving such treatment describe anticipatory nausea and other symptoms when a repeat course is due to begin. Medical management to treat the nausea together with behavioural methods is useful in enabling patients to continue with essential treatment.

Radiotherapy This is often associated with anxiety and depression, both because of the unpleasant physical side effects and because it is used to treat life-threatening illnesses.

Additional information Medications reported to cause depression

Cardiovascular drugs	Alpha-methyldopa
	Reserpine
	Propranolol
	Guanethidine
	Clonidine
	Thiazide diuretics
	Digitalis
Hormones	Oral contraceptives
	ACTH (corticotropin) and glucocorticoids
	Anabolic steroids
Psychotropics	Benzodiazepines
	Neuroleptics
Anticancer agents	Cycloserine
Antiinflammatory	Non-steroidal antiinflammatory agents (NSAIDs)
Antiinfective agents	Ethambutol
	Sulfonamides
Others	Cocaine (withdrawal)
	Amphetamines (withdrawal)
	L-dopa
	Cimetidine
	Ranitidine
	Disulfiram
	Metoclopramide

Additional information Medication reported to cause other psychiatric symptoms

Delirium	CNS depressants
	Digoxin
	Cimetidine
	Anticholinergic drugs
Psychotic symptoms	Hallucinogenic drugs
	Appetite suppressants
	Sympathomimetic drugs
	Corticosteroids
Elation	Antidepressants
	Corticosteroids
	Isoniazid
	Anticholinergic drugs

Surgical treatment Most patients are anxious before major surgery; those who are most anxious before surgery are also most distressed afterwards. Anxiety can be reduced by a clear explanation of the operation, its likely consequences, and the plan for post-operative care, including the effective treatment of pain. In addition, a written handout is helpful since anxious people do not remember all that they have been told.

When surgery leads to changes to the body's appearance (e.g. mastectomy) or function (e.g. colostomy) there may be additional psychological problems. These patients benefit from psychological support which may be given by a specially trained nurse.

Effects on families

Close relatives may suffer as much, or even more, distress than patients. It is important to involve relatives in discussions about the patient's treatment and consider ways of helping relatives with their distress and any practical problems caused by the patient's illness.

Determinants of psychiatric consequences of physical illness

Physical illness and treatment as a direct cause of psychiatric symptoms Most anxiety and depression following physical illness is part of a psychological reaction. However, several medical disorders also cause anxiety and depressive symptoms directly, presumably through some physiological mechanism. They include some neurological disorders (e.g. Parkinson's disease and some strokes) some infections, several endocrine disorders, and several forms of malignancy (Table 11.3). As explained above, some drugs have psychiatric side effects.

Determinants of psychological impact The impact depends on the interaction of the nature, unpleasantness, and significance of the illness and treatment with factors in the patient's personality and circumstances (Table 11.4).

Some types of illness (Table 11.5) are especially likely to cause psychiatric problems, while patients with histories of psychiatric disorder or of previous difficulties in coping with stresses and those in adverse social circumstances are especially likely to suffer distress.

Psychiatric assessment of a physically ill patient

Among severely ill patients, distress is often seen as understandable and inevitable and no help is offered. Since most people cope remarkably well with the most severe medical problems, distress is abnormal and requires assessment and treatment (psychiatric disorder is always abnormal by definition).

The psychiatric assessment of a physically ill patient is similar to that of a patient presenting solely with psychiatric symptoms (described in Chapter 2) except that it requires knowledge of the nature and prognosis of the physical illness. The key questions are outlined in Table 11.6. It is especially important to be aware that:

(1) some symptoms, such as tiredness and malaise, may occur in both physical and psychiatric disorder;

Table 11.3.

Associations between physical disorders and psychiatric symptoms

Depression
Carcinoma, infections, neurological disorder, endocrine disorder

Anxiety
Hyperthyroidism, hyperventilation, hypoglycaemia, drug withdrawal

Fatigue
Anaemia, sleep disorder, chronic infection, hypothyroidism, diabetes, carcinoma, radiotherapy

(2) some physical disorders and some drugs are especially likely to cause psychological symptoms;

(3) it is important to speak to relatives: (1) because they can provide extra information about the patient, and about other problems which may also be causing distress; and (2) also because families frequently require help themselves.

Table 11.4.

Determinants of the psychological impact of physical illness

1. *Illness factors*	Pain
	Threat to life
	Course
	Duration
	Disability
	Conspicuousness
2. *Treatment factors*	Pain
	Side effects
	Uncertainty of outcome
	Self-care demands
3. *Patient factors*	Psychological vulnerability
	Social circumstances
	Other stresses (chronic and acute)
	Reactions of others

Table 11.5.

Factors associated with a particularly high risk of psychiatric problems

1. *Severe illness*	Unpleasant, threatening, acute, relapsing, or progressive illness
2. *Unpleasant treatment*	Major surgery
	Radiotherapy
	Chemotherapy
3. *Vulnerable patients*	History of previous psychiatric problems
	Current psychiatric disorder
	Adverse social circumstances
	Lack of personal and emotional support

Management

Although some emotional distress is an almost inevitable accompaniment of the stress of physical illness and its treatment, even in those who are coping well, it

Table 11.6.
Recognition of emotional disorder in the physically ill

1. *Screening questions for psychiatric symptoms*
   How have you been feeling in yourself?
   Have you been very worried about your health?
   How have you been sleeping?

2. *Screening questions about the psychiatric history*
   Are you taking any sleeping tablets or tablets for your nerves?
   Have you ever suffered from tension or nerves?
   Have you ever consulted a doctor about your nerves?

3. *Screening questions about social factors*
   Any problems recently that have upset you?
   Any problems at home or at work?

4. *Observation of the patient*
   Mood and behaviour during the interview

5. *If emotional disorder is suspected*
   Take a full psychiatric history
   See other informants

can often be reduced by appropriate treatment. Advice, explanation, and discussion of anxieties are always helpful.

The treatment of any specific psychiatric disorder is similar to that of the same condition occurring in a physically healthy person although particular attention should be paid to adverse consequences of the side effects of antidepressant and other drugs, and to drug interactions.

- *Adjustment disorder* patients need further opportunities for discussion, explanation, and problem solving and also follow-up to review progress.

- *Anxiety disorder.* Psychological treatment (as described in Chapter 7) may be required for anxiety disorders, especially if they are persistent. In the short term, brief treatment with a benzodiazepine as a hypnotic during daytime can be helpful.

- *Depressive disorder.* Less serious depression can often be helped by support or problem-solving counselling, but more severe disorder requires antidepressant medication. The choice of antidepressant may be affected by side effects and by medical contraindications; for example, tricyclic antidepressants are generally contraindicated for those with cardiac disorders, glaucoma, and prostate disorders.

Psychological problems associated with specific medical disorders
Cancer

Although some doctors are reluctant to tell patients that they have cancer, most patients prefer to know the diagnosis and how it will affect their lives. The doctor needs to set aside adequate time to explain the prognosis and what treatment can be offered, following the general lines described above.

Although psychological problems are common in patients with cancer and can often be treated successfully, many remain undetected.

The diagnosis, the treatment, and the relapse of cancer may all be associated with severe distress in the form of an adjustment disorder or, in over a third of patients, a psychiatric disorder, usually an anxiety or a depressive disorder. Persistent problems occur most often in those with pre-existing social problems or psychological vulnerability and who lack a supportive family. They are particularly common after mastectomy, mutilating surgery, and radiotherapy. Recurrence or progression of the disease may lead to further affective disorder and in some cases to an organic brain syndrome (Table 11.7).

Table 11.7.
Psychiatric consequences of cancer

1. Emotional reaction on diagnosis or recurrence
2. Emotional reactions to surgery, radiotherapy, or chemotherapy
3. Anticipatory nausea with chemotherapy
4. Organic mental disorder due to metastases, metabolic changes, or chemotherapy
5. Neuropsychiatric syndromes
6. Depressive and other reactions to terminal illness

Additional information **Psychological problems associated with some medical disorders**

Accidents and trauma

Psychological factors are important contributory causes of accidents. Their factors include: in children, overactivity and conduct disorders; in younger adults, alcohol and drug abuse, and mood disorder; and in the elderly, organic mental disorders.

Following accidents, anxiety and depressive symptoms are common especially when there is injury to the head. Such symptoms are not closely related to the severity of the accident or to the physical injuries. Some road accident victims develop *phobic travel anxiety* or, less frequently, *post-traumatic stress disorder*.

The term *compensation neurosis* (or accident neurosis) has been used for physical or mental symptoms caused psychologically and occurring when there is an unsettled claim for compensation. There is little evidence that such symptoms are caused solely by compensation proceedings, although these proceedings may sometimes be one of several psychological and social factors prolonging disability.

Myocardial infarction

Acute problems The sudden onset of severe chest pain and accompanying physical symptoms frequently causes *anxiety*. In severe infarcts, *delirium* is frequent. In contrast, a sizeable minority of patients show *denial* with little distress. Such patients are often slow to consult doctors, and seem remarkably unconcerned about being in hospital. Such denial is usually a temporary and useful way with coping with a threatening illness. However, if denial persists it may lead to non-compliance with treatment.

Convalescence In the weeks after an infarct patients frequently describe *depressive* symptoms, including lack of interest and energy, poor memory, poor sleep, poor concentration, irritability. Some worry excessively about *non-cardiac chest pain* and other pains. Such problems usually improve, and most patients return to full activities over a period of weeks. A few patients develop a depressive illness and this is associated with increased mortality in the ensuing months.

The *management* of patients with myocardial infarction should include information about common psychological problems and about the importance of progressive graded increase in activities. Cardiac aftercare and rehabilitation concentrates on physical fitness and activity but it should also take into account anxiety about physical activity, sexual problems, and work difficulties, as well as any depressive disorder.

HIV Infection

Testing for HIV infection inevitably causes anxiety, which is often as severe in those eventually found to be HIV negative as in those who were HIV positive. Although knowledge that HIV infection is present is inevitably distressing, psychological symptoms are usually temporary, and usually do not return as long as the patient is free from symptoms. Psychiatric disorder during this asymptomatic period is most likely in patients with previous psychiatric disorder or major social problems.

The appearance of one of the physical syndromes of HIV infection may cause further anxiety or depression as well as delirium and dementia. In the advanced stages of the disease, psychiatric problems are similar to those of other terminal illness.

Diabetes

Diabetes is associated with psychiatric and behavioural problems because its complications may be disabling and because it demands meticulous self-care which may interfere with everyday life. Many patients with diabetes have *unsatisfactory glycaemic control*. While this is partly poor understanding of advice, it is more often due to psychological factors which make it harder for the patient to fit the requirements of diabetes care into the pattern of everyday life. Since poor glycaemic control is associated with acute complications, such as hypoglycaemic attacks and with an increased risk of longer-term complications, it is important that management takes full account of psychological factors.

Some diabetic patients (nearly always women) have *associated eating disorders*. These disorders do not seem to be more common than in people without diabetes, but they are more difficult to treat than they would be in non-diabetics.

In advanced diabetes, cerebrovascular disease, and perhaps the cerebral consequences of poor glycaemia control, may lead to cognitive impairment.

Endocrine disorders

A number of endocrine disorders may directly cause psychiatric syndromes, principally **organic mood disorder** and **organic anxiety disorder**. See *Additional information*.

Movement disorders

A number of movement disorders cause symptoms which may be misdiagnosed as signs of psychiatric disorder; in addition, they may also be associated with psy-

Additional information **Psychological problem associated with endocrine disorders**

Hyperthyroidism Restlessness, irritability, and distractibility which may resemble an anxiety disorder. Medical treatment usually results in improvement in psychological symptoms.

Hypothyroidism In infancy this leads to retardation. In adult life there is mental slowness, apathy, complaints of poor memory. Occasionally, there may be an organic mental disorder or severe depression. Paranoid symptoms are common. The condition may be mistaken for primary dementia or a depressive disorder. Early treatment usually reverses the psychiatric symptoms but prognosis is less good in chronic, long-established cases.

Cushing's syndrome (Hyperadrenalism) Depressive symptoms are frequent and a minority develop a severe depressive disorder. Treatment of the medical condition usually results in improvement in psychiatric disorder.

Corticosteroid treatment The symptoms are similar to those of Cushing's syndrome but a manic disorder is more common. The syndrome is not clearly related to the size of the dose and the aetiology is uncertain. Symptoms usually improve when the dose of corticosteroid is reduced but antidepressant drugs may be required. Lithium prophylaxis should be considered for patients who need to continue steroid treatment after treatment of the affective disorder.

Phaeochromocytoma A rare adrenaline and noradrenaline secreting tumour which can cause episodic attacks of anxiety with blushing, sweating, palpitations, headache, and raised blood pressure. Between attacks blood pressure is usually continuously raised. The attacks may be precipitated by physical exertion or, occasionally, by emotion.

Additional information **Psychological problems associated with movement disorders**

Parkinson's disease In this disorder, there is an increased incidence of dementia and of depression, and the anticholinergics used to treat parkinsonism drugs may cause excitement, agitation, delusions, and hallucinations. Levodopa (L-dopa) may cause delirium.

Spasmodic torticollis In this rare condition there are repeated, purposeless movements of the head and neck, sustained abnormal postures, and muscle spasm. The onset is usually between the ages of 30 and 50 years. The course is variable, but there is usually a slow progression over many years. Psychological factors can increase the symptoms and the condition has been thought to be psychogenic. However, it is more likely to have an organic cause. Many treatments have been tried but none is effective.

Tics These are purposeless, stereotyped, and repetitive jerking involuntary movements occurring most commonly in the face and neck. Usually there is a single kind of movement. They are much more common in childhood than in adult life, the peak age of onset being about 7 years. They are more common in boys than girls. Tics sometimes begin at a time of emotional upset and they are worsened by anxiety. Tics occurring in childhood often last only a few weeks; and all but a few improve within five years. There is no effective treatment.

Gilles de la Tourette syndrome In this rare condition, multiple tics are accompanied by sudden vocalisations in the form of grunting, snarling, the uttering of obscenities ('coprolalia'). There may be stereotyped movements resembling jumping and dancing. Other features include overactivity, difficulties in learning, and emotional disturbance. The condition usually starts at about age 5, and nearly always before age 16 years. The tics usually precede the other features.

The *cause* is uncertain, although it may be organic, involving the basal ganglia. The most satisfactory *treatment* is haloperidol. The long-term *prognosis* is uncertain, but is probably poor.

Writer's and occupational cramps In *writer's cramp*, attempts at handwriting are accompanied by painful spasms of the muscles controlling fine movements of the fingers. *Occupational cramps* are similar disorders in which a particular motor skill is impaired. They occur, for example, in pianists, violinists, and typists.

These conditions are thought by some to be psychogenic and psychological treatments have been tried though without benefit. The cause is more likely to be predominantly organic. No treatment is of proven value.

Table 11.8.
Some common physical symptoms which may have psychological causes

Pain syndromes
- abdominal pain
- non-cardiac chest pain
- headache
- atypical facial pain
- muscular pain
- low back pain
- pelvic pain

Chronic fatigue

Non-ulcer dyspepsia

Irritable bowel

Palpitations

Dizziness

Tinnitus

Dysphonia

Premenstrual tension

Psychological food intolerance

chiatric symptoms. Specialist assessment by both a neurologist and a psychiatrist is often required. See *Additional information*.

Psychological causes of physical symptoms

Some physical symptoms occur without any physical cause and a psychological cause is suspected. These symptoms are listed in Table 11.8. *Medically unexplained symptoms* are frequent in the general population and are common reasons for seeking treatment. Most of these symptoms are short-lived, resolving either spontaneously or after an explanation of their benign origin, but a minority persist.

Aetiology

Misinterpretation of physiological or emotional changes Medically unexplained physical symptoms may arise in several ways, as is shown in Fig. 11.2. Symptoms and disability can result from the meaning that the person attributes to bodily sensations arising from normal physiological processes such as tachycardia of exercise, or from emotional arousal or from minor physical pathology. Patients who mistakenly attribute these sensations to pathological causes experience them as physical symptoms, may believe that they are seriously ill and become disabled.

Once symptoms have been experienced their subsequent course is affected by:

(1)   the patient's continuing understanding of their meaning;

(2)   the reactions of family and others;

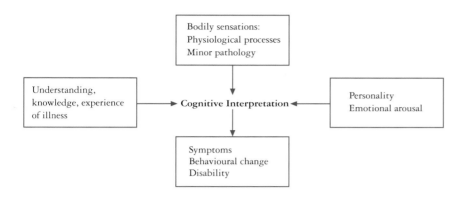

Fig. 11.2 Aetiology of medically unexplained symptoms.

(3)   the response of doctors—unclear, contradictory, or overcautious medical advice can prolong the symptoms.

Medically unexplained symptoms may also complicate a physical disorder, for example, non-cardiac chest pain of psychological origin may follow myocardial infarction. It is important to identify and treat such symptoms because they cause unnecessary disability.

Psychiatric disorder is a common cause of non-specific physical symptoms and may also be secondary to them or be secondary and then exacerbate and maintain the physical symptoms. There are two main groups:

1.   **Psychiatric disorders causing physical symptoms** (Table 11.9) The commonest psychiatric disorders causing physical symptoms are *adjustment disorder*, *anxiety disorders of all kinds*, *and depressive disorder*.

2.   **Somatoform disorders.** This poorly defined group of conditions is characterized by **persistent** concern about physical health, and unexplained physical symptoms without an underlying psychiatric disorder or emotional arousal. The central feature of these conditions is abnormal concern about health. The subclassification is not particularly useful in everyday clinical practice but is summarized for reference in *Additional information*.

Management

General measures

Assessment After appropriate physical examination, the patient's views about the causes of his symptoms should be elicited and discussed. Attention should be directed to thoughts and behaviours that accompany the physical symptoms, and to reactions of the relatives or friends. It is often useful to interview other informants as well as the patient.

A search should be made for a psychiatric disorder. A psychiatric diagnosis should be made only on the same positive grounds that would be used if there were no unexplained physical symptoms. In particular, *it should not be assumed that physical symptoms*

Table 11.9.

Psychiatric disorders associated with non-organic physical symptoms

- Adjustment disorder
- Anxiety disorders (generalized, panic, or phobic)
- Depressive disorder
- Somatoform disorder
- Others
    - schizophrenia
    - organic mental disorder
    - personality disorder

Additional information **Somatoform disorders**

Somatization disorder	Multiple recurrent and changing physical symptoms not accounted for by physical pathology. It begins in adolescence or early life and has a chronic and often fluctuating onset. Patients usually consult many doctors seeking reassurance and further investigation.
Hypochondriasis	Essential feature is anxiety about ill health and conviction of disease despite negative medical investigations and appropriate reassurance.
Dysmorphophobia	A persistent, inappropriate concern about the appearance of the body (e.g. about the shape and size of the nose or the breasts). Some patients demand cosmetic plastic surgery. Although surgery can be helpful in those with clear and reasonable expectations, a specialist opinion from a psychiatrist should always be requested.
Somatoform pain disorder	In this poorly defined condition, pain cannot be accounted for by any primary physical or mental disorder.
Undifferentiated somatoform disorder	A large residual category of unexplained physical symptoms in spite of negative investigation and medical reassurance.

are of psychological origin merely because the patient is experiencing stressful events. Such events are common and may coincide with physical disease.

Treatment of unexplained physical symptoms in general practice and in out-patient clinics is summarized in Table 11.10. There are general points that are important:

1. Avoid contradictory advice, unnecessary investigation, and inappropriate referral to other doctors.

2. Ensure that the patient understands that although the symptoms are not due to physical illness, they are recognized as real and are being taken seriously.

3. Explain the origin of the symptoms and discuss the patient's concerns.

The results of the assessment and investigations should be discussed and it should be explained why no further investigation is required. It should be explained that psychological factors can contribute to the causation of physical symptoms, alone or in combination with physical pathology, and that it is important to consider them as carefully as physical causes. Many patients who do not fully accept that their symptoms have psychological causes are willing to agree that psychological factors might influence their perception of these symptoms, and that psychological interventions may have a part in helping them to cope with the symptoms.

When the physical symptoms have a recent onset, reassurance about their benign nature may be effective; when physical symptoms have been present for a long time, further help is usually needed. This additional help depends on the

Table 11.10.

Management of unexplained physical symptoms

1. **Presenting for the first time**

   Assessment
   - Appropriate physical investigations
   - Review possible psychological causes and the patient's concerns
   - Look for a psychiatric disorder

   Treatment
   - Acknowledge reality of the symptoms
   - Explain the symptoms; discuss the patient's concerns
   - Give help with any psychological problems
   - Treat any psychiatric disorder
   - Follow-up to check progress

2. **Persistent symptoms**

   Assessment
   - Review the need for further physical investigation
   - Take a psychiatric history, review evidence for a depressive or other psychiatric disorder

   Treatment
   - Repeat the explanation of the causes of the symptoms and discussion of cancer
   - Treat any psychiatric disorder
   - Discuss with relatives
   - Consider the value of:
     - graded increase of activities
     - anxiety management
     - cognitive therapy

3. **Failure to improve**
   - Reconsider the physical assessment
   - Consider referral to a psychiatrist or clinical psychologist

associated problems: antidepressant medication when there is evidence of underlying depressive disorder, problem-solving or specific behavioural techniques of anxiety management (p. 372) and cognitive therapy (p. 367) for persistent symptoms in which health anxiety is prominent.

Some specific symptoms and syndromes

The treatment of some symptoms and syndromes which are commonly encountered in primary care and hospital practice is described next.

Chronic fatigue syndrome

Symptoms of depression, fatigue, and malaise are common following influenza, hepatitis, infectious mononucleosis, and other viral infections but usually improve over days and weeks.

Chronic fatigue syndrome is characterized by persistent fatigue, aching limbs, and muscle and joint pains. Mild physical exertion is often followed by increased fatigue and pain so that patients alternate between brief periods of activity and prolonged rest. Many patients are convinced that their symptoms are caused by a chronic virus infection or another, as yet, undetected medical condition. However, few cases are found to have a specific medical cause after thorough investigation.

In most cases, the causes are neither wholly psychological nor wholly organic, but a variable mixture of the two, with psychological factors being increasingly common over time. Inactivity and the resultant lack of physical fitness play a reinforcing role in chronic cases. Some patients have clear symptoms of depressive disorder, and may improve with antidepressant treatment.

Treatment It is explained that the syndrome is real, common, and familiar and that although there is no specific medical treatment, there are ways of achieving a good outcome. A graded programme of slowly increasing activity should be started with regular monitoring. Considerable effort is needed to ensure that patients practise progressively rather than alternating erratically between excessive activity and resting in bed. It is often appropriate to seek specialist advice for these patients.

Chronic pain (Table 11.11)

The treatment of chronic pain is difficult, and several specialist pain clinics have been established. Many patients attending these clinics have organic disease, but experience more pain than can be accounted for by the organic pathology. Analgesia should be made as effective as possible; patients should be encouraged to try ways of coping better with the pain. Procedures include distraction and reducing any behaviour that focuses attention on the pain (e.g. repeatedly rubbing or checking the area). Antidepressant medication is sometimes helpful even in patients who have no depressive disorder (Table 11.11).

Multiple chronic symptoms (somatization disorder)

Patients who have *multiple unexplained symptoms* over long periods (somatization disorder) are difficult to treat. The aim of management (Table 11.12) is usually to limit distress and unnecessary investigation rather than cure. The general approach described above (see p. 217) is used, with emphasis on avoiding inappropriate investigation and ensuring a consistent approach used, if possible by a single doctor, usually the general practitioner. A psychiatric assessment may be useful in establishing a treatment plan although specialist psychiatric treatment is seldom of much value for these patients.

Additional information **Unexplained symptoms**

Headache and atypical facial pain

The term *tension headache* is often used to describe headache for which no physical cause can be found and which is not migraine. It is a dull generalized feeling of pressure or tightness extending around the head. Such headache may be associated with anxiety and with depression. Antidepressant medication is widely used, even when there are no symptoms of depression, and is often successful.

Atypical facial pain is deep and throbbing. It is frequently encountered in dental practice where it may be attributed to an abnormal bite or other minor physical disorders. If persistent, the role of psychological factors should be assessed. In some cases, the pain is relieved by antidepressant drugs even when there is no evidence of depressive disorder.

Non-cardiac chest pain and benign palpitations

Non-cardiac chest pain is often associated with complaints of breathlessness and palpitations, sometimes with episodes of hyperventilation, and generally with limitation of activities. In some cases, symptoms are due to an anxiety disorder (especially panic disorder) or, less often, to a depressive disorder. More frequently, a patient misinterprets sensations from a source other than the heart (often the chest wall or oesophagus) as evidence of heart disease. Some check the pulse repeatedly.

Benign palpitations are due to an excessive awareness of sinus rhythm or of normal ectopic beats. Anxiety disorders are a frequent cause.

Treatment involves explanation, the management of associated anxiety and hyperventilation (see p. 372), and advice on graded increase of activities.

Irritable bowel syndrome and abdominal pain

In irritable bowel syndrome there is abdominal pain or discomfort, usually with a change of bowel habit, persisting for longer than three months in the absence of any demonstrable organic disease. The condition is common although not all those with the symptoms seek medical help. Psychological factors seem to determine whether sufferers seek help. Careful assessment and thorough explanation of the benign nature of the condition may reduce the patients distress and increase tolerance of any remaining symptoms. Anxiety management (see p. 372) may help some patients.

Acute abdominal pain of psychogenic origin is seen frequently in the emergency department and may lead to admission as suspected appendicitis. There is often an improvement with rest, but a high proportion of surgically removed appendices are normal. In the absence of physical signs, conservative medical treatment is appropriate.

Table 11.11.
Treatment of chronic pain

1. Acknowledge the reality of the symptoms
2. Explain the origin of the pain and discuss the patient's concerns
3. Treat any cause if possible
4. Agree a regime of analgesia with the patient
5. Discuss how the patient might cope better with the pain
6. Involve the family in the management plan
7. Consider antidepressant medication

Table 11.12
Management of multiple somatic symptoms

1. Take a full history and interview relatives
2. Review medical notes; discuss with doctors currently involved
3. Attempt to simplify the medical care (negotiating with others involved):
   - Perform only essential investigations
   - Limit the number of staff involved
   - Agree who has primary responsibility
   - Minimize the use of psychotropic drugs
4. Arrange brief regular appointments
5. Avoid repeating reassurance about the symptoms
6. Focus on coping with disability and psychosocial problems
7. Encourage graded return to normal activities

A conversion (or dissociative) symptom is one that suggests physical illness but occurs in the absence of relevant physical pathology and is produced through unconscious psychological mechanisms. There are two obvious practical difficulties in applying this concept:

1. It is seldom possible to exclude physical pathology completely at the time when a patient is first seen.

2. It is difficult to be certain that the symptoms are produced by unconscious mechanisms rather than consciously and deliberately. (The deliberate feigning of symptoms is known as *malingering*.)

Dissociative and conversion disorders

An alternative name for these disorders is **hysteria**. This term is not now used because the word *hysteria* also has a lay pejorative meaning as an extravagant display of emotion. Conversion disorder refers to unexplained sensory and unclear symptoms; dissociate disorder refers to unexplained amnesia, fatigue, stupor, or identity disorder see (see *Additional information*).

Unfortunately, classification differs in DSM-IV and ICD-10. In the former, *conversion disorder* is listed among somatoform disorders and there is a separate category for *dissociative disorder*. In ICD-10, both are grouped together in a single category *dissociative disorder*.

Conversion and dissociative symptoms occur in many psychiatric disorders other than conversion and dissociative disorders, notably in anxiety, depressive, and organic mental disorders. It is important to recognize this fact and to search carefully for symptoms of these other disorders before concluding that a conversion (or dissociative) symptom is part of a conversion (or dissociative) disorder. (See differential diagnosis, p. 224).

Additional information **Hysteria**

- Very long complex history as a physical explanation of obscure complaints. The word dates from ancient Greek concepts of aetiology (hysteria = wandering womb).

- Said by Freud to be due to 'conversion' of anxiety into physical symptoms, with resultant reduction of distress ('primary gain').

- Often believed to be associated with 'la belle indifférence' (lack of concern) and 'secondary gain' (social advantages).

- Frequently confused with now obsolete category of hysterical (histrionic) personality (now called histrionic).

- Now replaced by operationally defined syndromes of conversion and dissociation.

- Closely related to dissociative disorders. (A term which derives from a 19th-century explanation as due to separation of feelings from conscious awareness).

The **prevalence** of conversion and dissociative disorder varies between countries, being reported more often in less industrialized societies. In Western societies the prevalence is between 3 and 6 per 1000 for women, and substantially less for men.

General clinical features

Although conversion and dissociative symptoms are not produced deliberately, they are nevertheless shaped by the patient's concepts of illness. Sometimes, the symptoms resemble those of a relative of friend who has been ill. Sometimes they originate in the patient's previous experience of ill health; for example, dissociative memory loss may appear some years after head injury. Usually there are obvious **discrepancies between signs and symptoms** of conversion and dissociative disorder and those of organic disease; for example, a pattern of sensory loss which does not correspond to the anatomical innervation of the part. These discrepancies are important in diagnosis.

Motor disorders These disorders include paralysis of voluntary muscles, tremor, tics, and abnormalities of gait. **Paralysis** of this type is an inability to move a part due to simultaneous action of extensor and flexor muscles neither of which is actually paralysed. Reflexes are not altered (in particular the plantar response is flexor) and there is no wasting except exceptionally in very chronic cases, in which disuse atrophy has been reported. Conversion **disorders of gait** are usually of a striking kind, unlike the gait disorder of any known neurological condition and are worse when the patient is observed.

Psychogenic **tremor** is coarse and involves the whole limb. It worsens when attention is drawn to it, but so do many tremors with neurological causes. Psychogenic tics also occur. Disease of the nervous system should be considered carefully in all cases and the advice of a neurologist sought when there is any doubt.

Conversion disorders with **aphonia** and **mutism** are not accompanied by any disorder of the lips, tongue, palate, or vocal cords, and the patient is able to cough normally.

Psychogenic **convulsions** differ from epilepsy in three ways. First, the patient does not become unconscious, although he may appear inaccessible; second, the pattern of movements does not show regular and stereotyped form of a seizure; and third, there is no incontinence, cyanosis, or injury, and the tongue is not bitten.

Sensory disorders Sensory symptoms of conversion disorder include anaesthesiae, paraesthesiae, hyperaesthesiae, pain, deafness, and blindness. In general, the sensory changes are distinguished from those in organic disease by: a distribution that does not conform to the known innervation of the part; their varying intensity; and their responsiveness to suggestion.

Hyperaesthesia and **paraesthesia** may be described as painful or burning. Sometimes the description is in extravagant terms but this is not a safe diagnostic point because some patients describe symptoms of organic disease in an equally florid manner. Anaesthesia does not follow anatomical patterns.

Psychogenic **tunnel vision** may occur. Psychogenic **blindness** takes the form of a report of inability to see. The blindness is not accompanied by changes in pupillary reflexes, visual evoked responses are normal. There may be indirect evidence that the person can see more than he reports; for example, he may avoid bumping into furniture. Similar considerations apply to psychogenic **deafness**.

Dissociative symptoms Dissociative **amnesia** starts suddenly. Patients are unable to recall long periods of their lives and sometimes deny any knowledge of their previous life or personal identity.

In a dissociative **fugue** the patient loses his memory and wanders away from the usual surroundings. When found he denies memory of his whereabouts during the period in which he was wandering, and may also deny knowledge of his own personal identity.

In **dissociative stupor**, the patient is motionless and mute and does not respond to stimulation, but he is aware of the surroundings. Before diagnosing psychogenic stupor, it is essential to exclude other causes of stupor (i.e. schizophrenia, depressive disorder, mania, and organic brain disorder).

Multiple personality is an exceedingly rare condition in which there are sudden alterations between the patient's normal state and another complex pattern of behaviour (a second personality). Each is 'forgotten' by the patient when the other is present.

Epidemic hysteria Occasionally, dissociative or conversion disorders spread as an epidemic within a group of people; for example, in closed groups of young women. The epidemic begins, usually at a time of heightened anxiety for the group, sometimes when there is the possibility of being involved in an epidemic of actual physical disease already present in the outside community. The symptoms are variable but fainting and dizziness are common.

Prognosis

Most dissociative and conversion disorders of recent onset seen in general practice or hospital emergency departments recover quickly. Those that persist for longer than a year are likely to continue for many years more. As has already been noted, organic disease may be present but undetectable when these patients are first seen, becoming obvious later. For this reason patients should be followed up most carefully.

Differential diagnosis

An important differential diagnosis is from biological disorder. This depends on careful physical assessment highlighting any discrepancies in the physical signs which are unlikely to have a physical basis. Frequently, the clinical picture is such as to be inconsistent with physical condition, but in others it may be difficult to reach a definite conclusion and it is important to keep an open mind. It is important to remember that conversion symptoms are common accompaniments to physical disorder.

Another differential diagnosis, especially in those who may have advantages from illness, such as those seeking compensation, such as prisoners and military servicemen, is the exaggeration or feigning of physical symptoms. Again, a detailed history and examination is required.

Diagnosis is not solely dependent on the exclusion of physical causes, but also on psychological assessment to identify psychological reasons for the onset and course of the symptoms.

Treatment

Acute disorders seen in general practice or hospital emergency departments, respond usually to:

- efforts to **resolve the stressful circumstances** that provoked the reaction;
- strong **suggestion** that the symptoms will recover;
- **assessment** of personal or social problems should lead to an offer of continuing assessment and help for these.

For *persistent cases*, the general approach is similar, although the results are less satisfactory. It should be explained to the patient that the disability (as in remembering, or moving an arm) is not caused by a physical disease but an interference with conscious control over action, perception, or memory. Otherwise, attention is directed away from the symptoms and towards problems that have provoked the disorder. Staff should show sympathetic concern for the patient, but at the same time encourage self-help and avoid reinforcing the disability, for example a patient with a conversion disorder of gait should be encouraged to walk, not offered a wheelchair.

The main emphasis should be to try and concentrate the patient's attention on understanding problems and methods of solving them. Although patients with dissociative and conversion disorders often engage well in **exploratory psychotherapy**, psychological exploration seldom produces results better than those of the simple measures described above. Indeed, such exploration may deflect attention from the patient's current difficulties, and lead to dependency.

Self-inflicted and simulated illness

Factitious disorder

The term **factitious disorder** refers to the intentional production of physical pathology or the feigning of physical or psychological symptoms, with the apparent aim of being diagnosed as ill. Factitious disorder differs from malingering in that it does not bring any external reward such as avoidance of duties, or financial compensation. Common symptoms include skin lesions ('dermatitis artefacta') and pyrexia of unknown origin. Sometimes the patient deliberately worsens an existing physical disorder, for example, preventing the healing of varicose ulcers or neglecting the care of diabetes. At other times the whole condition is induced, for example by self-inflicted damage to the skin. There is no specific treatment, supportive counselling is often offered, and helps some patients but many do not take up the treatment.

Munchausen syndrome is an extreme and uncommon form of factitious disorder in which a patient gives a plausible and often dramatic history of an acute illness, with feigned symptoms and signs. Symptoms may be of any kind, including psychiatric symptoms. These patients often attend a series of hospitals, giving different names to each. Frequently, strong analgesics are demanded for pain. Patients often obstruct efforts to obtain additional information about them and may interfere with diagnostic investigations. The cause of the condition is unknown except that these patients have abnormal personalities. The prognosis is poor, and patients almost invariably discharge themselves before psychological treatment can be given.

The term *Munchausen syndrome by proxy* refers to a form of child abuse in which a parent (or occasionally another adult, such as a nurse) gives a false account of symptoms in a child, and may fake physical signs see p. 420).

Malingering

Malingering is the fraudulent simulation or exaggeration of symptoms with the intention of gaining of financial or other rewards. It is the obvious external gain that distinguishes malingering from factitious disorder (see above). When malingering occurs it is most often among prisoners, the military, and people seeking compensation for accidents. Malingering should be diagnosed only after a full investigation of the case. When the diagnosis is certain, the patient should be informed tactfully of this conclusion and encouraged to deal more appropriately with any problems that contributed to the behaviour.

Practical issues

A number of practical clinical problems are particularly likely to occur in the general hospital where the responsibility of the immediate management is likely to be with non-specialists rather than psychiatrists.

Patients who refuse to accept advice about treatment

Occasionally, patients are unwilling to accept their doctor's advice about treatment that is essential for a serious medical condition. There are many reasons for such refusal. Commonly it is because the patient is frightened or angry, or does not understand fully what is happening. Discussion and explanation are often effective.

Occasionally, the cause of refusal is a mental illness that interferes with the patient's ability to make an informed decision and this should be treated.

It has to be accepted that mentally healthy patients may refuse treatment even after a full and rational discussion of the reasons for carrying it out and it is the right of a conscious, mentally competent adult to do so (see Chapter 21).

Psychiatric emergencies in general hospital practice

However urgent the problem, the successful management of psychiatric emergency, like any other medical emergency, depends greatly on a thorough clinical assessment. The aims are to establish a good relationship with the patient, to take a brief history, observe behaviour, and assess the mental state. When the patient's behaviour is very disturbed, the history may have to be obtained from other people such as relatives or nurses. Although time pressures often make it difficult to follow the usual systematic scheme of history taking and examination, mistakes will be avoided and time saved if the assessment is as complete as the circumstances permit.

Acute disturbed behaviour and violence The conditions most often leading to behaviour requiring immediate action in a general hospital (or in primary care) are delirium, schizophrenia, mania, agitated depression, and alcohol and drug-related problems. Among in-patients delirium is the most common. If the patient's behaviour is very disturbed and his manner is threatening, the first task is to assess the risk of violence.

The potentially violent patient When a patient is potentially or actually violent, it is essential to arrange for adequate but unobtrusive help to be available. When approaching the patient the doctor should appear calm and helpful, avoid confrontation, and try to persuade the patient to talk about the reasons for his anger.

If the patient responds so aggressively that restraint cannot be avoided, it should be accomplished quickly by an adequate number of people using the minimum of force. Single-handed attempts at restraint should be avoided. Apart from these rare circumstances, physical contact (including physical examination) should not be attempted unless the purpose has been clearly understood by and agreed with the patient. Extreme caution is, of course, required with a patient thought to possess any kind of offensive weapon. At such times the help of the police may be required.

Drug treatment of disturbed or violent patients If a patient is very frightened, and simple reassurance fails, oral or parenteral diazepam (5–10 mg) is useful. If the patient is more disturbed, rapid calming can usually be achieved with 2–10 mg of haloperidol injected intramuscularly. Chlorpromazine (75–150 mg intramuscularly) is a more sedating alternative to haloperidol, but more likely to cause hypotension. When the patient is calm, haloperidol may be continued in smaller doses usually three to four times a day, preferably by mouth, using a syrup if the patient will not swallow tablets. The dosage depends on the patient's weight and on the initial response to the drug. Careful observation, by nurses, of the physical state and behaviour are necessary during this treatment. Extrapyramidal side effects may require treatment with an antiparkinsonian drug.

Psychiatric services for a general hospital

General practitioners are responsible for all aspects of their patients' care: physical, psychological, and social. Similarly, in a general hospital, psychological aspects of illness are part of the consultant's responsibilities. In most cases, these aspects of care will be provided by the nurses and others in the consultant team but, in other instances, psychiatric advice is needed. In larger hospitals this advice may be from a special **consultation liaison** service. This service is staffed by psychiatrists, nurses, and psychologists usually with a social worker. The consultant liaison service may provide:

- an emergency service for patients admitted after deliberate self-harm;
- emergency consultation for other accident and emergency department attenders;
- a consultation service for in-patients;
- out-patient care for patients referred with psychiatric complications of physical illness or functional somatic symptoms;
- regular liaison visits to selected medical and surgical units in which psychiatric problems are especially common (e.g. neurology, renal dialysis, terminal care).

In many hospitals the management of deliberate self-harm takes up most of the time of the psychiatric team, but in better staffed units some or all of the other functions are carried out.

The consultation Consultations should be briefly recorded in the medical notes together with copies of any correspondence with physicians or primary care. They should avoid jargon and concentrate on practical issues relevant to treatment. The main headings should be:

(1) reason for referral;

(2) psychiatric diagnosis;

(3) previous personality and social circumstances;

(4) significant aspects of the patient's attitude and behaviour to their symptoms or physical illness;

(5) any relevant features of previous or current medical management and attitude and behaviour to the patient;

(6) list of immediate conclusions and actions;

(7) information passed on by others;

(8) summary of further actions to be taken by the psychiatric consultant.

Review of clinical syndromes

The remainder of this chapter is concerned with a number of common psychiatric problems associated with medical illness or encountered in general hospital. (The management of organic cognitive disorders and deliberate self-harm are described in Chapters 10 and 12, respectively.)

Disorders of eating

Anorexia nervosa is a disorder usually among women, and onset is usually during school age years, whereas *bulimia nervosa* is more common and occurs in a wider age range, mainly among women. At least a third of those needing treatment for eating problems have an atypical eating disorder described in DSM-IV (Eating Disorder Not Otherwise Specified, EDNOS). These conditions are regarded as the product of the interaction of physical, psychological, and social risk factors.

Anorexia nervosa

The main clinical features of anorexia nervosa are low body weight, an intense wish to be thin and, in women, amenorrhoea. Most patients are young women who have a distorted image of the body, believing themselves to be fat even when severely underweight. The condition generally begins with ordinary efforts at dieting by a person who was somewhat overweight at the time, and progresses to a relentless attempt to achieve an abnormally low body weight. Most cases of anorexia nervosa begin between the ages of 16 and 17, and a few after the age of 30.

Epidemiology Anorexia nervosa occurs largely among school age girls where the prevalence is between 0.1% and 0.5%. Nearly all (95%) of patients are female and the condition is more common in the upper social classes.

Clinical features The most striking features are excessive concern with shape and weight together with a pursuit of thinness which may take several forms (Table 11.13). Patients eat little and show a particular avoidance of carbohydrates. Some set daily calorie limits (often between 600 and 1000 calories). Some try to increase weight loss by self-induced vomiting (often by putting fingers in the throat), excessive exercise, or purging. Patients are often preoccupied with thoughts of food: some enjoy cooking elaborate meals for other people, and a few steal food.

Up to half of patients describe episodes of uncontrollable overeating (known as *binge-eating* or *bulimia*). During binges, the patients may eat very large amounts of the foods they usually avoid, for example, a whole loaf of bread with copious jam and butter. After overeating the patient feels bloated and may induce vomiting. Binges are also followed by remorse and intensified efforts to lose weight.

Amenorrhoea is an important feature. It occurs early in the development of the condition and in about a fifth of cases it precedes obvious weight loss. Some patients ask for help for amenorrhoea rather than for the eating disorder.

Table 11.13.
Clinical features of anorexia nervosa

Excessive concern with shape and weight

Distorted body image

Pursuit of thinness with consequent low body weight
- dieting
- avoidance of carbohydrates
- self-induced vomiting
- excessive exercise
- purging

Preoccupation with food (binge-eating in some patients)

Amenorrhoea

Low mood

Lack of sexual interest

Consequences of starvation
- emaciation
- constipation
- low blood pressure
- bradycardia
- sensitivity to cold
- hypothermia

Consequences of vomiting and laxative abuse
- alkalosis
- hypokalaemia

Depressive symptoms, lability of mood, and social withdrawal are all common. Lack of sexual interest is usual.

Physical consequences Patients are emaciated and often have cold, blue extremities. Some have signs which are secondary to the low food intake, namely constipation, low blood pressure, bradycardia, sensitivity to cold, and hypothermia. In most cases, amenorrhoea is secondary to weight loss but, as mentioned above, it is occasionally the first sign of the disorder. Vomiting and abuse of laxatives may lead to alkalosis and hypokalaemia and these abnormalities may cause epilepsy or, rarely, death from cardiac arrhythmia.

Aetiology Anorexia nervosa appears to result from a combination of individual genetic predisposition and social factors that encourage dieting. Many school-children and female college students diet at one time or another but most stop without difficulty. Those progressing to anorexia are more likely to have low self-esteem and a preoccupation with their appearance. The prevalence of anorexia nervosa is increased in ballet students and others strongly concerned with weight and appearance. When the disorder has started, concern and overprotection by the family and arguments about food and meals may help to perpetuate it.

Course and prognosis In its early stages, anorexia nervosa often runs a fluctuating course with periods of partial remission. The long-term prognosis is variable:

- about a fifth of patients make a full recovery;

- another fifth remain severely ill;

- the remaining three-fifths have a chronic, fluctuating course.

There is an *increased mortality* both from the effects of starvation and from suicide. Among those with improved weight and menstrual function, some continue to have abnormal eating habits, some become overweight, and some others develop bulimia nervosa (see p. 231). The most useful *predictor of poor outcome* is a long history at the time the patient is first seen by a doctor.

Assessment Although specialist treatment is usually necessary, most patients with anorexia nervosa are reluctant to see a psychiatrist, and thus many are assessed by general practitioners and physicians.

1. A thorough **history** should be taken of the development of the disorder, the present pattern of eating and weight control, and the patient's ideas about body weight.

2. In the **mental state examination**, particular attention should be given to depressive symptoms. More than one interview may be needed to obtain this information and to gain the patient's confidence.

3. Whenever possible the parents or other informants should be interviewed.

4. Assess family interactions and especially attitudes and behaviour in relation to food and meals.

5. In the **physical examination**, particular attention should be paid to the distribution of body hair (normal in anorexia nervosa, abnormal in pituitary failure—see below), the degree of emaciation, signs of vitamin deficiency, and the state of the peripheral circulation. A search should also be made for evidence of any other wasting disease, such as malabsorption, endocrine disorder, or cancer. Electrolytes should be measured if there is any possibility that the

Table 11.14.
Starting treatment of anorexia nervosa

Assess
- the severity of the condition (see text)
- the presence of depressive disorder
- family problems

If evidence of severe weight loss or severe emotional problems, refer to a psychiatrist, otherwise proceed to:
- Take time to establish working relationships with the patient and family
- Give advice about healthy eating, and the hazards of extreme dieting
- Agree a target for weight gain, and a plan for achieving this
- Treat depressive disorder if present
- Help with personal and family problems
- Arrange regular follow-up

patient has been inducing vomiting or abusing purgatives, because of the risk of potassium depletion.

Starting treatment (Table 11.14) If weight loss is severe, or decreasing rapidly, specialist help should be obtained urgently, otherwise treatment can be initiated by the primary care physician. Success largely depends on making a good relationship with the patient, and gaining her collaboration. The patient and family should be told about the nature of the disorder, and the hazards of extreme dieting, and should understand the nature and purpose of the proposed treatment. It should be made clear that the maintenance of adequate weight is an essential first priority. It is important to agree with the patient a reasonable dietary plan and to set this out clearly, together with a medially reasonable, but not overambitious, target weight. At the same time, help should be offered with any psychological problems. Simple supportive measures are usually enough to increase the patient's sense of personal effectiveness. When there are serious family problems which seem to be maintaining the disorder, family interviews may be helpful.

Patients referred to a specialist will be treated in a similar way, as out-patients. Rarely, the patient's weight loss is so severe as to pose an immediate threat to life. If such a patient cannot be persuaded to enter hospital (or remain there), compulsory powers have to be used.

Treatment in hospital Admission to hospital may be needed if the patient's weight is dangerously low (less than 65% of standard weight), if weight loss is rapid, or if there is severe depression. It is also indicated when out-patient care has failed.

In hospital there should be an understanding that the patient will stay until an agreed target weight has been reached. Usually, this target has to be a compromise between the ideal weight (from height and weight tables) and the patient's idea of what her weight should be. The plan should be understood clearly by all those treating the patient. A balanced daily diet of at least 3000 calories is provided as three to four meals a day. Eating is supervised by a nurse, who has three important roles: (1) to reassure the patient that she can eat without the risk of losing control over her weight; (2) to be firm about the agreed targets; and (3) to ensure that the patient does not induce vomiting or take purgatives. It is reasonable to aim for a weight gain of between a half and one kilogram each week. This is a satisfactory weight gain in hospital in about four patients out of five; the treatment of the others is very difficult and requires further long-term effort to establish a relationship with the patient that will help her to begin to eat more and also be a basis for trying to solve other personal and social difficulties.

Treatment in hospital usually lasts between two and three months. Patients often demand to leave hospital before their treatment is finished, but with patience the staff can usually persuade them to stay.

Bulimia nervosa

The term 'bulimia' refers to episodes of uncontrolled excessive eating, sometimes called 'binges' (Table 11.15). As mentioned above, the symptom of bulimia occurs in some cases of anorexia nervosa, but it also occurs without preceding anorexia nervosa in a syndrome known as *bulimia nervosa*. This syndrome has two principal components: bulimia, and behaviour intended to prevent weight gain, usually rules about diet and self-induced vomiting but also the abuse of purgatives and excessive exercising. The balance between these behaviours is such that patients are usually of normal weight. Most patients are female and they have normal menses. Like patients with anorexia nervosa, patients with bulimia nervosa are excessively concerned with their shape and weight. Unlike patients with anorexia nervosa most bulimic patients accept the need for treatment.

The episodes of bulimia may be precipitated by stressful events or by the breaking of self-imposed dietary rules, or they may be planned. It is this extreme lack of control over eating that distinguishes bulimia nervosa from anorexia nervosa. During the episodes, enormous amounts of food are consumed: for example, a loaf of bread, a whole pot of jam, a cake, and biscuits. This voracious eating takes place alone. At first it brings a pleasurable relief from the urge to eat and other kinds of from tension, but relief is soon followed by guilt and disgust. The patient induces vomiting, at first often by putting fingers in the throat, but later by an effort of will. There may be many episodes of bulimia and vomiting each day.

Depressive symptoms are common. Usually, they are secondary to the eating disorder, but a few patients have an associated a depressive disorder.

Physical consequences Repeated vomiting leads to several complications. *Potassium depletion* is particularly serious, resulting in weakness, cardiac arrythmia, and renal damage. Urinary infections, tetany, and epileptic fits may occur. *The teeth may be pitted* by the repeated vomiting of acid gastric contents, and the *parotid glands may become swollen.*

Epidemiology Bulimia nervosa has a prevalence of between 1% and 2% in women aged 15–40. It is more frequent in developed countries.

Prognosis is uncertain since there have been no long-term studies. Many patients continue with abnormal eating habits for many years, although the severity varies.

Aetiology Unlike anorexia nervosa, genetic factors do not seem to be important, although low self-esteem and perfectionism are predisposing factors. Two important types of risk factor are those that increase the likelihood of dieting and those for psychiatric disorder in general.

Assessment The assessment of bulimia nervosa is similar to that described for anorexia nervosa, but is usually easier because the patient recognizes the need for treatment.

Table 11.15.
Clinical features of bulimia nervosa

Excessive concern with shape and weight
Binge-eating
Behaviours to prevent weight gain
• dietary restraint
• self-induced vomiting
• excessive exercise
• purging
Consequent normal body weight
Consequences of potassium depletion
• weakness
• cardiac arrythmia
• renal impairment
Other consequences of repeated vomiting
• swollen parotid glands
• pitted teeth

The mental state is examined for an associated depressive disorder needing treatment with antidepressant drugs. The patient's physical state should be assessed.

Treatment The treatment of choice is cognitive-behaviour therapy designed to reduce dietary restraint and increase control over eating and vomiting and which results in a full and lasting recovery in between a half and two-thirds of patients. Patients keep records of their food intake and episodes of vomiting, and attempt to identify and avoid any emotional changes that regularly provoke episodes of bulimia.

Since specialized treatment is demanding and not widely available, there has been increasing interest in simpler and briefer forms of treatment for use in primary care. Cognitive-behaviour self-help programmes appear to be effective on their own and especially if they are accompanied by a limited amount of support and encouragement from a non-specialist (guided self-help). These programmes include educational material which aims to correct misconceptions about eating and weight control, detailed self-monitoring of eating habits so that patients can characterize their problems, behaviour measures to help regain control over eating, and simple cognitive procedures which are designed to improve the ability to solve problems and to reduce concerns about shape and weight.

Only those patients who fail to benefit from this type of intervention need to be referred for full specialist treatment. Options for those who fail to respond to this treatment include adding an SSRI (specific serotonin reuptake inhibitor antidepressant), or changing to a different form of psychotherapy.

Psychogenic vomiting

Psychogenic vomiting is repeated, episodic vomiting without an organic cause. The diagnosis is made only after most careful physical investigation. It commonly occurs after meals and without nausea. It should be distinguished from the more common syndrome of bulimia nervosa in which *self-induced* vomiting is accompanied by abnormal ideas about body weight and shape. In *treatment* a clear explanation of the cause is often helpful. The habit of repeated vomiting can often be modified by taking regular small meals. At the same time, any associated stressful circumstances should be attended to.

Obesity

By convention, obesity is diagnosed when body weight exceeds standard weight by 20%. Most obesity is probably caused by a combination of constitutional factors and social factors that encourage overeating. In most cases, psychological causes are not of great importance in causing the obesity, although once established obesity can have psychological consequences of low self-esteem and lack of self-confidence.

Treatment Most mildly obese people need nothing more than advice about diet. Others (and the moderately obese) require more help. Many of these obese people do not eat more than other people, and of those who do, few have obvious psychological causes. It is not surprising therefore that the long-term results are disappointing. Weight groups, whether supervised or self-help, produce short-term benefit but do not improve long-term results. The role of the newer appetite-suppressing drugs remains unclear although they may be of use as a part of specialist treatment. Behavioural methods designed to change eating habits have short-term benefits but their long-term value in uncertain. Advice should be obtained from a physician experienced in treating obese patients.

Screening for physical disorder or risk

Screening procedures for physical disorders, such as hypertension or early cancer or for major risk factors, such as high blood lipid levels, are used increasingly. Screening causes little distress if it is explained clearly. However, a few subjects are made anxious by the screening, whether the result is positive or negative. For these people extra help is needed.

Genetic counselling

Counselling about the risk of hereditary disease is mainly given to couples contemplating marriage or planning or expecting a child. It includes providing information about risks, help with worry about increased risk, help in taking well-informed decisions about family planning (including sterilization) and treatment. Genetic counselling is usually provided in obstetric and genetic clinics, but there is also a need for advice by family doctors.

Information about increased risk is particularly distressing for parents who have experienced a previous abnormal pregnancy. Unfortunately, counselling is more effective in imparting knowledge than in changing behaviour and many couples ignore warnings that future children will be at high risk.

Psychiatric aspects of obstetrics and gynaecology

Pregnancy

Psychiatric disorder is more common in the first and third trimesters of pregnancy than in the second. In the first trimester, unwanted pregnancies are associated with anxiety and depression. In the third trimester, there may be fears about the impending delivery, or doubts about the normality of the fetus. Psychiatric symptoms in pregnancy are more common in women with a history of previous psychiatric disorder, although some women with chronic psychiatric disorders may improve during pregnancy. Women with chronic psychiatric problems often attend irregularly for antenatal care and consequently have more than the average of obstetric problems (see Table 11.16 for some psychological problems of pregnancy).

Treatment of psychiatric disorder during pregnancy During pregnancy great care must be taken in the use of psychotropic drugs, because of the possible risk of fetal malformations, impaired growth, and perinatal problems (see p. 334). **Benzodiazepines** should be avoided throughout pregnancy, and also during breast-feeding because of the danger of depressed respiration and withdrawal symptoms in the neonate. **Lithium** should be stopped throughout the first trimester of pregnancy. It but can be restarted later if there are pressing reasons but should be stopped again at the onset of labour. Mothers taking lithium should not breast-feed. It is preferable to avoid **tricyclic antidepressants** and **neuroleptics** during pregnancy unless there are compelling clinical indications. Abuse of **alcohol, opiates,** and **street drugs** may affect the fetus and should be strongly discouraged, especially in the first trimester when the risk to the fetus is greatest.

Loss of a fetus and stillbirth

Loss of a fetus during pregnancy or stillbirth can be expected to have a substantial and immediate psychological impact for a mother and also for the father. The bereavement is associated with significant depression which may continue for a

Table 11.16.
Some psychological problems of pregnancy

Unwanted pregnancy   Most medical decisions about termination are now made by the family doctor and gynaecologist without involving a psychiatrist. In a small proportion of patients with psychiatric disorder, a specialist opinion should be obtained.

Hyperemesis gravidarum   This syndrome of severe and repeated vomiting is rare. It appears to have primary physiological causes but the psychological reaction may exacerbate the severity and duration of the symptoms and result in greater difficulty in management.

Pseudocyesis   A rare condition in which a woman believes she is pregnant when she is not and develops amenorrhoea, abdominal distension, and other changes resembling early pregnancy. It usually resolves quickly following diagnosis. It may be recurrent.

Couvade syndrome   A rare condition in which the husband of a pregnant woman experiences symptoms of pregnancy.

number of weeks. The stress is likely to be greatest when the pregnancy was particularly wanted and when there is a history of previous miscarriages or stillbirths.

Spontaneous abortion at any stage of pregnancy causes distress and depression is frequent.

Termination of pregnancy for medical reasons is especially likely to cause distress, depression, and feelings of guilt which usually improve over a period of two to three months.

Stillbirth is associated with even greater distress than loss of the pregnancy at an earlier stage.

After abortion, termination, or stillbirth, mothers and fathers should be encouraged to grieve the loss as they would the death of an infant.

Post-partum mental disorders
There are several kinds of post-partum psychiatric disorder:
- maternity 'blues';
- puerperal psychosis;
- other depressive disorders.

Maternity 'blues'
Between a half and two-thirds of women delivered of a normal child experience a brief episode of irritability, lability of mood, muddled thinking, and tearfulness. Of these symptoms, lability of mood is particularly characteristic. All these symptoms reach their peak on the third or fourth post-partum day.

Both the frequency of the emotional changes and their timing suggests that maternity 'blues' may be related to readjustment in hormones after delivery, but there is no direct evidence to support this idea. The patient and her partner should be reassured that the condition is common and short-lived. No other treatment is needed.

Puerperal psychosis

There are three types of puerperal psychosis: (1) delirium; (2) affective; and (3) schiz-ophrenic. The clinical features of each of these syndromes are similar to those of the corresponding syndromes occurring outside the puerperium. Delirium used to be common before antibiotics were introduced to treat puerperal sepsis. Now it is rare.

Affective syndromes are more common than schizophrenic ones. Puerperal psy-chosis begins, typically, two to three days after delivery and nearly always in the first one to two post-partum weeks.

Puerperal psychosis occurs in about 1 in 500 births. It is more frequent among primiparous women, those who have suffered previous serious major psychiatric disorder, and those with a family history of psychiatric disorder. Puerperal psy-chosis is not more common after complicated deliveries.

Assessment As well as taking a *history* and examining the *mental state* in the usual way, it is essential to ascertain the mother's *ideas concerning the baby*. Severely depressed patients may have delusional ideas that the child is malformed or other-wise imperfect. Some patients with puerperal psychosis may attempt to kill the child to spare it from future suffering. A*ssessment of suicidal intent* is also important.

Treatment is as described for affective disorder and schizophrenia occurring outside pregnancy. For depressive disorders of marked or moderate severity, *ECT* is often the best treatment because its rapid effect enables the mother to resume the care of her baby quickly. When the disorder is not severe and the mother has no ideas of harm-ing herself or the baby, treatment can be at home with appropriate help to ensure the safe care of the baby. When the disorder is more severe, or there are ideas of harm to self or baby, the mother should usually be admitted to hospital, if possible to a special mother and baby unit. If antidepressant or antipsychotic drugs or lithium have to be prescribed, then breast-feeding will have to be stopped.

Prognosis Most patients recover fully from a puerperal psychosis but a few (most-ly those with a schizophrenic psychosis) remain chronically ill. At a subsequent birth, the recurrence rate for puerperal depressive illness is between 1 in 2 and 1 in 3 (compared with 1 in 500 for those without a previous puerperal psychosis). At least half the women with a puerperal depressive illness go on to develop a depressive illness unrelated to childbirth.

Treatment during subsequent pregnancies Women who have had a puerperal psychosis should be referred to a psychiatrist and monitored closely during sub-sequent delivery. Patients who have a history of bipolar disorder may require lithium prophylaxis, avoiding the first trimester and stopping soon after delivery.

Other puerperal depressive disorders

Depressive disorders of mild and moderate severity are much more common than puerperal psychoses, occurring in 10–15% of recently delivered women. This prevalence is little different to that in the general population of young women. Tiredness, irritability, and anxiety are often more prominent than depressive mood and there may be prominent phobic symptoms.

These disorders are caused mainly by the psychological adjustments required after childbirth, by loss of sleep, and by the hard work involved in the care of the baby. Some of these women have a history of psychiatric illness and some have experienced stressful events near the time of onset of the disorder.

Treatment Additional help with child care may be needed, together with counselling about any marital problems in looking after the infant. Antidepressant drugs are prescribed if there are 'biological' symptoms of depression.

Menstrual disorders

Premenstrual syndrome

This term denotes psychological and physical symptoms starting a few days before, and ending shortly after the onset of a menstrual period. The psychological symptoms include anxiety, irritability, and depression; the physical symptoms include breast tenderness, abdominal discomfort, and a feeling of distension. Estimates of the frequency of the premenstrual syndrome in the general population vary widely from 30% to 80% of women of reproductive age depending on the diagnostic criteria used. The cause is uncertain. Psychological factors may exacerbate distress and disability originating from physiological changes around menstruation.

Treatments Many have been tried, including progesterone, oral contraceptives, bromocriptine, diuretics, and psychotropic drugs. There is no convincing evidence that any of these treatments is generally effective, and randomized trials indicate a high placebo response. Psychological support and cognitive-behaviour treatment can be helpful in enabling women to cope with symptoms and the consequences in a positive way that enables them to feel more in control of their everyday life.

The menopause

Some menopausal women complain of physical symptoms of flushing, sweating, and vaginal dryness, and of headache, dizziness, and depression. Although there is a widespread belief that emotional problems are an inevitable part of the menopause, it is not certain whether psychological symptoms are more common in menopausal women than in other women of similar age. Depressive and anxiety-related symptoms around the time of the menopause could be related to hormonal changes but this has not been proved. Alternatively, or additionally, the symptoms could result from changes in the woman's role as her children leave home, her relationship with her husband alters, and her own parents become ill or die.

Treatment Oestrogens have been used but the results have been disappointing. Hormone replacement therapy (HRT) should not be seen as a treatment of depressive illness in those of menopausal age. Psychiatric disorders around the menopause should be treated as at other times of life.

Hysterectomy

It has been claimed that hysterectomy is more likely than other operations to be followed by depressive disorder. However, patients who are free from psychiatric symptoms before hysterectomy seldom develop them afterwards while most of those who are depressed after hysterectomy were depressed beforehand. Also, some who were depressed before the operation, recover afterwards. There is no reason, therefore, to withhold the operation for fear that it will cause depressive disorder, but it is important to detect depressive disorder in those seeking the operation, and treat this appropriately before making the final decision about surgery.

Sleep disorders

Insomnia

Insomnia is a common problem complained of by between 10% and 30% of the adult population. People vary in the amount of sleep they need, and many of those who complain of insomnia may be having as much sleep as others who do not complain and as much as they require physiologically. Some take 'catnaps' in the day often through boredom and still expect to sleep as long at night. In some, it is frequently secondary to other disorders, notably *painful physical conditions*, *depressive disorder*, *anxiety disorder*, and *dementia*. Other common causes are excessive use of *alcohol*, *caffeine*, or *tobacco*. Sleep may be disturbed for several weeks after stopping heavy drinking of alcohol (see Table 11.17).

Assessment In about 15% of cases of insomnia, no cause can be found ('*primary insomnia*').

The diagnosis of insomnia is usually based on the account given by the patient. Occasionally, EEG and other physiological recordings either in a sleep laboratory or at home are helpful when there is continuing doubt about the extent and nature of the insomnia. These observations often show that, despite the patient's complaint, sleeping time is within the normal range.

Treatment When insomnia is caused by a psychiatric or physical condition, the latter should be treated. When no such cause can be found it is useful to reassure the patient and emphasize the effectiveness of simple measures:

- encourage regular habits and exercise,
- discourage over-indulgence in tobacco, caffeine, and alcohol (especially before sleep);
- encourage a regular pattern of going to bed;
- avoid daytime sleep;
- advice on relaxation techniques for use if awake at night.

Although a hypnotic may be prescribed for a few nights at times of acute stress, demands for prolonged medication should be resisted. Withdrawal of hypnotics can lead to insomnia as distressing as the original sleep disturbance and continued use of hypnotics can impair performance during the day and lead to dependency.

Narcolepsy

This rare disorder usually begins between the ages of 10 and 20 years. Patients are extremely drowsy and have episodes of daytime sleep lasting about 15 minutes. Most patients have sudden temporary episodes of loss of muscle tone with paralysis (cataplexy), and a quarter experience episodes of paralysis on waking from sleep ('sleep paralysis'), and hypnagogic hallucinations. Some patients have secondary emotional and social difficulties which may be increased by other people's lack of understanding. Almost all cases of narcolepsy have the HLA type

Table 11.17.

Classification of sleep disorders

Insomnia
- related to a physical condition
- associated with a mental disorder
- associated with caffeine or alcohol
- primary insomnia

Hypersomnia
- Narcolepsy
- Hypersomnia related to a physical condition and medication (includes sleep apnoea, neurology)
- Primary idiopathic hypersomnia

Sleep–wake schedule disorder

Parasomnia*
- Nightmares
- Night terrors
- Sleepwalking

* See Chapter 19.

DR2 (compared with about a quarter of the general population), but it is not known how this relates to the cause of the condition.

There is no effective treatment. Patients should be referred to a specialist and encouraged to follow a regular routine with planned short periods of sleep during the day.

Idiopathic hypersomnia

Patients complain that they are unable to wake completely until several hours after getting up. During this time they feel confused and may be disorientated. They usually report prolonged and deep night-time sleep. The cause of the condition is unknown. Many patients respond to small doses of stimulant drugs. Specialist advice should be obtained.

Sleep apnoea

In this condition, daytime drowsiness occurs in association with excessive snoring and disturbed respiration at night, usually associated with upper airways obstruction. The typical patient is a middle-aged overweight man. Treatment consists of relieving the cause of the respiratory obstruction or the obesity. If this is not successful, continuous positive pressure ventilation using a face mask may be needed.

Sleep–wake schedule disorder

It is well known that fatigue and transient difficulty in sleeping accompany changes in bodily rhythms after travel across time zones or changes in shift work. Repeated changes from day to night work may lead to persistent poor sleep, fatigue, and impaired concentration. Management consists in organizing timetables and sleeping patterns as far as possible in an attempt to obtain fuller and more regular sleep. There is a role for melatonin in selected cases.

Parasomnias

Parasomnias are disturbances of behaviour occurring during sleep. These are: nightmares, night terrors, and sleepwalking. Since all are mainly problems of childhood they are discussed in Chapter 19.

Further reading

Fairburn, C. G. (1995). *Overcoming Binge Eating*. Guilford Press New York.
A practical account of the treatment of eating disorders.

Guthrie, E. and Creed, F. (1996). *Seminars in Liaison Psychiatry*. Gaskell.
Contains good reviews of all the main issues with an emphasis on treatment.

Creed, F., Mayou, R., and Hopkins, A. (1992). *Medical Symptoms Not Explained by Organic Disease*. Gaskell.
A practical account of general principles and common syndromes.

Wessely, S., Hotopf, M., and Sharpe, M. (1998). *Chronic Fatigue Syndromes*. Oxford University Press.
An authoritative review of physical, psychological, and social aspects of chronic fatigue syndrome.

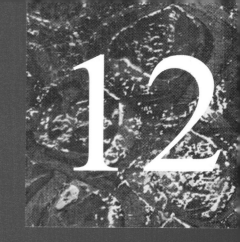

Suicide and deliberate self-harm

- Suicide and suicidal risk

- Deliberate self-harm

Suicide and deliberate self-harm

Many patients deliberately take drug overdoses or harm themselves in other ways. Some die (suicide); others survive (attempted suicide, parasuicide, or deliberate self-harm). The characteristics of those who kill themselves and those who harm themselves are rather different, although they overlap. The main clinical issues are the assessment of suicide risk and the management of deliberate self-harm.

Suicide accounts for about 1% of deaths. It is rare among children and uncommon in adolescents. Rates increase with age and are higher in men than in women. There are two sets of interacting causes: social factors, especially social isolation, and medical factors, among which depressive disorder, alcoholism, and abnormal personality are particularly important. **The assessment of suicide risk** depends on evaluating: (1) the presence of suicidal ideas; (2) presence of psychiatric disorder; (3) factors known to be associated with increased risk of suicide.

Referral is usually appropriate when the suicidal intentions are strong, associated psychiatric illness is severe, and the person lacks social support. If the risk does not seem to require hospital admission, their management depends on ensuring good support, telling the patient how to obtain help quickly if needed, and ensuring that all those who need to know are informed.

Deliberate self-harm is usually by drug overdose, but may be by self-injury, lacerations and also more dangerous methods such as jumping from a height, shooting, drowning.

The incidence of deliberate self-harm is commonest among young people but has been increasing in recent years at all ages. Predisposing factors include childhood difficulties, adverse social circumstances, and poor health. Precipitating factors such as stressful life events, including quarrels with spouses or other close relationships, are frequent. Only a minority have psychiatric disorder. The motives are complex and often uncertain. The act is frequently compulsive with no particular wish to die.

Up to a quarter of people who harm themselves do so again in the following year and the risk of suicide is about 1–2%, a hundred times the risk in the general population.

Assessment must include: (1) the risk of suicide; (2) the risk of further deliberate self-harm; (3) current medical and social problems. Those with severe psychiatric disorder require admission and others need continuing help from a psychiatric out-patient clinic, general practitioner, or other therapist. About a quarter require no special treatment.

Suicide and suicidal risk

Most completed suicides are planned and precautions against discovery are often taken. About one in six leaves a **suicide note**. Some notes are pleas for forgiveness. Other notes are accusing or vindictive, drawing attention to failings in relatives or friends. In most cases, some warning of intention is given to relatives or

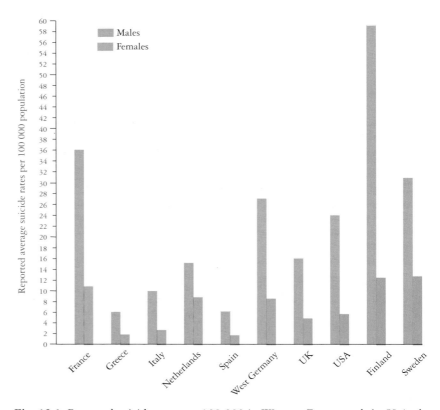

Fig. 12.1 Reported suicide rates per 100 000 in Western Europe and the United States (ages 25–44): 1986–8. (Reprinted with permission from Charlton *et al*. *Population Trends*, 71, 34–42, 1993.)

friends, or to doctors. There is a history of deliberate self-harm in between a third and a half of completed suicides.

It is important to understand the epidemiology and causes of suicide for several clinical reasons:

- As a basis for assessing suicidal risk.
- To help the relatives and others in the aftermath of suicide.
- As a guide to suicide prevention.

Epidemiology

In the UK where the suicide rate is about 10 per 100 000 per year (which is in the lower range of rates reported for Western countries see Fig. 12.1). Suicide accounts for about 1% of all deaths. However, official suicide statistics almost certainly underestimate the numbers of actual suicides because uncertain cases are not counted.

Suicide rates are highest in older people, in men, and those who are divorced or unmarried. In most countries, *drug overdoses* (especially analgesics and antidepressants) account for about two-thirds of suicides among women and about a third of those among men. The remaining deaths are by a variety of *physical means*: hanging, shooting, wounding; drowning, jumping from high places, and falling in front of moving vehicles or trains.

Causes of suicide

The large international, regional, and temporal variations in the prevalence of suicide reflect the importance of social causes. These interact with individual psychiatric and medical factors (Table 12.1). Psychiatric disorder is an important cause (in contrast to its lesser importance in deliberate self-harm). (see Table 12.2.)

Social causes

Social isolation Compared with the general population, people who have died by suicide are more likely to have been divorced, unemployed, or be living alone. Social isolation is a common factor among these associations.

Stressful events Suicide is often precipitated by stressful events, including bereavement and other losses.

Social factors influencing the method Social factors also influence the means chosen for suicide: thus a case that has attracted attention in a community or received wide publicity in newspapers or on television may be followed by others using the same method.

Table 12.1.
Causes of suicide

Social
- Old age
- Living alone
- Lack of family and other support
- Stressful events
- Publicity about suicides

Medical
- Depressive disorder
- Alcohol abuse
- Drug abuse
- Schizophrenia
- Personality disorder
- Chronic painful physical illness and epilepsy

Table 12.2.
Comparison of those who die by suicide and of those who harm themselves

	Suicide	Deliberate self-harm
Age	Older	Younger
Sex	More often male	More often female
Psychiatric disorder	Common, severe	Less common, less severe
Physical illness	Common	Uncommon
Planning	Careful	Impulsive
Method	Lethal	Less dangerous

Psychiatric and medical causes

Many of the people who die from suicide have some form of *psychiatric disorder* at the time of death, most often a depressive illness or alcohol dependence. Some have chronic, painful *physical illness*.

Depressive disorder The rate of suicide is increased in patients with depressive disorder with a lifetime risk of about 15% in severe cases. Depressed patients who commit suicide differ from other depressed patients in being older, more often *single, separated, or widowed* and having made more *previous suicide attempts*.

Alcohol abuse also carries a high risk of suicide. The risk is particularly great among: (i) older men with a long history of drinking, a current depressive disorder, and previous deliberate self-harm; and (ii) people whose drinking has caused physical complications, marital problems, difficulties at work, or arrests for drunkenness offences

Drug abuse also carries an increased risk of suicide.

Schizophrenia has a high risk of suicide with a lifetime risk of about 10%. The risk is particularly great in younger patients who have retained insight into the serious effect which the illness is likely to have on their lives.

Personality disorder is detected in a third to a half of people who die by suicide. Personality disorder is often associated with other factors that increase the risk of suicide, namely, abuse of alcohol or drugs and social isolation.

Chronic physical illness is associated with suicide, especially among the elderly.

Causes among special groups

Rational suicide Suicide is sometimes the rational act of a mentally healthy person. However, even if the decision appears to have been reached rationally, given more time and more information the person may change his intentions. For example, a person with cancer may change a decision to take his life when he learns that there is treatment to relieve pain. Doctors should try to bring about this change of mind, but some rational suicides will take place despite the best treatment.

Children and young adolescents Suicide is rare among children, and uncommon in adolescents although rates in older adolescents have increased recently. In adolescence, suicide is associated with broken homes, social isolation and depression, and also with impetuous behaviour and violence.

Doctors The suicide rate among doctors is greater than that in the general population. The reason is uncertain although several factors have been suggested, such as the ready availability of drugs, increased rates of addiction to alcohol and drugs, the extra stresses of work, reluctance to seek treatment for depressive disorders, and the selection into the medical profession of predisposed personalities.

Suicide pacts In a suicide pact, two people, usually in a close relationship in which one is dominant and the other is passive, agree that at the same time each will die by suicide. Such pacts, which are uncommon, have to be distinguished from murder followed by suicide (occurring sometimes when the murderer has a severe depressive disorder), and when one person survives. Suicide pact has to be distinguished from the aiding of suicide by a person who did not intend to die.

The assessment of suicide risk

Every doctor will encounter at some time, patients who express suicidal intentions and must be able to assess the risk of suicide (Table 12.3). This assessment requires:

- Evaluation of suicidal intentions.
- Assessment of any previous act of deliberate self-harm (see p. 252).

Table 12.3.

Risk factors for suicide

Intention	Evidence of intent to die
Psychiatric	Depression
	Schizophrenia
	Personality disorder
	Alcohol and drug dependence
Social and demographic	Older age
	Severe social and interpersonal stressors
	Isolation
Medical	Chronic painful illness and epilepsy

- Detection of psychiatric disorder.
- Assessment of other factors associated with increased risk of suicide.
- Assessment of factors associated with a reduced risk.
- In some cases, assessment of associated homicidal ideas.

Evaluation of intentions Some people fear that asking about *suicidal intentions* will make suicide more likely. It does not if the enquiries are made sympathetically. Indeed, if the person has thought of suicide he will feel better understood when the doctor raises the issue, and this feeling may reduce the risk. The interviewer can begin by asking whether the patient has thought that life is not worth living. This question can lead to more direct ones about thoughts of suicide, specific plans, and preparatory acts such as saving tablets. Table 12.4 shows a useful standard instrument—the Beck suicide intent scale—which combines these and other informative questions.

When suicidal intentions are revealed they should be taken seriously. There is no truth in the idea that people who talk of suicide do not enact it; on the contrary, two-thirds of people dying by suicide have told someone of their intentions. A few people speak repeatedly of suicide so that they are no longer taken seriously, but many of these people eventually kill themselves. Therefore their intentions should be evaluated carefully on every occasion.

Previous deliberate self-harm of any kind is an indicator of substantially increased risk of suicide. Certain features of previous self-harm are particularly important; these are summarized on p. 252 and in Table 12.8.

Detection of psychiatric disorder is an important part of the assessment of suicide risk. If possible an informant should be interviewed. *Depressive disorder* is highly important especially when there is severe mood change with hopelessness, insomnia, anorexia, weight loss, or delusions. It is important to remember that suicide may occur during recovery from a depressive disorder in patients who, when more severely depressed, had thought of the act but lacked initiative to carry it out. *Schizophrenia*, *personality disorder*, and *alcohol and drug dependence* also carry an increased risk of suicide.

Table 12.4.

Beck suicide intent scale

Circumstances related to suicidal attempt

1. Isolation	0 Somebody present
	1 Somebody nearby or in contact (as by phone)
	2 No one nearby or in contact
2. Timing	0 Timed so that intervention is probable
	1 Timed so that intervention is not likely
	2 Timed so that intervention is highly unlikely
3. Percautions against discovery and/or intervention	0 No precautions
	1 Passive precautions such as: avoiding others but doing nothing to prevent their intervention (alone in a room with unlocked door)
	2 Active precaution such as: locked door
4. Acting to gain help during/after attempt	0 Notified potential helper regarding the attempt
	1 Contacted but did not specifically notify potential helper regarding the attempt
	2 Did not contact or notify potential helper
5. Final acts in anticipation of death	0 None
	1 Partial preparation or ideation
	2 Definite plans made (changes in will, giving of gifts, taking out insurance)
6. Degree of planning for suicide attempt	0 No preparation
	1 Minimal preparation
	2 Extensive preparation
7. Suicide note	0 Absence of note
	1 Note written but torn up
	2 Presence of note
8. Overt communication of intent before act	0 None
	1 Equivocal communication
	2 Unequivocal communication
9. Purpose of attempt	0 Mainly to change environment
	1 Components of '0' and '2'
	2 Mainly to remove self from environment

Self-report

10. Expectations regarding fatality of act	0 Patient thought that death was unlikely
	1 Patient thought that death was possible but not probable
	2 Patient thought that death was probable or certain
11. Conception of method's lethality	0 Patient did less to himself than he thought would be lethal
	1 Patient wasn't sure, or did what he thought might be lethal
	2 Act equalled or exceeded patient's concept of its medical lethality

Table 12.4.

Beck suicide intent scale

12. 'Seriousness' of attempt	0	Patient did not consider act to be a serious attempt to end his life
	1	Patient was uncertain whether act was a serious attempt to end his life
	2	Patient considered act to be a serious attempt to end his life
13. Ambivalence towards living	0	Patient did not want to die
	1	Patient did not care whehter he lived or died
	2	Patient wanted to die
14. Conception of reversibility	0	Patient thought that death would be unlikely if he received medical attention
	1	Patient was uncertain whether death could be averted by medical attention
	2	Patient was certain of death even if he received medical attention
15. Degree of premeditation	0	None; impulsive
	1	Suicide contemplated for 3 hours or less prior to attempt
	2	Suicide contemplated for more than 3 hours prior to attempt

Reprinted with permission from Beck, A. T. *et al.* (1974). *The Prediction of Suicide.* Charles Press, Maryland.

Assessment of other general factors associated with increased risk of suicide These factors have been described above and summarized in Table 12.1 and include old age, loneliness, severe and intractable current life problems, and chronic painful illness or epilepsy.

Factors may be associated with a reduced risk These include the availability of good support from the family and others to assist with social, practical, and emotional difficulties.

Homicidal ideas in suicidal patients A few severely depressed suicidal patients have homicidal ideas; for example, the idea that it would be an act of mercy to kill the spouse or a child, in order to spare that person intolerable suffering. If present, such ideas should be taken extremely seriously since they may be carried into practice. It is especially important to be aware of the dangers with mothers of small children.

Management of a patient at risk of suicide

The risk of suicide should be considered in any patient who is depressed or whose behaviour or talk gives any suggestion of the possibility of self-harm. In hospital, in-patient or emergency departments, evidence of suicidal intent should normally lead to obtaining advice from a specialist. However, other medical staff need to be aware of the general principles of assessment, especially with patients who are reluctant to stay and who are medically fit.

In primary care, *referral* to a psychiatrist is usually appropriate when:

- suicidal intentions are clearly expressed;
- associated psychiatric illness is severe;
- the person lacks social support.

Exceptions to the general principles of admission may be made when the patient lives with reliable relatives, who wish to care for the patient, understand their responsibilities, and are able to fulfil them. In these circumstances, a psychiatric opinion is very often useful. If hospital treatment is essential but the patient refuses it, compulsory admission will be necessary.

A number of patients remain a *long-term suicidal risk* but despite specialist assessment and treatment and in whom there are no indications that hospital treatment would be of benefit. An example would be a patient with long-standing problems who has had intensive psychiatric and social help, and in whom it is evident that hospital admission would do nothing to help with the long-term problems in everyday life. Such a decision requires a particularly thorough knowledge of the patient and his problems and should generally be made by a psychiatrist in conjunction with the general practitioner.

The main principles of treatment are:

1. **Prevention of harm** The obvious first requirement is to prevent the patient from self-harm by preventing access to methods of harm and appropriately close observation.

    Most patients at serious suicidal risk require *admission to hospital*. The first requirement is the safety of the patient. To achieve this requires an adequate number of vigilant nursing staff, an agreed assessment of the level of risk and good communication between staff. If the risk is very great, nursing may need to be continuous so that the patient is never alone.

    If *out-patient treatment* is chosen the patient and relatives should be told how to obtain help quickly if the strength of suicidal ideas increases, for example an emergency telephone number. Frustrated attempts to find help can make suicide more likely.

2. **Treatment of any associated mental illness** should be initiated without delay.

3. **Reviving hope** However determined the patient is to die, there is usually some remaining wish to live. These positive feelings can be encouraged and the patient helped towards a more positive view of the future. One way of doing this is to show concern for the problems.

4. **Problem solving** Initially, overwhelming problems can be dealt with one by one.

Help after a suicide

When a person has died by suicide, help is required by surviving relatives and friends who may need to deal with feelings of loss, guilt, or anger. They should have a full explanation of the nature and reasons for medical and other actions to assess the suicidal risk, to treat the causes and prevent harm. They should also have an opportunity to discuss their own feelings, including guilt that if they had behaved differently the suicide could have been prevented. Those most directly involved in the previous care of the dead person should offer to meet the relatives as soon after the suicide as possible and to meet again at a later stage if the family and friends believe it would be helpful. The relatives' distress may be considerable and may be expressed indirectly in complaints about medical care. Some relatives suffer from longstanding or psychiatric or other problems which deserve treatment in their own right.

The doctor should also support other professional staff who had been closely involved with the patient. After suicide, the case should be reviewed carefully to determine whether useful lessons can be learnt about future clinical practice. This review should not be conducted as a search for a person at fault; some patients die by suicide however carefully the correct procedures have been followed.

Suicide prevention

There are two main approaches to prevention, *early recognition* and *help for those at risk* and modification of predisposing social factors.

• *Identifying high-risk patients*. Many people who commit suicide have contacted their doctors shortly beforehand, and many of these have a psychiatric disorder, or alcohol dependence. Doctors can *identify some high-risk patients*, and offer help.

• *Supporting those at risk*. Helping agencies like the Samaritans give *support to lonely and hopeless* people who express suicidal ideas, but it has not been shown convincingly that they reduce suicide.

• *Reducing the means* may help reduce suicide (e.g. providing safety rails at high places, prescribing cautiously). However, people determined on suicide can find other means, such as overdoses of non-prescribed drugs.

• *Education* might be provided for teenagers about the dangers of drug overdosage and discussion of ways of coping with common emotional problems. However, there is little evidence that such education is effective.

• *Public health or social and economic policy.* Isolation and other social factors which increase the risk of suicide cannot be prevented by the medical profession they require public policy decision.

Deliberate self-harm

Deliberate self-harm is not usually failed suicide. Only about a quarter of those who have deliberately harmed themselves say they wished to die; most say the act was impulsive rather than premeditated. The rest find it difficult to explain the reasons or say that:

• they were *seeking* unconsciousness as a temporary escape from their problems;

• they were trying to *influence* another person (e.g. making the partner feel guilty for threatening to end the relationship);

• that they are uncertain whether or not they intended to die—they were 'leaving it to fate'.

When behaviour is carried out to influence another person or as a general signal of distress it is sometimes referred to as a 'cry for help'.

Epidemiology Deliberate self-harm is common and rates have risen progressively over the last thirty years. It now accounts for about 10% of acute medical *admissions* in the UK. A further smaller number are seen by general practitioners but not sent to hospital because the medical risks are low, or attend emergency departments but are not admitted.

Epidemiological studies have shown the kind of people who are more likely to harm themselves and the methods that are common. Deliberate self-harm is more common among:

- **Younger adults** the rates decline sharply in middle age. (They are also very low in children under the age of 12 years.)
- **Women**, particularly those aged 15–25 years (the sex difference is less marked in older people).
- **People of low socioeconomic status**.
- **Divorced individuals, teenage wives, and younger single people**.

Methods of deliberate self-harm

Drug overdosage In the UK, about 90% of the cases of deliberate self-harm treated by general hospitals are by a drug overdose. The drugs taken most commonly in overdose are **anxiolytics, non-opiate analgesics**, such as salicylates and paracetamol, and antidepressants. Paracetamol is particularly dangerous because it damages the liver and may lead to the delayed death, sometimes in patients who had not taken the drugs with the intention of dying. **Antidepressants** are taken in about a fifth of cases: of these drugs, tricyclics are particularly hazardous in overdosage since they may cause cardiac arrhythmias or convulsions. Despite these and other dangers, most deliberate drug overdoses do not present a serious threat to life.

The use of alcohol About half the men and a quarter of the women who harm themselves have taken alcohol in the six hours before the act. This often precipi-

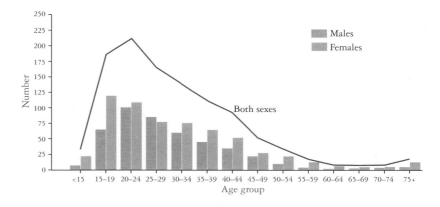

Fig 12.2 Self-harm. Age groups of DSH patients by gender (1986). (Reproduced by permission of Professor K. E. Hawton, Oxford University.)

tates the act by resulting in lack of restraint. Subsequently, its effects interact with those of the drugs.

Self-injury In the UK, between 5% and 15% of all deliberate self-harm treated in general hospitals are self-inflicted injuries. Most of these injuries are lacerations, usually of the forearm or wrists. Most patients who cut themselves are young, have low self-esteem with impulsive or aggressive behaviour, unstable moods, difficulty in interpersonal relationships, and often problems of alcohol or drug abuse. Usually, the self-laceration follows a period of increasing tension and irritability, which is relieved by the self-injury. The cuts are usually multiple and superficial, often made with a razor blade or a piece of glass.

Less frequent forms of self-injury are medically more serious lacerations, jumping from heights or in front of a moving train or motor vehicle, shooting, or drowning. These highly dangerous acts occur mainly among people who intended to die but have survived.

Causes

Deliberate self-harm is usually the result of multiple social and personal factors (Table 12.5), including national and local attitudes. Overall, rates are clearly affected by awareness of the occurrence and methods of self-harm in a population; for example, television and press reports and local knowledge of suicide and attempted suicide in the neighbourhood. Psychiatric disorder is less important than in suicide.

Social and family factors

Predisposing factors Evidence of childhood emotional deprivation is common. Many patients who harm themselves have long-term marital problems, extramarital relationships, or other relationship problems, and may have financial and other social difficulties. Rates of unemployment are greater than in the general population.

Precipitating factors Stressful life events are frequent before the act of self-harm, especially quarrels with or threats of rejection by spouses, or sexual partners.

Association with psychiatric disorder

Although many patients who harm themselves are anxious or depressed, relatively few have a psychiatric disorder other than an acute stress reaction, adjustment disorder, or personality disorder. The latter is found in about a third to a half of self-harm patients, and dependence on alcohol is also frequent. (In contrast, psychiatric disorder is common among patients who die by suicide, see p. 245.)

The difference between factors associated with suicide and deliberate self-harm are summarized in Table 12.2 (p. 243).

Outcome

Since deliberate self-harm results from long-term adverse social factors and is associated with personality disorder, it is not surprising that a significant proportion of subjects have a poor overall outcome in terms of the personal and social adjustment (Table 12.6). More specifically, outcome is assessed in terms of repetition of self-harm and of suicide. Between 15% and 25% of people who harm themselves

Table 12.5.
Causes of deliberate self-harm

Psychiatric disorder
Personality disorder
Alcohol dependence
Predisposing social factors
Early parental loss
Parental neglect or abuse
Long-term social problems: family, employment, financial
Poor physical health
Precipitating social factors
Stressful life problems

Table 12.6.
Outcome in self-harm

- In-patient psychiatric care
- Continuing psychiatric and social out-patient care
- Repetition of deliberate self-harm
- Subsequent suicide
- Long-term psychiatric problems
- Long-term impaired quality of life

Table 12.7.

Factors predicting the repetition of deliberate self-harm

- Deliberate self-harm before the current episode
- Previous psychiatric treatment
- Alcohol or drug abuse
- Antisocial personality disorder
- Criminal record
- Low social class
- Unemployment

do so again (Table 12.7) in the following year and 1–2% commit suicide. Of those who harm themselves again:

- some repeat the act only once;
- some repeat several times within a period in which there are continuing severe stressful events;
- a few repeat many times over a long period as a habitual response to minor stressors.

The factors associated with repetition of deliberate self-harm are shown in Table 12.7.

People who have deliberately harmed themselves have a much increased risk of later suicide. In the year after the self-harm, the risk of suicide is about 1–2%, that is, about 100 times the risk in the general population. The risk factors are shown in Table 12.8.

It is important to note that a *non-dangerous method of self-harm does not necessarily indicate a low risk* of subsequent suicide (although the risk is higher when a violent or dangerous method has been used).

Table 12.8.

Factors predicting suicide after deliberate self-harm

Evidence of intent	Evidence of serious intent (see Table 12.9)
	Continuing wish to die
	Previous acts of deliberate self harm
Psychiatric disorder	Depressive disorder
	Alcoholism or drug abuse
	Antisocial personality disorder
Social and demographic	Social isolation
	Unemployment
	Older age group
	Male sex

Assessment

Every act of deliberate self-harm should be assessed thoroughly. In many cases, for patients seen in general practice, the consequences of the act and concern about the result of repetition will lead to hospital referral. In some cases, referral may not be necessary, for instance, when the act was not reported until some time later, where there is good evidence of lack of medical seriousness and of suicidal intent, and where the patient and family are known to the doctor.

All deliberate self-harm patients seen in hospital emergency departments should have a psychiatric and social assessment. This assessment can be carried out by a psychiatrist, by general medical staff, or by psychiatric nurses or social workers with appropriate special training, or by a psychiatrist. All patients found on this assessment to be suffering from psychiatric disorder or with a high risk of further self-harm should be seen by a psychiatrist. Since many patients who are medically fit may not wish to stay for specialist assessment, it is essential that all emergency department medical staff are competent to assess risk.

Steps in assessment

The assessment should be carried out in a way that encourages the patient to undertake a constructive review of his problems and of the ways he can deal with them. If the patient can resolve his present problems in this way, he may do so again in the future instead of resorting to self-harm again.

When to assess When the patient has recovered sufficiently from the physical effects of the self-harm he should be interviewed, if possible, where he will not be overheard or interrupted. After a drug overdose, the first step is to determine whether consciousness is impaired; if so, the interview should be delayed until the patient has recovered further and can concentrate on the questions.

Sources of information Information should be obtained also from relatives or friends, the general practitioner, and any other person (such as a social worker) already involved in the patient's care. Such information frequently adds significantly to the account given by the patient. The following issues should be considered.

Information required

1. What were the patient's intentions before and at the time of the attempt? Patients who intended to die as a result of the act of self-harm are at greater risk of a subsequent fatal act of self-harm (see Table 12.9 and Fig. 12.3).

- Was the act *planned* or carried out on impulse?

- Were *precautions* taken against being found?

- *Did the patient seek help?*

- *Was the method dangerous?* Not only should the objective risk be assessed, but also the risk anticipated by the patient, which may be different (e.g. if he believed that he had taken a lethal dose of a drug when in fact he had not).

- *Was there a 'final act'* such as writing a suicide note or making a will?

2. Does the patient now wish to die? The interviewer should ask directly whether the patient is pleased to have recovered or wishes to die. If the act suggested serious suicidal intent, but the patient denies such intent, the interviewer should try to find out by tactful but thorough questioning whether there has been a genuine change of resolve.

3. What are the current problems? Many patients will have experienced a mounting series of difficulties in the weeks or months leading up to the act of self-harm. Some of these difficulties may have been resolved by the time the patient is interviewed, but if serious problems remain, the risk of a fatal repetition is greater. This risk is particularly great if the problems are of loneliness or ill-health. Possible problems should be reviewed systematically covering: *intimate relationships* with the spouse or another person; *relations with children and other relatives; employment, finance,* and *housing; legal problems; social isolation; bereavement,* and *other losses.*

Table 12.9.
Circumstances of self-harm suggesting high suicidal intent

- Planning in advance
- Precautions to avoid discovery
- No attempts to obtain help afterwards
- Dangerous method
- 'Final acts'

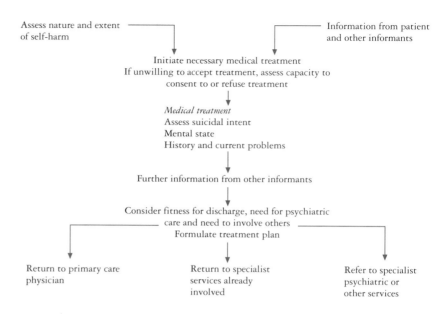

Fig. 12.3 Self-harm: action in the emergency department.

4. Is there psychiatric disorder? This question is answered with information obtained from the history, from a brief but systematic examination of the mental state, and also from other informants and medical notes.

5. What are the patient's resources? These include the capacity to solve problems; material resources; and the help that others may provide. The best guide to future ability to solve problems is the past record of dealing with difficulties such as the loss of a job, or a broken relationship. The availability of help should be assessed by asking about the patient's friends and relatives, and about support available from medical services, social workers, or voluntary agencies.

6. Is treatment required and will the patient agree to it?

Management

Management aims to:

- treat any psychiatric disorder;
- manage high suicide risk;
- enable the patient to *resolve difficulties* that led to the act of self-harm; and
- *deal with future crises* without resorting to self-harm.

Of the patients referred to hospital for treatment of deliberate self-harm:

(1)   About 1 in 10 need immediate in-patient psychiatric treatment, usually for a depressive disorder or alcohol dependency; or for a period of respite from overwhelming stressors.

(2)   About two-thirds need care from a psychiatric out-patient team or from the general practitioner (but many do not accept this help).

(3)   About a quarter require no special treatment because their self-harm was a response to temporary difficulties and carried little risk of repetition.

The mainstay of treatment is *problem solving* (see p. 365) based on the list of problems compiled during the assessment. The patient is encouraged to consider what steps he could take to resolve each of these problems, and to formulate a practical plan for tackling one at a time. Throughout this discussion, the therapist helps the patient to do as much as possible to help himself. When there are interpersonal problems, it is often helpful to have a joint or family discussion.

The results of treatment

Successful treatment of a depressive or other psychiatric disorder reduces the risk of subsequent self-harm. The evidence is less strong that problem solving and other psychological methods reduce repetition, although they do reduce personal and social problems. This lack of strong evidence may be due, in part, to the methodological difficulties of randomized trials in this heterogeneous population.

Several controlled trials with subgroups of particular types of psychological or social problem have been shown to benefit from specific treatments, such as marital therapy for problems between couples, problem solving for practical and everyday difficulties, and cognitive-behaviour treatment for longstanding personal difficulties.

Management of special groups

There are a number of subgroups of patients who pose special management problems. In most cases, specialist advice should be obtained.

Mothers of young children Because there is an association between deliberate self-harm and child abuse, it is important to ask about any mother with young children about her feelings towards the children; and to enquire from other informants, as well as the patient, about their welfare. If there is a possibility of child abuse or neglect, appropriate assessment action should be carried out (see p. 420).

Children and adolescents Deliberate self-harm is uncommon among young children, but becomes increasingly frequent after the age of 12, especially among girls. The most common method is drug overdosage: and in only a few cases is there a threat to life. Self-injury also occurs, more often among boys than girls.

The motivation of self-harm in young children is difficult to determine, but it is more often to communicate distress or escape from stress—than to die. Deliberate self-harm in children and adolescents is associated with broken homes, family psychiatric disorder, and child abuse. It is often precipitated by difficulties with parents, boyfriends or girlfriends, or school work.

Most children and adolescents do not repeat an act of deliberate self-harm, but an important minority do so, usually in association with severe psychosocial problems. These repeated acts of deliberate self-harm carry a significant risk of suicide. Children or adolescents who harm themselves should be assessed by a child psychiatrist. Treatment is not only of the young person but also of the family.

Patients who refuse assessment and treatment Some patients try to leave hospital before emergency gastric lavage and other treatment. Others seek to do so slightly later before psychological assessment can be completed.

In most countries, there is a legal power to detain those who require potentially life-saving treatment and whose competence or capacity to take an informed decision about discharge is likely to be impaired by their mental state. The doctor should obtain as much information as time allows. The patient should only be allowed to leave hospital when serious suicidal risk has been excluded.

In taking decisions about emergency treatment, the doctor is likely to be helped by relatives, in-patient medical notes, by telephoning the primary care doctor and any other doctor, social worker, or person who has been involved in the past. It is essential to write detailed notes and to be aware of the legal requirements.

Frequent repeaters Some people take overdoses repeatedly often at times of stress in circumstances that suggest that the behaviour to reduce tension or gain attention. These people usually have a personality disorder and many insoluble social problems. Although sometimes directed towards gaining attention, repeated self-harm may cause relatives to become unsympathetic or hostile, and these feelings may be shared by professional staff as their repeated efforts at help are seen to fail. Usually, neither counselling nor intensive psychotherapy is effective, and management is limited to providing support. Sometimes a change in life circumstances is followed by an improvement, but unless this happens the risk of death by suicide is high.

Deliberate self-laceration It is difficult to help people who lacerate themselves repeatedly. These patients often have low self-esteem and experience extreme tension. The patient often has difficulty in recognizing feelings and expressing them in words. Efforts should be made to increase self-esteem and to find an alternative simple way of relieving tension, for example, by taking exercise. Anxiolytic drugs are seldom helpful and may produce disinhibition. If drug treatment is needed to reduce tension, a phenothiazine is more likely to be effective.

Further reading

Hawton, K. and Catalan, J. (1987). *Attempted Suicide: A Practical Guide to its Nature and Management*. Oxford University Press.
Chapters 1–3 include a review of the nature and causes of the condition: Chapter 4 discusses assessment: the remaining chapters consider treatment.

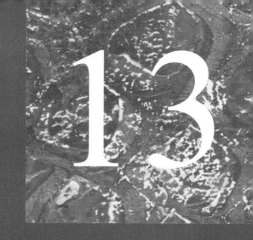

13

Problems due to use of alcohol and other psychoactive substances

- Problems due to the use of alcohol

- Treatment of the problem drinker

- Problems due to use of psychoactive substances

Problems due to use of alcohol and other psychoactive substances

This chapter is about the medical conditions caused by the use of alcohol, psychoactive drugs, and certain other chemical substances. Health problems may arise following substance use due to:

- **Intoxication** The psychological and physical effects of the substance which disappear when the substance is eliminated.
- **Withdrawal** Symptoms and signs occurring when the substance is reduced or stopped. The nature, time to onset, and course of the symptoms vary for different substances.
- **Tolerance** The state in which repeated administration leads to decreasing effect.
- **Dependence** A syndrome that includes withdrawal states, sometimes tolerance, and other features such as persistent use despite harmful effects. Dependence may be both *physical* (physiological tolerance occurs) and *psychological*. A person is said to have a *dependence syndrome if* they have experienced three of the following characteristics in the past twelve months:

  1. A strong desire or sense of compulsion to take the substance.

  2. Difficulties in refraining from using the substance, stopping using it, or limiting the amount taken.

  3. A physiological *withdrawal* state when substance use has stopped or been reduced. Withdrawal symptoms may be avoided by further use of the substance.

  4. Evidence of *tolerance*, a state in which increasing doses of the substance are required to produce the effect originally produced by lower doses.

  5. Progressive neglect of alternative pleasures or interests due to the use of the psychoactive substance and in the time needed to obtain supplies, or to recover from its effects.

  6. Persistent use of the substance despite clear evidence of harm.

Problems due to substance use are very common. Doctors in all branches of medicine need to know how to recognize and manage its the various manifestations.

Problems due to the use of alcohol

Terminology

Although the term *alcoholism* is widely used in everyday speech, it has too broad a meaning to be clinically useful. It can refer to excessive consumption of alcohol, to dependence on alcohol, or to the damage caused by excessive use. The following terms define more useful categories:

- **Harmful use of alcohol** refers to a pattern of use that has caused actual mental or physical damage to the user.
- **Dangerous use** refers to a level of consumption which increases the risk of future harm (see below).
- **Problem drinking** is drinking that has caused mental, physical, or social harm but not necessarily dependence.

Central to these categories is the concept of **alcohol-related disability**, which refers to any mental, physical, or social harm resulting from excessive alcohol consumption. Both **harmful** and **dangerous** use may exist together; for example, a drinker who has already damaged his health may continue to drink heavily in a way that will cause more damage in the future. We will refer collectively to dangerous use, harmful use, and alcohol dependence as **alcohol problems.**

What is a safe level of alcohol consumption?

The relation between alcohol consumption and harm is not straightforward. Low levels of alcohol consumption may protect older people against coronary heart disease. So what is a safe level of alcohol consumption? Despite the difficulties in assessing the relation between level of intake and harmful effects, certain 'safe levels' are widely accepted. These are expressed in terms of **units** of alcohol; one unit is 8 grams of ethanol, and corresponds to the following measures in which alcohol is usually consumed:

- half a pint of beer
- a wine glass of wine
- a sherry glass of sherry or other fortified wine
- a standard measure of spirits.

These measures are clinically useful but should not be regarded as precise because the strengths of different beers and wines vary.

In these terms, the 'safe level' of alcohol consumption is:

- *Men*:   up to **21 units** per week;
- *Women*:   up to **14 units** per week (lower because of the lower average body weight of females;

provided that the whole amount is not taken on one occasion and that there are occasional drink-free days. This level is equivalent, for example, to an average of three half pints of beer a day for a man. These limits should be modified in some patients, for example, pregnant women should be advised to abstain from alcohol.

Dangerous levels of drinking (i.e. levels of consumption at which harm is likely) are:

- *Men*:   over **50 units** per week
- *Women*:   over **35 units** per week

Levels of drinking between the safe and dangerous amounts are called **hazardous**. In this chapter, for simplicity, we will refer to hazardous and dangerous use as dangerous use.

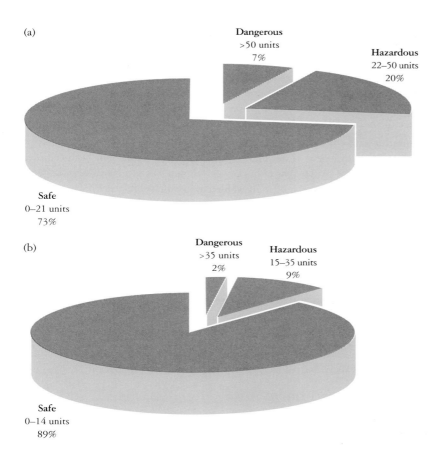

Fig. 13.1 Reported alcohol consumption in England and Wales: (a) men; (b) women. (Source: *General Household Survey*, HMSO, London 1996.)

Alcohol consumption in the population

Reliable epidemiological data are difficult to obtain because people tend to be evasive about the amount they drink and the consequences of their drinking. However, the General Household Survey in the UK includes questions on alcohol consumption (Fig. 13.1). The majority of the population report safe levels of consumption with a minority drinking more heavily. Records of the national consumption of alcohol reveal marked international variations in alcohol consumption per capita. European countries such as France and Italy have higher levels of consumption than countries such as the USA and UK—although the differences are decreasing with time. Countries with higher alcohol consumption have higher death rates from cirrhosis of the liver. Dangerous use of alcohol has increased among young women as their social roles have changed.

Factors associated with high alcohol consumption

Several factors are associated with the consumption of greater amounts of alcohol by individuals.

Population levels of consumption The higher the average consumption in a community, the greater the number of people who drink dangerous amounts of alcohol. This is because the consumption of alcohol in the general population is normally distributed—and the higher average is not due to a group of very heavy drinkers. This has an important practical implication. It means that population-based methods aimed at reducing everyone's level of alcohol consumption will reduce the number of people who drink dangerous amounts of alcohol (see below).

Age and sex The heaviest drinkers are among young men in their late teens and early twenties. In recent years, increased consumption of alcohol has been identified among 15- to 16-year-olds. Fewer women than men drink dangerous amounts of alcohol, but the rates in women are rising more quickly than in men. Women in professional and managerial employment are most likely to drink hazardous or dangerous amounts of alcohol.

Occupation The rates of dangerous consumption of alcohol are much increased among people working in occupations that provide easy access to alcohol, for example barmen, brewery workers, and kitchen porters. They are also higher among executives, salesmen, journalists, and actors, and others whose work is associated with social drinking. Doctors also have high rates of dangerous consumption.

Genetic factors Harmful drinking runs in families but this could be because of social factors. The evidence from twin studies is conflicting.

Personality factors such as anxiety and impulsiveness are suggested by clinical experience, but there is little good evidence for such an association.

Alcohol-related harm

Consumption of alcohol can lead to three types of harm (each of which is described later):

(1)   physical;

(2)   psychological; and

(3)   social.

This harm can occur whether or not the person has become dependent on alcohol, although very high levels of consumption are likely to cause dependency. The mechanisms of alcohol related harm are:

- **Intoxication** This includes a *direct toxic effect* on certain tissues, notably the brain and liver and an increased *risk of accidents* (particularly road traffic accidents and accidents in the home) and *public order offences*,

- **Chronic consumption** This may lead to poor diet and *deficiency of protein* and *B vitamins*, and *general neglect* which can lead to increased susceptibility to infection.

- **Dependence** When present, this may lead to serious withdrawal syndromes (see below).

Physical effects of alcohol abuse (Table 13.1)

The main physical consequences of dangerous use of alcohol (Table 13.1) are:

- **Gastrointestinal disorders** These are common, notably gastritis and peptic ulcer; damage to the liver; oesophageal varices and carcinoma;

Table 13.1.

Physical effects of excessive use of alcohol

Alimentary	Gastritis and peptic ulcer
	Oesophageal varices
	Oesophageal carcinoma
	Acute and chronic pancreatitis
	Hepatitis and cirrhosis
Neurological	Peripheral neuropathy
	Dementia
	Cerebellar degeneration
	Epilepsy
Other	Anaemia
	Episodic hypoglycaemia
	Haemochromatosis
	Cardiomyopathy
	Myopathy
	Obesity

and acute or chronic pancreatitis. Damage to the liver includes fatty infiltration, hepatitis, cirrhosis, and hepatoma. A person dependent on alcohol has a 10-fold greater risk than average of dying of cirrhosis of the liver.

- **Disorders of the nervous system** These include peripheral neuropathy; dementia; cerebellar degeneration; and epilepsy; as well as several less common effects on the optic nerve, pons, and corpus callosum. Neuropsychiatric disorders are described below.

- **Other physical disorders** include anaemia; episodic hypoglycaemia; haemochromatosis; cardiomyopathy; and myopathy.

From these and other causes, the overall *mortality rate* of subjects consuming dangerous levels of alcohol is estimated to be about twice the expected level.

Effects on the fetus

Very heavy drinking during pregnancy may cause a syndrome of facial abnormality, low weight, low intelligence, and overactivity (*fetal alcohol syndrome*). It is uncertain whether such effects are seen only after very heavy drinking by the mother, or whether lesser degrees of damage are seen after less heavy drinking. Nevertheless, it is prudent to advise pregnant women to abstain from alcohol throughout pregnancy; if they will not accept this advice, they should be counselled strongly to avoid drinking in the first trimester, and to avoid heavy drinking.

Neuropsychiatric disorders (Table 13.2)

Alcohol-related psychiatric disabilities fall into four groups: (1) abnormal forms of intoxication; (2) withdrawal phenomena; (3) chronic or nutritional disorders; and (4) associated psychiatric disorders.

Table 13.2.

Neuropsychiatric effects of excessive use of alcohol

Intoxication states	Memory blackouts
	Idiosyncratic intoxication
Withdrawal states	Delirium tremens
Toxic and nutritional states	Korsakov's syndrome
	Wernicke's encephalopathy
	Alcoholic dementia
Associated states	Depressive disorder
	Anxiety symptoms
	Suicide and deliberate self-harm
	Personality change
	Pathological jealousy
	Sexual dysfunction
	Transient hallucinations
	Alcoholic hallucinosis

1. Abnormal forms of intoxication As well as the familiar picture of drunkenness, people who consume dangerous amounts of alcohol persistently may develop two syndromes.

1. **Memory blackouts** are losses of memory for events that occurred during a period of intoxication. Such episodes can occur after a single episode of heavy drinking in people who do not habitually abuse alcohol. When they occur regularly they indicate frequent heavy drinking; when they are prolonged, affecting the greater part of a day or whole days, they indicate sustained excessive drinking.

2. **Idiosyncratic intoxication** (or pathological drunkenness) is a marked change of behaviour occurring within minutes of taking alcohol in amounts that would not induce drunkenness in most people. Often, the behaviour is aggressive. The condition is rare although apparent cases may occur after a small further intake of alcohol in a person who already has a raised blood alcohol from unadmitted drinking.

2. Withdrawal phenomena These are described on p. 266.

3. Toxic and nutritional conditions There are three neuropsychiatric disorders of this kind: (1) *Korsakov's syndrome*; (2) *Wernicke's encephalopathy*; and (3) *alcoholic dementia*. (The first two are described in Chapter 11, pp. 195–6, because alcohol is not their only cause.)

Alcoholic dementia can arise after prolonged heavy intake of alcohol. Intellectual impairment is often associated with enlarged ventricles and widened cerebral sulci seen on a CT (computerized tomography) scan. After prolonged abstinence, some gradual improvement occurs in these changes, suggesting that the shrinkage is not wholly due to the loss of the brain cells. The *causes* of the dementia are uncertain but probably include a direct toxic effect of alcohol on the brain, and secondary effects of liver disease.

4. Associated psychiatric disorders

- **Depressive disorder** can be induced by prolonged dangerous use of alcohol, but depressed patients sometimes drink heavily to relieve their symptoms, so care needs to be taken to find out the sequence of changes.

- **Anxiety symptoms** occur commonly, especially during periods of partial withdrawal. However, some patients with an anxiety disorder with other causes, drink to relieve anxiety. So, as with depression, care is needed to determine the sequence.

- **Suicidal behaviour and deliberate self-harm** are more frequent among people who use alcohol heavily than among other people of the same age. Estimates of the proportion of harmful users of alcohol who eventually kill themselves vary from 6% to 20%.

- **Personality change** in heavy users of alcohol often includes self-centredness, lack of concern for others, and a decline in standards of conduct, particularly honesty and responsibility.

- **Pathological jealousy** is an infrequent but serious complication of heavy alcohol use. (It is described on pp. 179–81.) Non-delusional suspiciousness of the sexual partner is more common.

- **Sexual dysfunction** is common, usually as erectile dysfunction or delayed ejaculation. The causes include the direct effects of alcohol, and a generally impaired relationship with the sexual partner as a result of heavy drinking.

- **Transient hallucinations** of vision or hearing are reported by some heavy drinkers, generally during withdrawal, but without all the features of delirium tremens or alcoholic hallucinosis.

- **Alcoholic hallucinosis** is a rare condition characterized by distressing *auditory hallucinations*, usually of voices uttering threats, occurring *in clear consciousness*. Some patients argue aloud with the voices, others feel compelled to follow instructions from them. *Delusional misinterpretations* may follow, often of a persecutory kind, so that the clinical picture can resemble schizophrenia. The condition can arise while the person is still drinking heavily, or when intake has been reduced. It is of variable duration and when chronic needs to be distinguished from a primary schizophrenic disorder.

Social damage due to alcohol

Excessive drinking can cause serious **social damage** including:

1. Family violence.

2. Emotional and conduct problems in the patient's children.

3. Poor work performance and sickness absence.

4. Unemployment.

5. Road accidents. In the UK about a third of drivers killed on the road have blood alcohol levels above the statutory limit, and among those killed on a Saturday night the figure is estimated to be three-quarters.

6. Crime, mainly social disorder and petty offences, but also with fraud, sexual offences, and crimes of violence including murder.

The alcohol withdrawal syndrome

Withdrawal symptoms appear characteristically on waking, after the fall in blood alcohol concentration during sleep.

- The earliest and commonest feature is acute *tremulousness* affecting the hands, legs, and trunk ('the shakes'). The sufferer may be unable to sit still, hold a cup steady, or do up buttons. He is also *agitated* and easily startled, and often dreads facing people or crossing the road.

- *Nausea, retching, and sweating* are frequent. If alcohol is taken, these symptoms may be relieved quickly; it not, they may last for several days.

- As withdrawal progresses, *misperceptions and hallucinations* may occur, usually only briefly. Objects appear distorted in shape, or shadows seems to move; disorganized voices, shouting, or snatches of music may be heard.

- Later there may be *epileptic seizures*, and finally, after about 48 hours, *delirium tremens* may develop.

Delirium tremens This is a severe form of withdrawal syndrome which occurs when the patient is physically dependent on alcohol. The features are:

- *Those seen in any delirium*: clouding of consciousness, disorientation in time and place, impairment of recent memory, illusions and hallucinations (see below), fearfulness and agitation

- Special features of gross *tremor* of the hands (which gives the condition its name), *autonomic disturbance* (sweating, tachycardia, raised blood pressure, dilation of the pupils), and marked *insomnia*. There may also be *fever*.

- *Hallucinations* are characteristically visual and often frightening, involving people or animals. Auditory and tactile hallucinations also occur.

- *Dehydration and electrolyte disturbance* are characteristic. Blood testing shows leucocytosis, a raised erythrocycte sedimentation rate (ESR), and impaired liver function.

Delirium tremens usually last three to four days. As in other kinds of delirium (see pp. 187–9), the symptoms are characteristically worse at night. The condition often ends in deep and prolonged sleep from which the person awakes with no symptoms and little or no memory of the period of delirium. The **treatment** of delirium tremens is described on pp. 188–9.

Alcohol dependence syndrome

Heavy drinking can lead to an alcohol dependence syndrome with the general features described above (p. 259). The specific features of alcohol dependence are that in the late stages of dependence, due to liver damage, tolerance falls and the dependent drinker becomes incapacitated after only a few drinks. Since they can stave off withdrawal symptoms only by further drinking (**relief drinking**), many dependent drinkers take a drink on waking. In most cultures, early morning drinking is diagnostic of dependency. With increasing need to stave off withdrawal symptoms during the day, the drinker typically becomes secretive about the amount consumed, hides bottles or carries them in a pocket or handbag. Rough cider and cheap wines may be drunk regularly to obtain the most alcohol for the least money. A person dependent on alcohol develops a **stereotyped pattern of drinking**. Whereas the ordinary drinker varies his intake from day to day, the dependent person drinks at regular intervals to relieve or avoid withdrawal symptoms.

A severely dependent person who drinks again after a period of abstinence is likely to relapse quickly and totally, returning to his old drinking pattern within a few days (**reinstatement after abstinence**). The syndrome becomes established most often in the mid forties for men, and a few years later for women. It is now occurring increasingly among teenagers, and is sometimes seen for the first time in elderly people after retirement. Once established, the syndrome usually progresses steadily and destructively, unless the patient stops drinking or manages to bring it under control.

Preventing alcohol-related harm

Population-based approaches

As described above (p. 262), the population mean consumption predicts the number of problem drinkers. The aim of population-based approaches is to reduce the average level of consumption in the population and, by doing so, reduce the amount of problem drinking (see Fig. 13.2). This can potentially be achieved in several ways:

- **Raising the price** of alcoholic drinks by taxation.
- **Licensing laws** to limit the hours when alcohol is available.
- **Control of advertising and media portrayal of alcoholic drinks**. It is not certain how effective such measures would be: a ban on press and television advertising in British Columbia, Canada, made little difference.

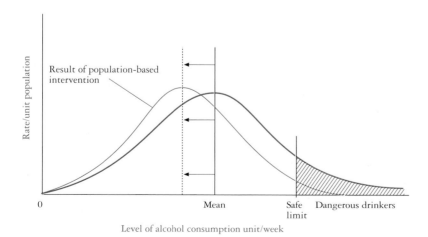

Fig. 13.2 Population-based approaches to reducing alcohol-related harm.

- **Controlling the sale** of alcohol by limiting sales in shops. It is known that relaxation of restriction on sales can lead to increased sales, but it is not certain that increasing restriction would reduce established rates of drinking.
- **Restrictions** on who may buy alcohol.
- **Health education** programmes aimed especially at schoolchildren. The effectiveness of these programmes is uncertain.

Individual approaches

Individual approaches focus on identifying individuals who are consuming hazardous or dangerous amounts of alcohol and intervening with the aim of avoiding or limiting alcohol-related harm. The actual treatment plan for each patient will need to be tailored to his indivual needs and will depend on the amount of alcohol being consumed and whether alcohol-related harm or dependence is present.

Recognition of dangerous use Treatment is more likely to be successful in early stages of dangerous use, and so it is important that such use of alcohol is recognized as soon as possible. General practitioners and hospital doctors are well placed to identify dangerous and harmful alcohol use: 10–30% of people admitted to general hospitals have alcohol problems—the higher rates being found in accident and emergency wards. Every patient should be asked how much alcohol he drinks each week. The possibility of dangerous levels of drinking should be considered particularly carefully in the *risk groups* shown in Table 13.3

The *medical conditions* that raise suspicion include: gastritis, peptic ulcer, liver disease, peripheral neuropathy, seizures especially those starting in middle life, and repeated falls among the elderly. *Psychiatric conditions* with the same significance

Table 13.3.
Identifying alcohol problems

1. Consider possible alcohol problems in the following high-risk groups:
   - medical or psychiatric conditions commonly associated with excessive use of alcohol (see text)
   - marital or sexual problems
   - trouble with the law
   - repeated absences or poor record at work
   - problems with the patient's children
2. Ask screening questions or use a screening questionnaire
   Ask for symptoms of alcohol dependence
3. Carry out a physical examination for alcohol-related medical conditions (see Table 13.1)
4. Arrange further investigations:
   - Alcohol diary
   - Laboratory tests (MCV, GGT)

MCV, mean corpuscular volume; GGT, gamma-glutamyltranspeptidase include anxiety, depression, erratic moods, poor concentration, memory impairment, and sexual dysfunction.

Questionnaires are useful methods of identifying heavy drinkers. In primary care, the *Alcohol Use Disorders Identification Test* (AUDIT; Box 13.1) can be used. In primary care, for detection of alcohol dependence, harmful use or dangerous intake, a cut-off point of 5 on this test has a sensitivity of 84%, a specificity of

Box 13.1 Alcohol Use Disorders Identification Test (AUDIT)

1. How often do you have a drink containing alcohol?
   - (0) never
   - (1) monthly or less
   - (2) 2–4 times a month
   - (3) 2 or 3 times a week
   - (4) 4 or more times a week

2. How many drinks containing alcohol do you have on a typical day when you are drinking?
   - (0) 1 or 2
   - (1) 3 or 4
   - (2) 5 or 6
   - (3) 7 to 9
   - (4) 10 or more

3. How often do you have six or more drinks on one occasion?
   - (0) never
   - (1) less than monthly
   - (2) monthly
   - (3) weekly
   - (4) daily or almost daily

4. How often during the past year have you found that you were not able to stop drinking once you had started?
   - (0) never
   - (1) less than monthly
   - (2) monthly
   - (3) weekly
   - (4) daily or almost daily

5. How often during the past year have you failed to do what was normally expected of you because of drinking?
   - (0) never
   - (1) less than monthly
   - (2) monthly
   - (3) weekly
   - (4) daily or almost daily

6. How often during the past year have you needed a first drink in the morning to get yourself going after a heavy drinking session?
   - (0) never
   - (1) less than monthly
   - (2) monthly
   - (3) weekly
   - (4) daily or almost daily

7. How often during the past year have you had a feeling of guilt or remorse after drinking?
   - (0) never
   - (1) less than monthly
   - (2) monthly
   - (3) weekly
   - (4) daily or almost daily

8. How often during the past year have you been unable to remember what happened the night before because you had been drinking?
   - (0) never
   - (1) less than monthly
   - (2) monthly
   - (3) weekly
   - (4) daily or almost daily

9. Have you or has someone else been injured as a result of your drinking?
   - (0) No
   - (2) Yes, but not in the past year
   - (4) Yes, during the last year

10. Has a relative or friend or a doctor or other health worker been concerned about your drinking or suggested that you cut down?
    - (0) No
    - (2) Yes, but not in the past year
    - (4) Yes, during the last year

Source: Piccinelli *et al.* (1997). *British Medical Journal*, 314, 420–4.

Box 13.2 **The CAGE questionnaire**

1. Have you ever felt you ought to Cut down your drinking ?
2. Have people Annoyed you by criticizing your drinking ?
3. Have you ever felt Guilty about your drinking ?
4. Have you ever had a drink first thing in the morning as an 'Eye opener'?

Two or more positive replies identify problem drinkers; one is an indication for further enquiry about the person's drinking.

Source: Mayfield *et al.* (1974). *American Journal of Psychiatry*, 131, 1121–3.

90%, and a likelihood ratio for a positive result of 8.4. The briefer CAGE questionnaire is probably less sensitive but more specific—a score of three or more has a specificity of almost 100% (Box 13.2).

If the screening questions raise the possibility of an alcohol problem, more detailed enquiries should be made:

- How much alcohol does the patient drink on a typical 'drinking day'? (Start by asking the amount drunk in the second half of the day, before asking about morning drinking.)

- How does the patient feel after going without alcohol for a day or two?

- How does the patient feel on waking?

- Questions should be asked about performance at work and in family life, and about any legal problems. Relevant questions about work include extended meal breaks, lateness, absences, declining efficiency, missed promotions, and accidents.

In appropriate cases, systematic enquiry should be made about features of the alcohol dependence syndrome and all the physical, psychological, and social disabilities described above.

There are several *laboratory tests* which may be useful in assessing the problem drinker:

- **Blood alcohol** concentration estimation using a breathalyser is the most direct measure, although this does not distinguish between a single recent episode of heavy drinking and chronic abuse.

- **Gamma-glutamyltranspeptidase** (GGT) levels are raised in about 80% of problem drinkers

- **Mean corpuscular volume** (MCV) is increased in about 60% of problem drinkers.

- **Urate levels** are raised in about half of all problem drinkers, but they are only useful as screening tests for men as they are poor discriminators in women

If other causes of abnormality can be excluded, abnormal MCV or GGT strongly suggest harmful drinking. They have the advantage that values do not return to normal for some weeks after the last period of heavy drinking.

Treatment of the problem drinker

The value of the assessment interview

A thorough enquiry into drinking habits and related problems is not only a way of detecting the harmful user of alcohol; it is also a first step in treatment because it helps the patient to recognize the extent and seriousness of his problem. This recognition is needed as a means of motivating the patient to control his drinking. Without such motivation, treatment will fail. Enquiries should be persistent to uncover the extent of the problem, but not judgemental. The assessment should normally involve the partner, for whom it may be a first opportunity to unburden feelings and obtain help.

The treatment plan (Table 13.4)

Treatment begins with a review of the extent of the drinking, the evidence for dependence, the effects of the patient's heavy drinking, and the likely consequences if it continues. Any urgently needed medical or psychiatric treatment is arranged and a decision is made about withdrawal (see below). The patient should be involved in formulating the treatment plan, and if possible the partner should take part. Specific and attainable goals should be set, and the patient given responsibility for reaching them. These goals should include control of drinking, collaboration with treatment for any associated medical condition, and resolution of problems in the family, at work, and with the law. These initial goals should be short term and achievable; for example, if the amount drunk is not too great to reduce consumption to the safe limit in the first two weeks. Unrealistic goals, especially in the early stages, will lead to failure, demoralization, and a return to drinking.

As treatment progresses, longer-term goals may be added concerned with improving marital relationships, or changing the use of leisure time. Potential obstacles to progress need to be identified; for example, the patient may work in a job in which drink is readily available, or may have social relations only with people who drink heavily. The patient should be helped to overcome these problems.

The plan will often include help for the family. The spouse or teenage children may need counselling about problems of their own that are consequent on the patient's heavy drinking. They may also need help in supporting the patient's efforts to reduce his drinking.

Abstinence vs. controlled drinking

It is important to decide whether to aim for total abstinence from alcohol or for controlled drinking. Abstinence remains the most appropriate goal for people with harmful use of alcohol, including dependence. Not all such patients will accept this goal; they either refuse treatment or report abstinence while continuing to drink alcohol. For those who drink dangerous amounts of alcohol but are not dependent, an appropriate goal can be the reduction of drinking to a safe level, provided that the person:

– has not incurred serious physical consequences of drinking which require abstinence;

Table 13.4

Treatment plan for a patient with an alcohol problem

1. *Review with the patient*
   - extent of drinking
   - evidence for dependence
   - alcohol-related disabilities
2. Arrange withdrawal of alcohol Treat urgent medical or psychiatric illness
3. *Set attainable goals for*
   - control of drinking*
   - treatment of medical disabilities
   - resolution of interpersonal problems
   - dealing with practical difficulties
   - establishing new interests (finance, employment, the law)
4. *Try to involve partner in treatment plan*
5. *Plan longer-term help*
   - individual or group counselling
   - AA meetings
   - help for the family

*Abstinence if evidence of harmful use.

— is not in a job (such as lorry driving) that carries a risk to others;

— is not pregnant.

The target can be the usual safe limit of 21 units per week for men and 14 for women. Reduction to these limits should be in achievable stages, say 5 or 10 units a week, but the process should not be so prolonged that motivation is lost.

Treatment of special groups

Women Despite the social changes that have led women to drink more alcohol, it is still difficult for them to admit to alcohol dependency or alcohol-related problems. For this reason treatment is often difficult. Compared with men, safe limits set in treatment should be lower (see p. 260). Drinking of alcohol by pregnant women carries risks for the fetus (see p. 263).

Doctors have higher than average rates of alcohol problems, and they too often have difficulty in admitting their problems and seeking help, especially from colleagues working in the same area. In some countries, including the UK, arrangements exist for doctors to obtain help outside their area of work, through a national scheme for sick doctors.

Withdrawal from alcohol—detoxification

When the patient is dependent on alcohol, a sudden cessation of drinking may cause severe withdrawal symptoms including delirium tremens or seizures. Since these complications may be dangerous, withdrawal (*detoxification*) should be carried out under medical supervision, whether at home or in hospital. In less severe cases, and where there is no significant physical illness of history of previous withdrawal seizures, withdrawal can be at home under the supervision of the general practitioner provided that there is someone to look after the patient. Community alcohol teams staffed by nurses can provide additional support for home detoxification and such psychological support is important for maintaining motivation.

Since dependent patients are unlikely to succeed in reducing alcohol gradually, it is usually best to stop the alcohol, replace it with a drug that will prevent delirium tremens or fits, and then withdraw this drug gradually. Benzodiazepines are the drugs of first choice. The choice of benzodiazepine should be made on the basis of speed of onset of action. For most planned withdrawals, a long-acting benzodiazepine, such as chlordiazepoxide or diazepam, is best at producing a smoother course of withdrawal and is less likely to be abused. For unplanned withdrawals, when withdrawal symtoms have already occurred, short-acting benzodiazepines may be preferable. Benzodiazepines should not be continued for longer than 14 days because the patient may become dependent on them chlorpromazine and other neuroleptics are *not* suitable since they may provoke seizures; chlormethiazole is best *avoided* because of cross-dependence and respiratory depression.

A suggested regimen for withdrawal is shown in Box 13.3. If withdrawal is undertaken in hospital, lower doses of benzodiazepine can be used, tailored to the emergence of withdrawal symptoms rated by nursing staff.

Box 13.3 Suggested withdrawal regimen for detoxification from alcohol

Day 1: Chlordiazepoxide 80–100mg in split doses
Day 2–5: Gradual and complete reduction of dose of chlordiazepoxide
- Advise consumption of fruit juices and soft drinks
- Course of vitamins orally
- If history of seizures, use phenytoin
- Monitor symptoms, blood pressure, and fluid intake

Psychological treatment

Brief interventions consisting of assessment of the quantity of alcohol consumed (by asking the patient to keep a diary of his consumption) and the provision of information about the hazards of alcohol and advice about safe limits are effective in reducing dangerous alcohol consumption. Such brief interventions can be provided in primary care and general hospital settings. Problem-solving counselling (pp. 365–6) can be provided by the general practitioner or a member of a specialist team. The patient can keep a diary of his alcohol consumption, and of the circumstances of any relapse. Diary keeping is helpful because relapses occur in many patients and, if dealt with constructively, provide opportunities for finding out how to avoid further relapse.

In patients who do not respond to the brief interventions described above, more intensive psychological interventions are available that are directed at: (1) sustaining motivation; (2) avoiding relapse; and (3) relieving psychological problems that contributed to the development of the alcohol problem.

Group therapy is probably the most widely used treatment in specialist units, because patients often accept support and advice more readily from other patients with similar problems than from doctors. Advice should be provided about *developing new activities* with the family or as hobbies or other interests. Factors that led to or maintained the alcohol problem may need specific treatment. For example, marital problems may require marriage guidance counselling; whereas difficulty in dealing with angry feelings in other relationships might require short-term psychotherapy.

Medication to maintain abstinence

Disulfiram (Antabuse: 100–200 mg/day) is used, usually in specialist practice, as a deterrent to impulsive drinking. It interferes with the metabolism of alcohol by blocking one of the enzymes involved. As a result, when alcohol is taken acetaldehyde accumulates, with consequent flushing, headache, choking sensations, rapid pulse, and anxiety. These unpleasant effects discourage the patient from drinking alcohol while taking the drug.

Treatment with disulfiram carries the occasional risks of cardiac irregularities or, rarely, cardiovascular collapse. Therefore, the drug should not be started until at least 12 hours after the last ingestion of alcohol. Disulfiram has unpleasant side-effects, including a persistent metallic taste in the mouth, gastrointestinal symptoms, dermatitis, urinary frequency, impotence, peripheral neuropathy, and toxic confusional states. It should not be used in patients with:

- recent heart disease;
- significant suicidal ideation;
- severe liver disease.

Potential drug interactions should also be identified by consulting the manufacturer's literature or a work of reference.

Self-help groups and voluntary services

Self-help groups can be very useful for helping to maintain motivation. They also provide a valuable means of support. Patients with alcohol problems often find it easier to talk to others who have had similar problems.

Alcoholics Anonymous (AA) hold group meetings at which members obtain support from one another. If in crisis between meetings, they can obtain support from other members by telephone. Not all problem drinkers are willing to join the organization because it requires total abstinence and because the meetings involve repeated confession of each person's faults and problems. Those who remain in the organization are usually helped, and anyone with a drink problem should be encouraged to try it.

Al-Anon is a parallel organization providing support for the spouses of excessive drinkers. **Al-Ateen** does the same for their teenage children.

Councils on alcoholism are voluntary agencies that advise problem drinkers where to obtain help, provide social activities for those who have recovered, train counsellors, and co-ordinate services.

Hostels for homeless problem drinkers are provided in some places, often by voluntary organizations. Usually, abstinence is a condition of residence, and counselling and rehabilitation are provided.

When to obtain specialist help

Most problem drinkers can be treated in primary care using brief interventions. The general practitioner knows the patient and the family, and can carry out the treatment of the problem drinking in the context of the patient's general health, an approach that is often acceptable to the patient. The family doctor will often be able to withdraw the patient from alcohol—community alcohol teams are increasingly being developed to support general practitioners in this task.

The main reasons for referral to a specialist are:

- Severe withdrawal symptoms, especially fits or delirium tremens which should be treated as emergencies.
- Planned withdrawal from alcohol when home withdrawal is inappropriate.

- Medical or psychiatric complications requiring specialist assessment (see Tables 13.1 and 13.2).

- Complex personal or interpersonal problems requiring more intensive psychological treatment than simple counselling.

The results of treatment

For the majority of problem drinkers, brief interventions are as effective as more intensive treatments. The results of treatment for patients with serious drinking problems are poor and so the aim should be for the early detection and treatment of alcohol problems. It is important to maintain a helpful and non-judgemental attitude. Relapses should be viewed constructively and further help offered. The general practitioner is in a good position to patiently watch, waiting for opportunities to help.

In early stages of dangerous drinking, the patient is more likely to have characteristics which are related to good outcome:

- good insight

- strong motivation

- a supportive family

- a stable job

- the ability to form good relationships

- control of impulsivity

- the ability to defer gratifications.

Problems due to the use of psychoactive substances

The term *psychoactive substance* is often used instead of the term *drug* because some people use substances that are not generally regarded as drugs, for example, organic solvents or mushrooms with psychedelic properties. We use the term *psychoactive substance* when the broad meaning is required, while retaining the word *drug* for other purposes. The substances that are used commonly fall into six groups:

1. Opioids

2. Anxiolytics and hypnotics

3. Stimulants

4. Hallucinogens

5. Cannabis

6. Organic solvents.

In this chapter, we focus on the harmful effects of these substances of the user's health. The use of many of these substances is illegal in many countries. The use of others (e.g. nicotine) is legal despite the harmful medical consequences of smoking. It is important to distinguish between **harmful** use and **illegal** use of substances. The clinician's role should be directed at the former—to help the user overcome dependence and to avoid the adverse health consequences of psychoactive substance use.

The epidemiology of psychoactive substance use

The extent of supply and consumption of drugs is often concealed because possession of many drugs is illegal or socially unacceptable. Therefore, there are no reliable estimates of the extent of drug consumption in the population. In the UK, indirect information has been collected about drug-related offences, hospital treatment, and cases reported to government agencies but none of these sources is reliable. Similar difficulties are encountered in different countries, so that no accurate international comparison can be made.

In the UK, at least 25% of schoolchildren have used illicit substances of solvents on at least one occasion by the age of 16 years. In most developed countries, the extent of drug use seems to be increasing.

The causes of the harmful use of psychoactive substances

Four kinds of cause are important:

1. **The pharmacological properties** of the substances themselves (see below).

2. **The availability of the substances.** The availability of most psychoactive substances is limited in one way or another psychoactive substances are usually obtained in one of three ways:

   (i) *Prescribed by doctors* (e.g. benzodiazepines);
   (ii) *Purchased legally* (e.g. nicotine, alcohol, and for adults, solvents);
   (iii) *Purchased illegally*. Most of the other drugs discussed in this chapter plus nicotine, alcohol, and solvents under certain age limits. Control of the availability of such drugs depends on political action and requires extensive activity by the police and other enforcement agencies to detect and control the importation and distribution of drugs.

3. **Personal factors** may determine why one person who has access to a drug uses it harmfully, while another with similar access does not. They include:

   • *personal vulnerability*: a lack of personal resources needed to cope with the challenges of life. This problem is often manifest in teenage years as difficulty in accepting authority, truancy or underachievement at school, or delinquency.

   • *disorganized family backgrounds*

4. **Social pressures** are important. Some social groups disapprove of drug taking, and this shared value helps to restrain its members; in other groups, drug taking is condoned or even encouraged, and it gives a young person status among his peers.

Types of dependence on psychoactive substances

Not all people who use psychoactive substances become dependent on them. Dependence may be pharmacological or psychological:

• **Pharmacological dependence** is caused by changes in the receptors and other cellular mechanisms affected by the substance. Substances vary in the degree to which thay cause pharmacological dependence: opioids and nicotine readily cause it, cannabis and hallucinogens are less likely to do so.

- **Psychological dependence** operates partly through conditioning: some of the symptoms experienced as a substance is withdrawn (e.g. anxiety) become conditioned responses which appear when withdrawal takes place again. Cognitive factors are also important: patients expect unpleasant symptoms and become distressed. For this reason, reassurance is an important part of the treatment of patients who are withdrawing from drugs.

Harm related to the use of substances

Substance related harm may be due to:

- The toxic properties of the substances themselves (see below).
- The method of administration (e.g. problems due to the intravenous use of substances, see Box 13.4).
- The social consequences of regular use of substances (see Box 13.5)

Diagnosis of dependence on substances

It is important to diagnose dependence early, at a stage when tolerance is less established, behaviour patterns are less fixed, and the complications of intravenous use have not developed. Dependent people may come to medical attention in several ways.

- Some declare that they are dependent on a substance
- Some conceal their dependency, asking instead for opioids to relieve pain or for powerful hypnotics to improve sleep. General practitioners and hospital

Box 13.4 The harmful effects of intravenous drug taking

Some drug abusers administer drugs intravenously in order to obtain an intense and rapid effect. The practice is particularly common with opioids, but barbiturates, benzodiazepines, and amphetamines are among other drugs that may be taken in this way. Intravenous drug use has important consequences, some local, some general.

Local effects include:

- Thrombosis of veins
- Infection at the injection site
- Damage to arteries.

General effects are due to transmission of infection, especially when needles are shared. They include:

- Bacterial endocarditis
- Hepatitis
- HIV infection.

Box 13.5 Social harm due to the use of psychoactive substances

There are three reasons why drug abuse has undesirable social effects:

1. *Chronic intoxication* may affect behaviour adversely, leading to a poor work record, unemployment, motoring offences, failures in social relations, and family problems including neglect of children.

2. *The need to finance the habit.* Most illicit drugs are expensive and the abuser may cheat or steal to obtain money. Women may adopt prostitution putting themselves at risk of sexually transmitted disease and other problems

3. *The creation of a drug subculture.* Drug users often keep company with one another, and those with previously stable social behaviour may be under pressure to conform with a *group ethos* of antisocial or criminal activity.

emergency department staff should be wary of such requests from temporary patients and if possible should obtain information about previous treatment (if necessary by telephone) before prescribing.

- Some dependent people ask for help with the complications of substance use such as cellulitis, pneumonia, hepatitis, HIV/AIDS, or accidents; or for the treatment of a drug overdose, withdrawal symptoms, or an adverse reaction to a hallucinogenic drug.

- A few dependent people are detected during treatment of an unrelated illness.

The doctor who is not used to treating substance-dependent people should remember that the patient may be trying to deceive him. Some overstate the dosage in the hope of obtaining extra supplies to use themselves, give to friends, or sell. Others take more than one substance but do not admit it. It is important, to check the patient's account for internal inconsistencies and to seek external verification whenever possible (e.g. by obtaining permission to contact another doctor who has treated the same patient).

Clinical signs lead to suspicion that drugs are being injected. These include:
- needle tracks and thrombosis of veins, especially in the antecubital fossa;
- scars of previous abscesses;
- concealing the forearms with long sleeves even in hot weather.

Intravenous drug use should be considered in any patient who presents with subcutaneous abscesses, hepatitis or HIV/AIDS, whether or not the person is asking for help with substance use.

Behavioural changes may suggest problem use. These include repeated absence from school or work, occupational decline, self-neglect, loss of former friends, and joining the 'drug culture'. Petty theft and prostitution are other indicators.

Laboratory tests should be used whenever possible to confirm the diagnosis. Most substances can be detected in the urine, the notable exception being LSD (lysergic acid diethylamide). Specimens should be examined as quickly as possible, with an indication of the interval between the last admitted drug dose and the collection of the urine sample. The laboratory should be provided with as complete a list as possible of drugs likely to have been taken, including those prescribed, as well as those obtained in other ways.

Principles of prevention

There are two main strategies of prevention of harm related to the use of psychoactive substances:

1. Reducing use

This includes:

- *Limiting availability.*
- *Health education*, particularly in schools, but also centred on locations with widespread drug use, such as clubs.
- *Media campaigns.*
- *Tackling social causes* such as poor social conditions, unemployment among young people, and lack of leisure facilities.

However, there is little evidence than any of these measures is effective: indeed, some health education and media campaigns may actually increase the extent of use.

2. Reducing harm associated with use of substances

The *harm reduction* approach became more accepted in the 1980s in response to the spread of HIV/AIDS through intravenous drug use and sexual intercourse. The main features of this approach include:

- education of drug-users about the dangers of intravenous use. Such advice is often more effective when given by ex-drug users than by doctors;
- schemes for providing clean syringes and needles in exchange for used ones in the hope of reducing the sharing of contaminated ones;
- prescription of oral maintenance drugs to avoid use of intravenous drugs (see pp. 282–3);
- free supply of condoms to reduce sexual transmission

These approaches are controversial since some of the measures can be seen to condone drug taking, but the danger of HIV infection is now generally considered greater than that of increasing drug abuse.

Principles of treatment and rehabilitation (Table 13.5)

The first part of treatment consists of:

- Assessment of the type, amount, and route of substance use, and the evidence for dependence.
- Provision of information about the dangers of continued use.
- Assessment of the motivation of the user to change his own behaviour.

Table 13.5.

Treatment plan for a person using drugs harmfully

1. *Review with the patient*
   - the type of drug(s) and amounts taken
   - intravenous usage and its dangers especially HIV
   - evidence of dependence
   - consequences of drug taking
     - caused by the drug
     - related to intravenous use
     - social and psychological
   - The patient's personal and social resources and problems

2. *Arrange withdrawal*
   Treat urgent medical or psychiatric complications

3. *Set attainable short- and medium-term goals for:*
   - abstaining from drugs
   - parting from the drug culture
   - dealing with personal and financial problems
   - establishing new interests

4. *Plan longer-term help*
   - individual or group counselling
   - help for the family

- Clarification of the goals of treatment. These goals include: a defined period of abstinence, breaking contact with people who use substances and attempting to establish new relationships; starting to deal with debts or personal problems; and to take up new hobbies or interests so that time previously spend on obtaining and taking drugs does not remain unfulfilled.

The next step of treatment is to **withdraw the substance**. If the person is severely dependent or if withdrawal effects could be serious (e.g. seizures during withdrawal from barbiturates) withdrawal should be in hospital. Otherwise it can be at home under close supervision. Withdrawal is achieved by reducing the dose progressively over a period of one to three weeks depending on the initial dose. With opioids and benzodiazepines it is usual to begin by replacing the substance with an equivalent dose of a longer-acting compound of the same type, and then withdraw that substance. (A longer-acting compound is chosen because withdrawal effects are less acute.) As noted above psychological factors contribute to dependence, and strong and repeated reassurance is an important part of treatment.

Maintenance programmes

Maintenance refers to continued prescribing of a substance, usually an opioid drug, for a person who is unwilling to withdraw, combined with help with social problems and a continuing effort to bring the person to accept withdrawal. Maintenance is therefore more than merely providing drugs. The rationale for this procedure is to minimize harm in the following ways:

1. *Remove the need to obtain 'street' drugs*, and thereby reduce the need to steal, engage in prostitution, or associate with other drug users.

2. *Stop intravenous use*, thus reducing the spread of HIV.

3. The associated social and psychological help should bring the person to the point at which he will be *willing to give up* drugs.

Unfortunately, the available evidence does not suggest that these aims are achieved regularly: many patients continue in their previous way of life, many continue to take street drugs as well as the prescribed methadone, and few become willing to give up drugs. Despite these drawbacks, this treatment is in use in the hope that it may have some effect in reducing intravenous usage thereby limiting the spread of HIV.

Some patients on maintenance therapy attend a succession of general practitioners in search of supplementary supplies of drugs, posing as temporary residents. The doctor should not prescribe but should help the patient to return to the clinic where he is in treatment.

Rehabilitation

People who have abused drugs for a long time may need considerable help in making social relationships and in obtaining and retaining a job. When these problems are severe, treatment in a therapeutic community can be helpful. Less severe problems should be approached by counselling along the lines described on p. 273.

The effects and harmful use of specific substances

Opioids

This group of drugs includes morphine, heroin, codeine, and synthetic analgesics such as pethidine and methadone. As well as the desired effect of euphoria these drugs produce analgesia, respiratory depression, constipation, reduced appetite, and low libido. These drugs can be taken by mouth, intravenously, or by smoking. The most widely abused of these drugs is **heroin** which has a particularly powerful euphoriant effect. Although some people take heroin intermittently without becoming dependent, with regular usage dependence develops rapidly especially when the drug is taken intravenously.

Tolerance develops rapidly, leading to increasing dosage. When the drug is stopped, tolerance diminishes so that a dose taken after an interval of abstinence has a greater effect than it would have had before the interval. This loss of tolerance can result in dangerous—sometimes fatal—respiratory depression when a previously tolerated dose is resumed after a drug-free interval, for example, after a stay in hospital or prison.

Withdrawal symptoms The symptoms due to withdrawal from opioids are shown in Table 13.6.

Table 13.6.

The opioid withdrawal syndrome

- Intense craving for the drug
- Restlessness and insomnia
- Muscle and joint pain
- Running nose and eyes
- Sweating
- Abdominal cramps
- Vomiting and diarrhoea
- Pilo-erection
- Dilated pupils
- Raised pulse rate
- Instability of temperature control

With heroin, these features usually begin about 6 hours after the last dose, reach a peak after 36–48 hours, and then wane. These symptoms cause great distress which drives the person to seek further supplies but seldom threatens the life of a person in reasonable health.

The prognosis of opioid dependence After seven years only a quarter to a third of opioid-dependent people will have become abstinent, and between 10% and 20% have died from causes related to drug taking. Deaths are from accidental overdosage, often related to loss of tolerance after a period of enforced abstinence, and from medical complications such as infection with HIV. When abstinence is achieved, it is often related to changed circumstances of life, such as a new relationship with a caring person.

Pregnancy and opioid dependence The babies of opioid-dependent women are more likely than other babies to be premature and of low birthweight. Also, they may show withdrawal symptoms after birth, including irritability, restlessness, tremor, and a high-pitched cry. These signs appear within a few days of birth if the mother was taking heroin, but are delayed if she was taking methadone, which has a longer half-life. Later effects have been reported, these children being more likely as toddlers to be overactive and to show poor persistence. It is uncertain whether these late effects result from the unsuitable family environment provided by these mothers, or from a lasting effect of the exposure to the drug.

Treatment of opioid dependence Treatment of crisis Heroin-dependent people present in crisis to a general practitioner or casualty doctor in three circumstances.

1. *Seeking the prescription of drugs* either by requesting them directly, or by feigning a painful disorder. Although withdrawal symptoms are very unpleasant, they are not usually dangerous to an otherwise healthy person. Therefore, it is best not to offer drugs unless this is the first step of an agreed withdrawal or maintenance programme. (In the UK, only specially licensed doctors may legally prescribe heroin or certain related drugs to a drug-dependent person as maintenance treatment.)

2. *Drug overdose* requiring medical treatment, directed particularly to any respiratory depression produced by the drug.

3. *Complication of intravenous drug usage* such as an acute local infection, necrosis at the injection site, or infection of a distant organ usually the heart or liver.

Planned withdrawal of opioids (detoxification) The general principles of drug withdrawal have been outlined above. When heroin is withdrawn, psychological management is particularly important. Withdrawal is usually undertaken by substituting methadone (a longer-acting drug) for heroin. The main steps are shown in Box 13.6

Continued prescribing (maintenance) The principles of maintenance treatment for opiate dependence has been discussed. Methadone is prescribed and dispensed daily, usually in a liquid preparation formulated to discourage efforts to inject it. The equivalent dosage is difficult to determine since street drugs are adulterated to a varying degree. The treatment should be initiated by a specialist although care may be shared with the primary care physician. There is some evidence that drugs with a longer half-life, such as buprenorphine and levamethadyl

Box 13.6 **The planned withdrawal of opioids (detoxification)**

- When the starting dose is very high, withdrawal should be in hospital.
- It is often difficult to judge the starting dose because patients often take adulterated preparations of heroin (and may lie about the amount taken). For this reason treatment should be discussed with and often carried out by a specialist in drug dependence.
- The starting dose of methadone is usually 10–20 mg daily, increased in 10–20 mg steps until no signs of intoxication or withdrawal. The usual daily dose is 40–60 mg.
- The initial dose is reduced by about a quarter every two or three days, but a slower rate may be needed. However, very slow withdrawal should be avoided because it may lead to continued prescribing
- The regimen should be agreed with the patient as a contract that he will accept throughout the treatment.
- Urine tests for drugs should be carried out weekly after withdrawal until the doctor is confident that the patient is remaining drug-free.

acetate hydrochloride (LAAM) may be at least as effective as methodone. These drugs have the advantage that they can be taken less often than every day.

Rehabilitation This follows the general lines described on p. 281.

Results of treatment Although about 90% opioid-dependent patients can withdraw successfully, about 50% will recommence use by six months following withdrawal.

Anxiolytic and hypnotic drugs

The most frequently used drugs in this group are now benzodiazepines. The most serious health problems are presented by barbiturates which, although seldom used therapeutically, are widely available as street drugs. Other currently used drugs of this kind include chlormethiazole and glutethimide.

Barbiturates Barbiturates are taken by mouth and intravenously. Some elderly people are dependent on barbiturates prescribed originally many years ago as prescribed hypnotics. Younger dependent people use illegal supplies of barbiturates, and some dissolve capsules and inject intravenously—a particularly dangerous practice leading to phlebitis, ulcers, abscesses, and gangrene.

The symptoms of **barbiturate intoxication** resemble those of alcohol, with:

- slurred speech
- incoherence
- drowsiness
- depression of mood.

Younger intravenous users are often unkempt, dirty, and malnourished. *Nystagmus*, a useful diagnostic sign, is often present. Urine should be examined to investigate the possible simultaneous abuse of other drugs. Blood levels are generally useful only in acute poisoning.

Tolerance develops to barbiturates, although less quickly than to opioids. Tolerance to the psychological effects of barbiturates is greater than tolerance to their depressant effects on respiration, so increasing the risks of unintentional fatal overdosage.

Withdrawal Abrupt withdrawal of barbiturates from a dependent person can be followed by a withdrawal syndrome resembling that occurring with alcohol (see p. 266) and the *risk of seizures is high*. With longer-acting drugs, the withdrawal syndrome may be delayed for several days after the drug has been stopped; for this reason observation should be prolonged if dangerous consequences are to be avoided. The syndrome of barbiturate withdrawal begins with anxiety, restlessness, disturbed sleep, anorexia, and nausea. It may progress to tremulousness, disorientation, hallucinations, vomiting, hypotension, pyrexia, and to major seizures. If the withdrawal syndrome is not treated, some patients die.

When drugs are withdrawn as part of treatment, the patient should be supervised closely in hospital, unless: (1) the starting dose is small; and (2) there is no history of epilepsy. Phenothiazines should be avoided because they may lower the seizure threshold. Unless it is certain that the dosage is small the advice of a specialist should be obtained.

Benzodiazepines

Benzodiazepines cause symptoms of *intoxication* similar to those of barbiturates (see above). *Tolerance* and *dependence* develop when the drugs are prescribed continuously for a long period. The exact period is uncertain but 6–8 weeks is widely accepted as the limit that is without risk.

The **benzodiazepine withdrawal syndrome** is characterized by:

- irritability
- anxiety
- disturbed sleep
- nausea
- increased perceptual sensitivity
- tremor
- sweating
- palpitations
- headache
- muscle pain.

Seizures may occur when the dose of benzodiazepine taken has been high.

Planned withdrawal of benzodiazepines

- When benzodiazepines are withdrawn therapeutically, the dose should be reduced very gradually.
- Withdrawal symptoms are less pronounced with long-acting (e.g. diazepam) than with short-acting benzodiazepines (e.g. lorazepam) so a short-acting drug should be replaced with a long-acting drug in equivalent dose before starting withdrawal.
- The dose should be reduced gradually by about 10% every two weeks.

- If withdrawal symptoms appear during withdrawal, the dose can be increased slightly, and then reduced again by a smaller amount than before.

- As the dose decreases, it may not be possible to achieve the required dose reduction with the strengths of tablets available. At this stage the drug can be taken on alternate days or a liquid preparation (e.g. diazepam elixir or nitrazepam syrup) can be used.

- Anxiety management techniques (see pp. 372–3) help to reduce the distress caused by withdrawal symptoms. They have the advantage that they should reduce the need for anxiolytic medication if anxiety recurs in the future.

- Self-help groups (e.g. Tranx) can also be a valuable source of support during withdrawal.

Stimulant drugs

The stimulant drugs abused most often are amphetamines, cocaine, and 'ecstasy'.

- *Amphetamine sulphate* is taken by mouth or by intravenous injection.
- *Free-base amphetamine* (made by heating amphetamine sulphate) is usually smoked and absorbed through the lungs from which is absorbed rapidly.
- *Cocaine hydrochloride* is taken by sniffing into the nose (where it is absorbed through the nasal mucosa) or by injecting.
- *Free-base cocaine* ('crack') is usually smoked to give a rapid and intense effect.
- *Ecstasy* (3,4-methylenedioxymethamphetamine; MDMA) is taken orally. It has been used increasingly since the 1980s, especially at dances ('raves') and clubs. It produces an intense feeling of well-being and increased energy.

These drugs produce an elevation of mood, overactivity, overtalkativeness, insomnia, anorexia, and dryness of the mouth and nose. The pupils dilate, pulse rate and blood pressure increase and, with large doses, there may be cardiac arrythmia and circulatory collapse. The overactivity can cause dehydration: conversely overhydration can also occur as the user drinks large amounts of water to overcome dehydration. Occasionally, patients complain of an unusual feeling under the skin, as if insects were there ('formication').

Prolonged use of large quantities of these drugs may result in a disturbances of perception and thinking. Particularly with amphetamines, a **paranoid psychosis** may occur, closely resembling the paranoid form of schizophrenia, with persecutory delusions, auditory and visual hallucinations, and sometimes aggressive behaviour. Usually, the condition subsides within a week or two of stopping the drug, but occasionally persists for months. In some of these prolonged cases the diagnosis proves to be schizophrenia, not drug-induced psychosis.

Depression may also follow long-term use of stimulants. Ecstasy may be neurotoxic when taken repeatedly.

Stimulant drugs do not readily induce **tolerance**. The **withdrawal** syndrome is often troublesome and consists of low mood and reduced energy.

Treatment of *overdosage* requires sedation and the management of any hyperpyrexia or cardiac arrythmia. *Paranoid symptoms* can be controlled with an antipsychotic drug.

Hallucinogens

This group of drugs includes synthetic compounds such as *lysergic acid diethylamide* (LSD) and naturally occurring substances found in species of mushroom (e.g. *Psilocybe semilanceata*). Synthetic and naturally occurring *anticholinergic drugs* are also abused for their hallucinogenic effects.

The drugs produce distortions or intensifications of sensory perception, sometimes with 'cross-over' between sensory modalities so that, for example, sounds are experienced as visual sensations. Objects may seem to merge, or move rhythmically; time appears to pass slowly, and ordinary experiences to have a profound meaning. The body image may seem distorted or the person may feel as if outside his body. These experiences may be pleasurable, but at times they are profoundly distressing and lead to unpredictable and dangerous behaviour. The physical effects of hallucinogens are variable: LSD can cause a rise in heart rate and dilation of the pupils.

Frightening experiences can usually be controlled by strong reassurance; otherwise an anxiolytic such as diazepam should be given. Antipsychotic drugs are also effective but those with anticholinergic effects (such as chlorpromazine) must *not* be given if the patient has taken phencyclidine (PCP) which has anticholinergic properties, or an anticholinergic drug such as benzhexol.

'**Flashbacks**' are recurrences of experiences occurring originally during intoxication with hallucinogens, the recurrence occurring weeks or months after the drug was last taken. The experience may be distressing and require reassurance and treatment with an anxiolytic drug. Although flashbacks may recur, they subside eventually.

Phencyclidine

PCP or 'angel dust' is a synthetic hallucinogen with particularly dangerous effects. Intoxication with this drug can be prolonged and hazardous, with agitation, aggressive behaviour, and hallucinations, together with nystagmus and raised blood pressure. With high doses, there may be ataxia, muscle rigidity, and convulsions; and in severe cases, an adrenergic crisis with heart failure, cerebrovascular accident, or malignant hypothermia. In treatment, chlorpromazine should be avoided since it may increase the anticholinergic effects of PCP. Instead, haloperidol or diazepam may be given.

Cannabis

Cannabis, which derives from the plant *Cannabis sativa*, is consumed in two forms. The dried vegetative parts of the plant form marijuana ('grass'); the resin secreted by the flowering tops of the female plant form cannabis resin. In many parts of the world, cannabis is consumed widely, much as alcohol is consumed in the West. In most Western societies use of cannabis, although illegal, is widespread.

The effects of cannabis vary with the dose, the user's expectations, and the social setting. Like alcohol, cannabis seems to exaggerate the pre-existing mood, whether euphoria or dysphoria. It produces a feeling of enhanced enjoyment of aesthetic experiences, and distorts experiences of time and space. Cannabis intoxication can lead to dangerous driving. The physical effects of cannabis include reddening of the conjunctiva, dry mouth, and tachycardia.

Cannabis does not produce a **withdrawal syndrome**; and although **psychological dependence** can develop, physical dependence does not seem to occur. It is not certain whether cannabis causes a psychosis. Some patients develop an acute psychosis while consuming large amounts of cannabis, recovering quickly when the drug is stopped. In these cases it is uncertain whether cannabis caused the psychosis, or the increased use of cannabis was a response to the early symptoms of a psychosis with a different cause. Fortunately, this uncertainty seldom causes practical problems since the clinical management is unaffected: the drug should be stopped, the progress of the symptoms observed, and chlorpromazine or another antipsychotic drug prescribed if symptoms do not subside within a week.

Organic solvents

Use of volatile solvents occurs mainly among teenagers, usually as occasional experimentation. Serious problems arise in a minority who use solvents regularly, and any user may take an accidental overdose or become asphyxiated while taking the substance.

The solvents used most often are cleaning fluids, adhesives, and aerosols. Petrol and butane and other substances may also be used. The substance is inhaled from a partially closed container in which the concentration can build up, or from an impregnated cloth, or plastic bag.

Solvent intoxication is characterized by:

- slurring of speech
- disorientation
- uncoordination of gait
- nausea and vomiting
- coma
- Visual hallucinations (often frightening).

Psychological **dependence** occurs but physical dependence is unusual. Chronic heavy users may develop a transient psychosis.

Some of these substances have **neurotoxic effects** with resultant peripheral neuropathy and cerebellar dysfunction. Overdosage can be fatal, resulting from the direct effects of the drug, or from asphyxia or the inhalation of vomit.

Treatment is along the general lines of harmful use of drugs described on (pp. 279–81) with emphasis on improving any personal or family problems contributing to the abuse.

Further reading

Edwards, G., Marshall, J., and Cook, C. C. H. (1997). *The Treatment of Drinking Problems; A Guide for the Helping Professions* (3rd edn). Cambridge University Press.
A comprehensive account of the practical treatment of the problems due to the use of alcohol.

Robson, P. (1999). *Forbidden Drugs (2nd edn)*. Oxford University Press.
Reviews the effects of each group of illegal drugs, and considers why people take them and discusses the nature of addiction and approaches to treatment.

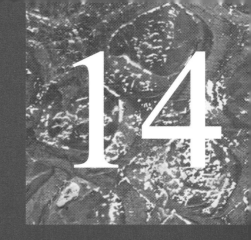

14

Problems of sexuality and gender

- Sexual behaviour in the population

- Sexual dysfunction

- Specific sexual disorders

- Disorders of sexual preference

- Disorders of gender identity: transsexualism

- Psychological problems of homosexual people

Problems of sexuality and gender

Problems of sexuality and gender are common. Doctors may be asked to give advice about four types of problem:

1. Sexual dysfunction—impaired or dissatisfying sexual enjoyment or performance.

2. Abnormalities of sexual preference—unusual sexual interests and activities that are preferred to heterosexual intercourse.

3. Disorders of gender identity—in which the patient is feels as if they are of the sex opposite to their biological sex.

4. Psychological problems encountered by homosexual people.

Of these, the first group are the most common. In this chapter, we describe the common sexual disorders and outline their treatment. After studying the chapter, the reader should:

- know the clinical features of the most common sexual problems;
- be able to take a history of a sexual problem; and
- understand how to formulate a sexual problem.

We assume that readers will have learnt about the physiology of the sexual response elsewhere—if not, we recommend reading the appropriate chapters of Bancroft's *Human Sexuality and its Problems* (Oxford University Press 1988). The main stages of the physiology of the sexual response are summarized in Tables 14.1 and 14.2.

Sexual behaviour in the population

A knowledge of the range of sexual behaviour in the general population will assist a doctor assess a patient's presenting problem. In many instances it can be helpful to offer reassurance that a patient's experiences lie within the normal range of sexual behaviour.

Age at first intercourse

Figure 14.1 shows the cumulative percentages of the age at first heterosexual intercourse in men and women. The figure shows that the age of first intercourse is dropping over time. This is probably due to a combination of a trend to earlier sexual maturity and a relaxation of social attitudes towards sexuality. At present, about 20% of females and about 30% of males experience heterosexual intercourse before the age of 16 years. Earlier age of first intercourse is associated with lower social class, lower levels of education, and lack of religious affiliation. The earlier first intercourse occurs, the less likely it is to be accompanied by adequate contraceptive use and the more it is felt by the subject, on retrospect, to have been too early.

Table 14.1
Male sexual response

	Excitement	Plateau	Orgasm	Resolution
Penis	Erection	Erection maintained	Urethra contracts repeatedly	Gradual detumescence
Scrotum	Skin thickens testes raised	Testes raised further	No change	Return to normal
Prostate, seminal vesicles			Contract with emission of seminal fluid to urethra	Return to normal
Pulse and blood pressure	Increase	Further increase	Further increase	Return to normal
Respiration		Rate increases	Rate increases further	Return to normal

Table 14.2.
Female sexual response

	Excitement	Plateau	Orgasm	Resolution
Breasts	Nipple erection in some	Enlargement areolar engorgement	No change	Return to normal
Labia		Engorgement	No change	Return to normal
Clitoris	Head swells	Head withdraws	No change	Return to normal
Vagina	Lubrication, expansion, distension of inner two-thirds	Outer third swells inner two-thirds distends further	Contractions of outer third	Return to normal
Uterus	Body and cervix raised	Further elevation	Contractions	Position returns to normal; os gapes open
Pulse and BP	Slight elevation	Further increase	Increase continues	Return to normal
Respiration		Rate increases	Rate increased further	Return to normal

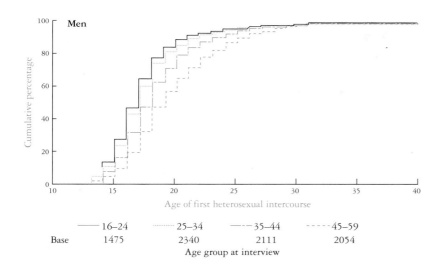

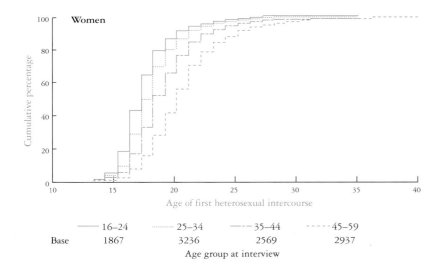

Fig. 14.1 Cumulative proportions of age at first heterosexual intercourse (after age 13) by age group when interviewed. (From Johnson, A. E., Wadsworth, J., and Field, J. (1994). *Sexual Attitudes and Lifestyles*. Blackwell, Oxford, with permission.) The British National Survey of Sexual Attitudes and lifestyle interviewed 18 876 people in 1990–91.

Frequency of sexual activity

Figure 14.2 gives estimates of the relative frequency of different sexual practices. **Fellatio** is the oral stimulation of the male genitals and **cunnilingus** is the oral stimulation of the female genitals. Oral sex is more common in younger age groups.

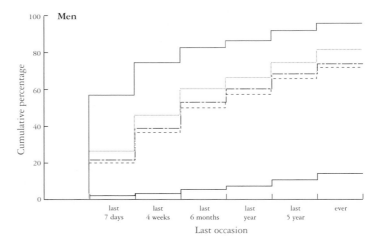

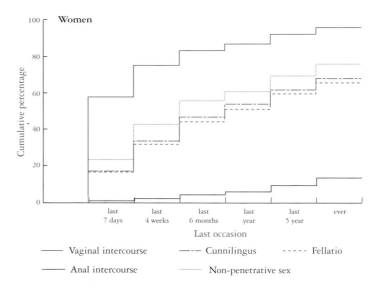

Fig. 14.2 Last occasion of different practices, cumulative percentages. (From Johnson, A. E., Wadsworth, J., and Field, J. (1994). *Sexual Attitudes and Lifestyles*. Blackwell, Oxford, with permission.) The British National Survey of Sexual Attitudes and lifestyle interviewed 18 876 people in 1990–91.

Homosexual orientation

Ninety-six per cent of men and 97% of women report mostly or exclusively **heterosexual** (a sexual orientation in which erotic thoughts and feelings are directed towards a person of the opposite sex) experience and attraction. One per cent of men and 0.25% of women report mostly or exclusively **homosexual** (a sexual orientation in which erotic thoughts and feelings are directed towards a person of the same sex) experience and attraction. However, 6% of males and 3% of females report some homosexual experience. Definite homosexual experience (one or more homosexual partners ever) is more common in people who attended single sex (only in males) or boarding school and who belong to non-manual social classes. There is some evidence that a minority of homosexual men report a larger number of sexual partners than heterosexual men.

Homophobic attitudes are widespread—about two-thirds of the population believe that homosexuality is always or mostly wrong.

Sexual dysfunction

It is difficult to establish the prevalence of sexual problems in the population because of the difficulties involved in carrying out surveys of people's sexual behaviour. The commonest kinds of problems presenting to a sexual dysfunction clinic are shown in Table 14.3.

The assessment of sexual dysfunction
(Boxes 14.1 and 14.2)

Patients with sexual problems often complain about other symptoms because they feel too embarrassed to reveal a sexual problem directly. For example, a patient may ask instead for help with anxiety, depression, poor sleep, or gynaecological symptoms. It is therefore important to routinely ask brief questions about sexual functioning when assessing patients with non-specific psychological or physical symptoms.

The interviewer should begin by explaining why it will be necessary to ask about intimate details of the patient's sexual life and should then ask questions in a sympathetic matter of fact way. Whenever possible both sexual partners should be interviewed, at first separately and then together. When obtaining an account of the problem, find out whether the problem has been present from the first intercourse, or started after a period of normal sexual functioning. Each partner

Table 14.3.

Relative frequency of sexual problems presenting to a sexual dysfunction clinic

Women	
Low sexual desire	50%
Orgasmic dysfunction	20%
Vaginismus	20%
Dyspareunia	5%
Men	
Erectile dysfunction	60%
Premature ejaculation	15%
Delayed ejaculation	5%
Low sexual desire	5%

Adapted from: Hawton, K. (1985). *Sex Therapy: A Practical Guide.* Oxford Medical Publications, Oxford University Press.

Box 14.1 Assessment of a sexual problem

- Define the problem
  - its nature
  - recent or longstanding
  - whether with this partner only
- Assess sexual drives of both partners
- Enquire about the marital relationship and social relationships in general
- Sexual development including traumatic experiences
- Previous and present psychiatric and medical illness and treatment; pregnancy, childbirth and abortion(s); alcohol and drug use
- Assess the mental state, especially for depressive disorder
- Assess motivation for treatment
- Physical examination and any relevant laboratory tests

Box 14.2 **Physical examination of men with sexual dysfunction**

1. *Is there evidence of diabetes mellitus or adrenal disorder?*

   Hair distribution; gynaecomastia
   Blood pressure, peripheral pulses
   Fundi for retinopathy
   Reflexes especially ankle
   Peripheral sensation

2. *Are there any abnormalities of the genitalia?*

   Penis: congenital abnormalities, foreskin, pulses, tenderness, plaques, infection, urethral discharge

   Testicles: size, symmetry, texture, sensation

should be asked, separately, whether the same problem has occurred with another partner, or during masturbation.

The *strength of sexual drive* should be assessed in terms of the frequency of sexual arousal, intercourse, and masturbation. *Motivation* for treatment should be assessed, starting with questions about who took the initiative in seeking treatment and for what reason.

Assess each partner's *social relationships* with the other sex, with particular reference to shyness and social inhibition. Enquiries are made about the partners' *feelings for one another*: partners who lack a mutual caring relationship are unlikely to achieve a fully satisfactory sexual relationship. Many couples say that their marital problems result from their sexual problems, when the causal connection is really the reverse. Tactful questions should be asked about commitment to the partner and, when appropriate, about infidelity and fears of sexually transmitted disease, including HIV.

When assessing *sexual development* and *sexual experience,* pay particular attention to experiences such as child abuse, incest, or sexual assault that may have caused lasting anxiety or disgust about sex. Enquiry should be made about homosexual as well as heterosexual feelings.

In the *medical history*, the most relevant things to look for are previous and present psychiatric and chronic physical disorders and their treatment; pregnancy, childbirth and abortion(s); use of alcohol or drugs, such as selective serotonin reuptake inhibitors (SSRIs). In the *mental state examination* look especially for evidence of depressive disorder. *Physical examination* is important because physical illness often causes sexual problems (see Box 14.2 and Table 14.4). Physical examination of women may require specialist gynaecological help. Further investigations may be necessary depending on the findings from the history and examination (e.g. if diabetes is suspected as a cause of sexual disorder).

Specific sexual disorders

Low sexual desire

This problem may occur in both sexes but is commoner in women. In some cases, sexual desire has always been low (**primary low sexual desire**): this may be the

Table 14.4.

Physical disorders and drugs causing low sexual desire

Physical disorders	Drugs
Hypogonadism	Hypnotics
Angina and previous myocardial infarction	Anxiolytics
Epilepsy	Antipsychotics
Renal failure and dialysis	
Hypothyroidism	
Mastectomy	
Oophorectomy	
Colostomy	
Ileostomy	

extreme of the range of biological variation, or it may be due to fears originating from adverse experiences in childhood, such as sexual abuse. In other cases, sexual desire has been normal in the past but has become impaired (**secondary low sexual desire**): the causes then include general problems in the relationship between the partners, physical disorders (Table 14.4), and depressive disorder (in which lack of sexual desire may continue for some weeks after other symptoms have resolved).

Treatment is of the cause if one can be identified. The relationship between the partners may improve with couple therapy (pp. 300–1); a depressive disorder should be treated in the usual way (see pp. 143–5); and fear or guilt caused by adverse experiences in early life may respond to psychotherapy (p. 375). Low sexual drive cannot be increased by giving hormones.

Male erectile dysfunction

Erectile dysfunction is the inability to reach erection or sustain it long enough for satisfactory coitus. Primary erectile dysfunction is rare and usually has a physical basis, such as neurological damage or leakage from the penile cavernous bodies. The common causes of secondary **erectile dysfunction** are:

- anxiety about sexual performance;
- alcohol abuse;
- drug side effects (see Table 14.5);
- diabetes;
- arteriosclerosis;
- other physical illness (see Table 14.5);
- age-related diminution of sexual function.

Assessment of erectile dysfunction should identify whether it is is invariable (suggesting a physical or drug cause) or present only in some circumstances (suggesting a psychological cause). Questions should be asked about erections on

Table 14.5.

Physical disorders and drugs causing erectile dysfunction

Physical disorders	Drugs
Diabetes mellitus	Antihypertensives
Arteriosclerosis	Beta-blockers
Hyperprolactinaemia	Diuretics
Pelvic autonomic neuropathy	Cimetidine
Rectal surgery	Tricyclic antidepressants
	MAOIs*
	Antipsychotics

*MAOI, monoamine oxidase inhibitor.

waking from sleep, and during masturbation: if they are present, a physical cause is unlikely.

Treatment of erectile dysfunction should combine psychological approaches with physical approaches as appropriate. If the disorder is caused by a drug or other physical cause, these should be stopped or treated if possible. Psychological treatment includes the use of sexual therapy techniques (see below) and anxiety management. Physical treatments of erectile dysfunction include intracavernosal injections of smooth muscle relaxants (e.g. papaverine or prostaglandin E_1), vacuum devices and, occasionally, surgical insertion of semi-rigid rods. A new development is a drug called sildenafil, a potent inhibitor of phosphodiesterase type V, which appears to be effective in the treatment of erectile dysfunction.

Conditions with discomfort or pain

Pain on intercourse occurs mainly among women, either as vaginismus or as dyspareunia.

Vaginismus

Vaginismus is painful spasm of the vaginal muscles during intercourse. This spasm may be due to aversion to intercourse or may result from painful scarring after episiotomy or other procedures. The condition may be made worse by an inexperienced or inconsiderate partner. Generally, the spasm begins when the man attempts penetration, but in severe cases it occurs even if the woman attempts to insert her own finger into the vagina. In such severe cases no intercourse can take place.

Treatment It should be explained to the patient that vaginismus is a form of muscle spasm which can be overcome by relaxation exercises. A graduated behavioural approach to treatment is used. At first, diagrams and mirrors are used to improve the patient's understanding of sexual anatomy and response. Once the woman is familiar and comfortable with her genitals, she is encouraged to introduce the tip of her finger into the vagina. She gradually inserts the whole of her finger and, once she can do this without discomfort, she should try inserting two fingers. In many women, this process will allow the woman to overcome the vaginismus. In situations where the woman finds it difficult to transfer from finger to penile penetration, graduated dilators can be used.

Vaginismus should be distinguished from **lack of vaginal lubrication** which is usually due to lack of sexual arousal, but may also be due to drug side effects and physical disorders (e.g. diabetes). It is more common following the menopause. **Treatment** consists of removing the cause or using additional lubrication.

Dyspareunia

Dyspareunia is pain on intercourse (see Table 14.6). When the pain arises after even partial penetration of the vagina, it may result from impaired lubrication with vaginal secretions (due to aversion to intercourse or inadequate foreplay) or from painful scarring. When pain is felt only during deep penetration, it may be due to pelvic pathology such as endometriosis, pelvic inflammatory disease, ovarian cyst, or tumour. Pain on deep penetration may also result from diminished lubrication in the later stages of prolonged intercourse.

Treatment of dyspareunia depends on the cause. When it is the result of psychological factors causing impaired sexual arousal, sexual therapy techniques can be used. Referral to a gynaecologist should be made if simple measures are ineffective

The few cases of dyspareunia among men involve **painful ejaculation**, an uncommon disorder usually caused by urethritis or prostatitis, but occasionally without detectable cause.

Orgasmic dysfunction

In men, orgasmic dysfunction is premature ejaculation or retarded ejaculation; in women it is inhibited orgasm.

Premature ejaculation

Premature ejaculation is habitual ejaculation before penetration or shortly afterwards, so that the woman gains no pleasure. It is common among young men during first sexual encounters, and usually improves with increasing sexual experience. The partner can assist by interrupting foreplay whenever the man feels himself becoming highly aroused (*stop–start technique*). This process prolongs the period during which the man can be highly aroused, but not ejaculate.

Retarded ejaculation

Retarded ejaculation may be part of a general psychological inhibition about relations with women. It can also be caused by drugs, notably antipsychotic drugs and monoamine oxidase inhibitors. If the condition is caused by drugs, the dose should be reduced if practicable. When the causes are psychological, psychotherapy can be tried although its results are uncertain.

Inhibited female orgasm

Inhibited female orgasm during intercourse is frequent although most women can achieve it through clitoral stimulation. In one survey, a quarter of women said they had not experienced orgasm during the first year of marriage. Whether treatment is requested depends on what the couple regards as abnormal. Failure of

Table 14.6.

Physical disorders and drugs causing pain and orgasmic dysfunction

Pain
1. *Dyspareunia*
   Episiotomy
   Endometriosis
   Pelvic inflammatory disease
   Pelvic cysts or tumours
1. *Painful ejaculation*
   Urethritis
   Prostatitis

Orgasmic dysfunction
Spinal cord injury

Drugs
Antipsychotics
MAOIs

female orgasm may be due to the man's incapacity to arouse his partner or show her affection and is a likely cause if the woman can experience orgasm by masturbation. Other causes are tiredness, depressive disorder, physical illness, and the effects of medication.

Treatment begins by dealing with any remediable cause. If no such cause if found, the woman is helped to express her sexual needs to the partner, and he is encouraged to respond to them (using sex therapy if necessary, see below). If the relationship between the couple is poor, marital therapy may be used (p. 379).

Sexual dysfunction among the physically handicapped

Physically handicapped people have sexual problems arising from several sources, including: direct effects of the handicap on sexual function (e.g. impairment of the autonomic nerves to the genitalia in disease of the spinal cord); general effects such as tiredness and pain; fears about the deleterious effects of intercourse on the handicapping condition; and lack of information about the sexual activities that are possible for people with the disability. It is helpful if the general practitioner can provide disabled individuals an opportunity to raise any sexual difficulties. When necessary, treatment is provided by adapting methods already described for treating sexual dysfunction in non-handicapped people.

Psychological treatment of sexual dysfunction

Specific treatment recommendations are give above in the sections on the individual disorders. Many disorders will respond to the steps outlined. However, treatment of a broad range of sexual dysfunction may need more structured psychological treatment. In this form of treatment the couple is seen together whenever possible. There are three stages: (1) improving communication; (2) education; and (3) 'graded activities'.

1. **Improving communication** has two main aims: (a) to help the couple to talk more freely about their problems; and (b) to increase each partner's understanding of the wishes and feelings of the other. These aims may be appropriate to various kinds of problems. For example, a woman may believe that her partner should know instinctively how to please her during intercourse; she may then interpret his failure to please as lack of affection rather than as the result of her not communicating her wishes to her partner. Alternatively, the man may wish the woman to take a more active role in intercourse but be unable to say this to her.

A further aim of this stage of treatment is to enable the couple to achieve a general relationship that is more affectionate and satisfying.

2. **Education** focuses on important aspects of the male and female sexual responses; examples are the longer time needed for a woman to reach sexual arousal, and the importance of foreplay, including clitoral stimulation, in bringing about vaginal lubrication. Suitably chosen books on sex education can reinforce the therapist's advice. Educational counselling is often the most important part of the

treatment of sexual dysfunction, and it may need to be repeated when the couple have made some progress with the graded activities described next.

3. 'Graded activities' begin by negotiating with the couple a mutually agreed ban on full sexual intercourse. The couple are encouraged instead to explore the pleasure that each can give the other in tender physical contact. The partners are encouraged to caress each other but not to touch the genitalia at this stage. When they can achieve caressing in a relaxed way that gives enjoyment to each partner, the next stage is genital foreplay without penetration. When genital foreplay can be enjoyed by both partners, the next stage is the resumption of full intercourse in a gradual and relaxed way, in which the partner with the greater problem sets the pace. In this stage a graduated approach starts with 'vaginal containment', in which the penis is inserted gradually into the vagina without thrusting movements. When this graded insertion is pleasurable for both partners, movement is introduced; usually by the woman at first. At each stage, each partner is encouraged to find out and provide what the other enjoys. The couple are advised to avoid checking their own state of sexual arousal. Such checking is common among people with sexual disorder, and has the effect of inhibiting the natural progression of sexual arousal to orgasm. Each partner should be encouraged to allow feelings and physical responses to develop spontaneously whilst thinking of the other person.

Hormones have *no place* in the treatment of sexual dysfunction except where there is a primary hormonal disorder.

The overall **results** of sex therapy are that about a third of cases have a successful outcome and another third have worthwhile improvement. Patients with low sexual drive generally have a poor outcome.

Disorders of sexual preference

Disorders of sexual preference are sometimes known as **paraphilias**. A sexual preference can be said to be abnormal by three criteria:

1. Most people in a society regard the sexual preference as abnormal.

2. The sexual preference can be harmful to other people (e.g. sadistic sexual practices).

3. The person with the preference suffers from its consequences (e.g. from a conflict between sexual preferences and moral standards).

Doctors may be concerned with these conditions in three circumstances. They may be asked for help by the person with the abnormal sexual preference; they may be approached by the sexual partner; or they may be asked for an opinion when a person has been charged with an offence against the law; for example, exhibitionism or a sexual act with a child. (These offences, and others unrelated to abnormal sexual preference, are considered in Chapter 21.)

Disorders of sexual preference are divided into: (1) abnormalities of the sexual 'object'; and (2) disorders of the sexual act (Table 14.7). The **aetiology** of these conditions is not known, and will not be discussed. **Treatment** is described after the descriptions of the disorders, on p. 304.

Table 14.7.
Abnormalities of sexual preference

1. *Abnormalities of the sexual object*
   - sexual fetishism
   - transvestism
   - paedophilia
2. *Abnormalities of the sexual act*
   - exhibitionism
   - voyeurism
   - sexual sadism
   - sexual masochism

Disorders of preference of the sexual object

Fetishism

In this condition, an inanimate object is the preferred or only means of achieving sexual excitement. Almost all fetishists are men and most are heterosexual. Among the many objects that can evoke arousal in different people, common examples are rubber garments, women's underclothes, and high-heeled shoes. The smell and texture of these objects is often as important as their appearance in evoking sexual arousal. Some fetishists buy the objects, but others steal them and so come to the notice of the police. Sometimes the behaviour is carried out with a willing partner or with a paid prostitute, but often it is a solitary accompaniment of masturbation.

Fetishistic transvestism

In this condition, the person repeatedly wears clothes of the opposite sex as the preferred or only means of sexual arousal. It can be thought of as a special kind of fetishism. Nearly all transvestites are men. The clothing varies from a single garment to a complete set of clothing. Cross-dressing nearly always begins after puberty. At first, the clothes are worn only in private; a few people, however, go on to wear the clothes in public, usually hidden under male outer garments, but occasionally without precautions against discovery. A few transvestites wear a complete set of female garments; the condition then has to be distinguished from transsexualism (see p. 304). The essential difference is that transvestites are sexually aroused by wearing the clothing, while transsexuals are not.

Paedophilia

Paedophilia is repeated sexual activity (or fantasy of such activity) with pre-pubertal children as the preferred or only means of sexual excitement. Most paedophiles are men. Of the few paedophiles who seek the help of doctors, most are of middle age although the behaviour has often started earlier. From the ready sale of pornographic material depicting sex with children, it is likely that paedophilic fantasies are not rare, although paedophilia as an exclusive form of sexual behaviour is infrequent.

The child is usually above the age of nine years but pre-pubertal, and may be of the same or opposite sex to the paedophile. The sexual contact may involve fondling, masturbation, or full coitus with consequent injury to the child.

Disorders of preference of the sexual act

The second group of disorders of sexual preference involves variations in the behaviour carried out to obtain sexual arousal. Generally, the acts are directed towards other adults but sometimes towards children (e.g. by some exhibitionists or sadists).

Exhibitionism

In this condition, sexual arousal is obtained repeatedly by exposure of the genitalia to an unprepared stranger. Nearly all exhibitionists are men. The act of exposure is usually preceded by a period of mounting tension which is released by the act. Usually, the exhibitionist seeks to shock or surprise a female. Most exhibitionists fall into two groups. The first consists of men with inhibited temperament who generally expose a flaccid penis and feel much guilt after the act. The second consists of men with aggressive personality traits who expose an erect penis while masturbating, and feel little guilt afterwards. In Britain, exhibitionists who are arrested are charged with the offence of *indecent exposure* (see p. 458).

When exhibitionism begins in middle or late life the possibility of organic brain disorder, depressive disorder, or alcoholism should be considered since these conditions occasionally 'release' this pattern of behaviour. In other people, the exhibitionism may start during a period of temporary stress.

Voyeurism

Voyeurism is observing the sexual behaviour of others as the preferred and repeated way of obtaining sexual arousal. Most voyeurs are inhibited heterosexual men. Some voyeurs spy on couples who are having intercourse, others on women who are undressing or naked.

Sexual sadomasochism

Sadomasochism is a preference for sexual activity that involves bondage or inflicting pain on another person. If the individual prefers to receive such stimulation, the disorder is called *masochism*. If the individual prefers to administer such stimulation, the disorder is called *sadism*. Beating, whipping, and tying are common forms of such activity. Sometimes the acts are symbolic and cause little actual damage, but occasionally the acts cause serious injuries from which the partner may die. Some people engage in solitary acts of self-injury; a particularly dangerous example is producing suffocation by covering the head with a plastic bag.

Mild degrees of sadomasochistic behaviour are common and are considered to be part of normal sexual activity. The disorder should only be diagnosed if sadomasochistic activity is the most important source of gratification or necessary for sexual stimulation.

Management of disorders of sexual preference

All cases of this kind should be referred to a specialist if possible, although the family doctor should first assess the problem as follows.

Assessment (Table 14.8)

The first step is to identify the problem and record its course. The second step is to *exclude any mental disorder* which may have released the sexual behaviour in a person who previously experienced sexual fantasies but did not act on them. Dementia, alcoholism, depressive disorder, and mania may each have this effect occasionally. It is particularly important to seek these causes when the abnormal sexual behaviour appears for the first time in middle or late life.

The third requirement is to *assess normal sexual functioning* since one of the main aims of treatment is to strengthen this. Whenever possible the patient's sexual partner should be interviewed as well. If normal sexual behaviour is inadequate, appropriate treatment is given (see pp. 300–1).

Next, an assessment is made of the *role of the abnormal behaviour* in the patient's life. As well as providing sexual arousal such behaviour may be used as a way of

Table 14.8.

Assessment of abnormalities of sexual preference

1. Identify the problem and its course

2. Exclude associated mental disorder (especially depressive disorder, alcoholism, and dementia).

3. Assess normal sexual functioning

4. Consider the 'role' of the abnormal sexual behaviour

5. Assess motivation for treatment

coping with loneliness, depression, or anxiety. If so, the patient should be helped to find adaptive coping mechanisms.

Finally, *motivation for treatment is assessed*. Often the patient has been urged to attend by another person: usually the wife or the police. In such cases the patient may have no wish to change. Other patients seek help when they become temporarily depressed or guilty, either because the sexual behaviour has caused a problem, or because of some other reason. Such people may lose their motivation quickly when their mood returns to normal.

Treatment

Counselling may help with any problems in forming relationships with the opposite sex. Any sexual dysfunction should be treated, using the methods described on pp. 300–1.

The patient should be encouraged to use distraction to control any fantasies of the abnormal sexual behaviour during masturbation, since such fantasies are likely to reinforce and maintain the sexual disorder. He should also stop the use of any pornographic materials used to stimulate these fantasies.

Counselling should be used to help with any problems consequent giving up the deviant sexual behaviour. Often, leisure time has been spent in seeking out abnormal sexual stimuli, and new interests may need to be developed. When the sexual behaviour has been used to cope with depression or anxiety, the patient should be helped to develop more adaptive ways of coping.

Antiandrogens and oestrogen have been used to reduce sexual drive, especially in patients whose abnormal sexual behaviour is potentially dangerous to other people. The benefits of such treatment have not been clearly established.

Some people with abnormal sexual preferences appear before the courts. Sanctions such as a suspended sentence or probation order sometimes help a patient to control his behaviour, provided that he is motivated to help himself.

Disorders of gender identity: transsexualism

In this rare disorder, the person has the conviction of being of the sex opposite to that indicated by the external genitalia. The person wishes to alter the external genitalia to resemble those of the opposite sex, and to live as a member of that sex. Most transsexuals are men; most women who cross-dress and imitate men are homosexual not transsexual. In transsexuals, the conviction of being a woman usually dates from before puberty, but medical help is not requested until early adult life, when most transsexuals have begun to dress as women. Unlike transvestites, they report no sexual arousal from cross-dressing; and unlike the homosexuals who dress as women, they do not seek to attract people into a homosexual relationship.

Many transsexuals go to great lengths in their attempts to appear as women. They practise female styles of speaking, gesturing, and walking; they remove body hair by electrolysis; they attempt to increase breast tissue by taking oestrogen or by obtaining a surgical implant; and they may seek an operation to remove the male external genitalia and form an artificial 'vagina'. Demands for such operations are often made in a most determined and persistent way, accompanied sometimes by threats of suicide or self-mutilation if surgery is not provided. Since such threats are carried out occasionally with serious consequences, a specialist opinion should be obtained.

It could be argued that the logical **treatment** of transsexualism would be a psychological procedure to alter the person's false beliefs about his gender identity. No form of psychotherapy, however, has been shown to succeed in this aim. Most transsexual patients reject such an approach, maintaining their determination to alter their bodies to conform more closely with their beliefs. In a few specialist centres operations with this purpose are carried out on selected patients (**gender reassignment**), and good results have been reported. However, there is no high quality evidence of the effectiveness of the procedure. Decisions about such treatment are therefore taken on an individual patient basis with thorough assessment and are made jointly by an experienced psychiatrist and surgeon, in consultation with the general practitioner.

Psychological problems of homosexual people

As described earlier (p. 294), there is no sharp dividing line between homosexual and heterosexual people. About 1% of men and 0.25% of women are exclusively homosexual throughout their lives, while a further proportion are overtly homosexual or bisexual for a few years but subsequently are predominantly heterosexual. This bisexual potential is greatest in adolescence, after which most people settle permanently into one or other sexual role. Homosexuality is not a psychiatric disorder, but homosexuals experience sexual and emotional problems for which they seek medical help. These problems are the subject of this section.

Helping homosexual people

Homosexual men consult doctors with four kinds of problem:

1. A sexually inexperienced young man who has homosexual thoughts and feelings may ask for advice on **whether he is homosexual**. The doctor should find out whether the young man has heterosexual as well as homosexual thoughts and feelings, and whether he has decided how he would prefer to develop. If the man has heterosexual feelings and wishes to develop them, he should be advised to avoid situations that stimulate homosexual feelings, and should be helped to develop social skills with women.

2. The second kind of problem is presented by young men who have realized correctly that they are predominantly homosexual and who ask for **counselling about the implications** for their lives. Such young men should be helped to think out the implications themselves, and may be put in touch with a self-help group of homosexuals.

3. The third problem is presented by the established homosexual who becomes **depressed or anxious** because of difficulties in his sexual relationships. Again, counselling is appropriate.

4. The fourth problem is presented by the homosexual who is **concerned about HIV and AIDS**. Such a patient requires appropriate medical investigation, treatment, and counselling.

Homosexual women ask for advice less often than homosexual men; when they do seek help, it is usually about problems in their relationship with the partner— often jealousy or depression. Married homosexual women may ask for advice about their relationships with the husband and family, or about dysfunction in heterosexual intercourse. Counselling is the appropriate treatment (pp. 365–6).

Further reading

Bancroft, J. H. J. (1998). *Human Sexuality and its Problems* (2nd edn). Churchill Livingstone, Edinburgh.
A comprehensive account of normal and abnormal sexual behaviour.

Hawton, K. (1985). *Sex Therapy: A Practical Guide.* Oxford University Press.
A practical account of simple kinds of therapy suitable for use by the non-specialist.

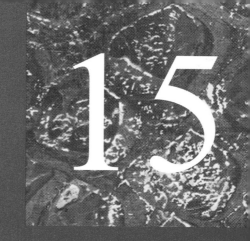

15

Psychiatry of the elderly

- Normal ageing

- Psychiatric disorder in the elderly

- Specific psychiatric disorders

- Appendix: Mini Mental State Examination

Psychiatry of the elderly

Psychiatric disorder, like medical illness, is especially prevalent in the elderly. This is reflected in the large proportion of time spent on the care of the elderly in primary care and the high proportion of hospital in-patient and out-patient attenders who are aged 65 or older. Although psychiatric disorders in old age have some special features, they do not differ greatly from the psychiatric disorders of younger adults.

Assessment should take account of the patient's physical state and of social circumstances, to decide whether the patient can be treated at home and if so what further practical help is necessary. It is important to obtain information from relatives or carers, especially where there is a possibility of intellectual impairment. **Treatment** must take account of the increased likelihood of concurrent medical disorders, social problems, and the needs of carers.

Delirium is much more frequent in the elderly than in younger people. It is frequently associated with major medical illnesses and treatments. When superimposed on dementia it leads to a major worsening of mental state and functioning.

The management of **dementia** is a major part of the psychiatry of old age. The most frequent causes of dementia at this age are Alzheimer's disease, vascular dementia, and Lewy body disease. Although it is important to consider the possibility of treatable causes, management is mainly concerned with assisting the patient and family to cope with the effects of dementia.

Affective disorder in the elderly is similar to that in younger patients. In treatment, particular care is needed in the dosages of antidepressant medication. It is often necessary to prescribe maintenance therapy.

Paranoid syndromes are not uncommon in the elderly. The most frequent causes are dementia, affective disorder, schizophrenia, and delusional disorder.

Normal ageing

In Western Europe, about 15% of the population is aged over 65 years. This proportion, especially the proportion of those aged over 85, will continue to rise in both developed and lesser developed countries (Fig. 15.1).

The following changes are seen in normal ageing:

- **Structural changes in the brain** The weight of the brain decreases, the quantity of nerve processes declines, and there is a minor and selective loss of cells with advancing age; senile plaques are increasingly common, and ischaemic lesions are present in brains from half of normal subjects aged over 65.

- **Psychological changes** From mid life there is a decline in intellectual functions as measured with standard intelligence tests together with deterioration of short-term memory and slowness. Also, there may be alterations in personality and attitudes, such as increasing cautiousness, rigidity, and 'disengagement' from the outside world.

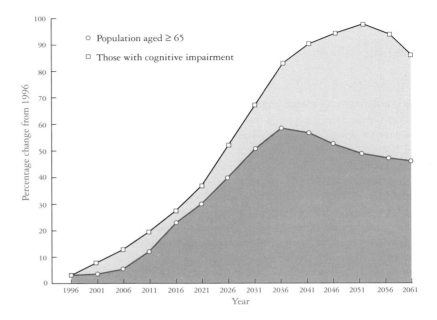

Fig. 15.1 Projected changes in the number of people aged ≥ 65 and in those with cognitive impairment in Britain by year from 1996. (Reproduced with permission from Melzer *et al.*, *British Medical Journal*, 315, 462, 1997.)

- **Social difficulties** Many elderly people have lower incomes and poorer accommodation than younger people. Most live at home; about half with their spouse, and about one in ten with their children. Some of those who live alone are very isolated. These unsatisfactory social circumstances are typical of most Western countries, but in some cultures, for example, the Chinese, the elderly are esteemed and most can expect to live with their children.

- **Use of medical services** The elderly consult their family doctors more often than younger people and they occupy a half of all general hospital beds. These demands are particularly great in those aged over 75. Treatment is often made difficult by the presence of more than one disorder and by increased sensitivity to drug side effects.

Psychiatric disorder in the elderly

The elderly suffer from all the psychiatric disorders described in other chapters of this book but dementia and delirium are particularly common. Since the prevalence of mental disorder and particularly dementia increases with age, there has been a disproportionate increase in the demand for psychiatric care for the elderly, and this trend is likely to continue (Fig. 15.2). Although mild in this age group, depression is the most frequent problem seen in primary care, dementia is the most serious.

General principles of assessment

Many elderly patients can be assessed in exactly the same way as younger people. However, even more careful consideration needs to be given to medical factors and social circumstances. After making a diagnosis there are three important practical issues that always need to be considered:

1. Can the patient's care be managed at home?

2. If so, what additional help is needed by the patient and family?

3. Can the patient manage his financial affairs?

Whenever possible the doctor should *interview any relatives or friends* who can give information about the patient and may be involved in care, especially if there is any possibility of intellectual impairment. The reasons for the request for treatment should be considered carefully, since this may reflect changes in the attitudes of the family and neighbours to the patient's longstanding problems rather than any change in the medical condition. When a specialist opinion is required it is often better to arrange this at the patient's home where patients can be observed in their usual surroundings.

History

The following specific information should be obtained during the assessment:

- Timing of onset of symptoms and their subsequent course.

- A description of behaviour over a typical 24 hours.

- Previous medical and psychiatric history.

- Living conditions and financial position.

- Ability for self-care and to manage finances and deal with hazards such as fire.

- Any behaviour that may cause difficulties for carers or neighbours.

- The ability of family and friends to help.

- Other services already involved in the patient's care.

Examination and investigation (Table 15.1)

Physical examination When there are medical indications and for all the more serious psychiatric problems, a thorough physical examination should be carried out, including an appropriately detailed neurological assessment with particular attention to vision and hearing.

Physical investigations If an organic cause of the psychiatric disorder is suspected, investigation may be required, guided by the diagnostic possibilities suggested by the history.

Psychological assessment Simple tests such as the Mini Mental State Examination (see Appendix, p.326) are valuable but must be used as part of a wider clinical examination. Regular clinical review and screening are valuable for older people. This should include search for possible psychiatric disorder, especially for early dementia and depressive disorder.

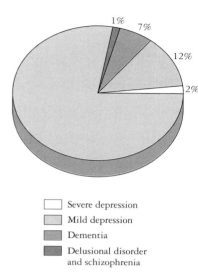

1%   7%
12%
2%

☐ Severe depression
▨ Mild depression
▨ Dementia
▨ Delusional disorder
   and schizophrenia

Fig 15.2 Prevalence of psychiatric disorder in the general population of those aged over 65 years (%).

Table 15.1.

Role of the primary care physician

- Reach the **correct diagnosis** and detect any remediable pathology
- Assess the patient's **functional state** and encourage optimum functioning
- Assess the role of the **primary health care team** in providing service
- Co-ordinate **social support** and make appropriate referrals to other agencies
- **Identify** the early stage of chronic disorders and help the patient and carers come to terms with diagnosis and prognosis
- Review **medication**
- Anticipate and **avert crises** by assessing social and domestic circumstances
- Monitor the **needs of carers** and support them

Principles of treatment

The treatment of psychiatric disorders in the elderly resembles that of the same conditions in younger adults, although there are some differences in emphasis:

- It is more often necessary to treat concurrent physical disorders.
- Special caution is needed in drug dosages.
- Social measures are even more important.
- Families need to be involved and supported, even more than with younger patients.

Treatment of physical illness Any physical disorder causing *organic mental disorder*, should be treated if possible. The treatment of other *physical disorders* may benefit the mental state in a non-specific way. *Mobility* should be encouraged, and is often helped by physiotherapy. A good *diet* should be ensured.

Place of treatment Although it may often be seem easier to treat more severe problems in hospital, *treatment at home* is usually preferable because most elderly people want to be at home and usually function better there. Plans should be responsive to changing needs, and discussed regularly with the family or other carers to ensure that home care does not place an unreasonable burden on them. *Short stays in hospital* may be needed for acute problems and to allow a holiday for the carers. *Long-term care* in a home or hospital is needed for a minority of the elderly.

Consent to treatment Older people, especially those with organic mental disorders, may be uncertain about or unwilling to accept medical and social care. It is usually possible to overcome these concerns by clear and repeated explanation and by involving family and others in the discussions. In some people the *capacity* to give informed consent has been impaired by dementia and mental health legislation has to be invoked to ensure essential treatment.

Use of psychotropic drugs

Drug-induced morbidity is common among elderly patients who may develop side effects at lower doses than do younger people. Some drugs may cause mental symptoms as side effects; most often those:

- used to treat cardiovascular disorders (hypotensives, diuretics, and digoxin);

- acting on the central nervous system (antidepressants, hypnotics, anxiolytics, antipsychotics, and antiparkinsonian drugs).

It is prudent to start treatment with small doses and increase these gradually to find the minimal effective dose. Response to the medication should be reviewed regularly. Despite the need for caution in prescribing, elderly patients should not be denied effective drug treatment, especially for depressive disorders.

Elderly patients may not take drugs as prescribed, especially when they are living alone, have poor vision, or are confused. For this reason, the drug regime should be as simple as possible, medicine bottles should be labelled clearly and easy to open, and the patient should be provided with memory aids (e.g. by containers with separate compartments for the drugs to be taken at each time of day). If possible, drug taking should be supervised by one of the carers or by a community nurse both of whom need to be adequately informed of the drug regime.

Many elderly people sleep poorly, and some take hypnotics regularly. Such drugs should be avoided since they may cause daytime drowsiness, confusion, falls, incontinence, and hypothermia. If a hypnotic is essential, the minimum effective dose should be used, the side effects monitored carefully, and the course of treatment made as short as possible. Dichloralphenazone, chlormethiazole, and medium- or short-acting benzodiazepines are used as hypnotics for the elderly.

Psychological treatment

Discussion and problem solving are as important in the care of the elderly as in the care of younger patients, and joint interviews with partners or carers are often valuable.

Memory aids Patients with memory disorder may be helped by simple measures such as the use of notebooks and alarm clocks to aid memory. In residential accommodation the use of colour coding of doors and similar features of design can help to reduce disorientation.

Interpretative psychotherapy is seldom appropriate for the elderly.

Social measures

Many patients can be helped to remain independent by attendance at a *club or day centre* as a way of encouraging self-care, domestic skills, and social contacts. *Domiciliary occupational therapy* may help patients who cannot travel to a day centre. More severely impaired patients may benefit from *residence* in an old people's home provided that their individual needs and dignity are respected.

Involving families

Families should be able to discuss problems and receive advice about the patient's care. If the patient is incontinent, relatives can be helped by the provision of laundry services. Day care or holiday admissions can allow carers periods of respite. With such help, many relatives can undertake the care of elderly people without undue burden.

Although most families care effectively for their elderly members, occasionally they *neglect or even abuse* the elderly person, or misuse their property. Elderly women are more often affected than elderly men, and those who have psychiatric disorder may be at greater risk.

Psychiatric emergencies

Psychiatric emergencies involving the elderly are relatively uncommon. There are three situations in which urgent action is required:

1. A confused person found *wandering*. A history should be obtained from a relative or neighbour and the patient medically examined. If the person is not well enough to go home, emergency medical, psychiatric, or residential care should be arranged.

2. Aggressive behaviour, usually in a patient with *dementia*. The nature and circumstance of the aggression should be reviewed and the possibility of *delirium* considered. Drug treatment (haloperidol or thioridazine) or admission for assessment may be required, or admission for assessment.

3. *Suicide attempt* or *self-harm*. Full assessment as described in Chapter 12 is required.

Specific psychiatric disorders

Delirium

The commonest causes of delirium in the elderly are infections of the urinary tract, chest, skin or ear, cardiac failure, iatrogenic side effects of drugs, and cerebrovascular ischaemia. The **clinical features** are summarized in Table 15.2 and

Table 15.2.
Clinical features of delirium

- Acute onset
- Fluctuating orientation
- Fluctuating alertness and disturbed sleep
- Impaired recent memory
- Abnormal perceptions, especially visual illusions or hallucination
- Perplexity or suspiciousness
- Irritability and agitation

Table 15.3.
Immediate treatment of delirium

Obtain information from informants and medical notes
Look for and treat the causes
↓
Maintain the patient's general physical condition
↓
Provide an appropriate environment:

Visual	–	adequate lighting, spectacles
Auditory	–	repeated, frequent explanations, hearing aids, minimal disturbance from others

↓
Maximise familiarity with the environment:

–	aid orientation by outside view, clock, etc.
–	visits by relatives
–	regular routine

↓
Consistent nursing

–	minimise medical interventions
–	avoid conflict
–	minimum number of staff involved

↓
Limited use of psychotropic drugs (see text)

delirium is more fully described in Chapter 10. Among elderly patients the central feature, impairment of consciousness, may not always be obvious, especially when the onset is gradual. When this happens delirium (a reversible disorder) may be misdiagnosed as dementia (an irreversible disorder). It is not uncommon for delirium to occur in patients with established dementia, resulting in considerable deterioration in cognitive function. In the absence of an obvious medical cause for delirium, look for occult urinary or other infection, or constipation. It is important not to miss alcohol-related cases, prescribed drug side effects or withdrawal, and head injury. Although the mental state improves when the cause of delirium is removed, many of the causes of delirium threaten life, and mortality is high.

Treatment is directed to the cause of the delirium but, until this has taken effect, drugs may be needed to control symptoms of agitation and disturbed behaviour and psychotic behaviour (see Chapter 10). The best choice is generally a small dose of an antipsychotic drug such as haloperidol which relieve symptoms without increasing confusion. If sleep is poor or disturbed a hypnotic can be useful; chlormethiazole or dichloralphenazone are often used, rather than benzodiazepines.

Dementia in the elderly

Dementia is common in the elderly. Most sufferers live at home, and in the UK about a quarter live alone. A primary care doctor with 2000 patients can expect to care for about 20 people. The main account of the syndrome of dementia is given in Chapter 10. This section is concerned with special points about dementia in the elderly. There are three common causes in this age group:

1. Alzheimer's disease

2. Vascular dementia

3. Lewy body disease

Alzheimer's disease

Prevalence The prevalence of moderate and severe Alzheimer's disease is about 5% of individuals aged 65 years and over, and 20% of those aged over 80 years. Therefore, as life expectancy increases in developing countries so the number of Alzheimer's patients increases (Fig. 15.3.). About 80% of these demented people live in the community rather than institutions. It is more common in women.

Pathology The brain is shrunken, with widened sulci and enlarged ventricles. There is cell loss, shrinkage of the dendritic tree, proliferation of astrocytes, and increased gliosis. Senile *plaques* and *neurofibrillary tangles* occur throughout the cortical and subcortical grey matter (Fig. 15.4.)

Aetiology Genetics factors play a role, especially in those with early onset of the disease. Pedigree studies of a small number of familes suggested inheritance which is consistent with autosomal dominance.

Recent evidence does not support the suggestion that excessive aluminium is a cause and other hypotheses about the role of slow viruses or abnormal immune mechanisms have not been confirmed.

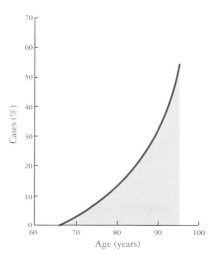

Fig. 15.3 Age-related prevalence curve for dementia (all types) derived from field studies in eight European countries: arithmetic scale Adapted with permission (Hofman *et al.* (1991). *International Journal of Epidemiology*, **20**, 736–40).

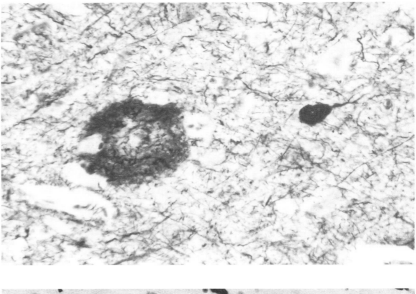

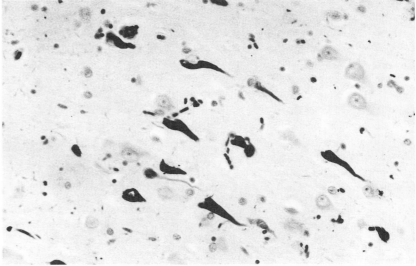

Fig. 15.4 (a) Amyloid plaque and neurofibrillary tangle from the brain of a patient who died of Alzheimer's disease. The plaque shows denser outer staining with an inner core. (b) Characteristic flame-shaped neurofibrillary tangles from the brain of a patient who died from Alzheimer's disease. The tangles are stained with an antibody to hyperphosphorylated tau protein. (Reproduced by permission of Professor Margaret Esiri.)

Table 15.4.

Clinical features of Alzheimer's disease and vascular dementia

Alzheimer's disease	Vascular dementia
Insidious decline	Stepwise progression
Poor memory	Poor memory
Progressive disorientation	Episodes of confusion
Mood change	Mood change
Restless activity	Personality change
Insomnia	Seizures
Decline in social behaviour	Neurological signs (see text)
Personality change	
Dysphasia, dyspraxia	

Clinical features Doctors are seldom consulted in the early stages of the disorder; help is often requested after a sudden worsening associated with an intercurrent physical illness.

The earliest feature is usually minor *forgetfulness*, which may be difficult to distinguish from the effects of normal ageing. *Disorientation* is usually an early sign and may be evident for the first time when the person is in unfamiliar surroundings, for example, on holiday. The *mood* varies; it may be predominantly depressed, euphoric, flattened, or labile. Many patients are *restless* by day, and some *sleep poorly* at night, waking disorientated and distressed. *Social behaviour declines* and self-care may be neglected although some patients maintain a good social facade despite severe cognitive impairment. *Personality change* may occur, often with an exaggeration of less favourable traits. *In the later stages* of the disorder, the above features progress, and signs of *parietal lobe dysfunction* (such as dysphasia or dyspraxia) may occur.

Course There is a progressive decline. Incidental physical illness may cause a superimposed delirium resulting in a sudden deterioration in cognitive function from which the patient may not recover fully. Death occurs usually within five to eight years of the first signs of the disease.

Vascular dementia

Vascular dementia is slightly more common among men than women. It begins usually in the late sixties or seventies, often more suddenly than Alzheimer's disease, sometimes after a cerebrovascular accident.

Pathology Vascular dementia is associated with multiple infarcts of varying size caused by thromboembolism from extracranial arteries or arteriosclerosis in main vessels. The brain is atrophic and the ventricles are dilated.

Clinical features The symptoms are characteristically fluctuating, and episodes of confusion are common, especially at night. Fits or episodes indicating cerebral

Table 15.5.
Causes of dementia

Alzheimer's disease

Vascular dementia

Lewy body disease

Mixed causes (e.g. Alzheimer's and vascular)

Parkinson's disease (see p. 215)

Vitamin B_{12} deficiency (see p. 192)

Normal pressure hydrocephalus (see p. 197)

Hypothyroidism (see p. 215)

Table 15.6.
Treatable causes apparent of dementia

- Depressive pseudodementia
- Delirium
- Slow-growing operable cerebral tumour
- Hypothyroidism
- Normal pressure hydrocephalus
- Vitamin B_{12} or folic acid deficiency
- Renal failure
- Severe anaemia

ischaemia occur at some stage in many cases. There may be neurological signs. In some cases emotional and personality changes may be apparent before impairment of memory and intellect

The diagnosis is difficult to make with certainty unless there is a clear history of stroke or neurological localizing signs. Suggestive features are patchy defects of cognitive function, stepwise progression of the condition, and the presence of hypertension and of arteriosclerosis in peripheral or retinal vessels. From the time of diagnosis the lifespan averages four to five years though the variations are wide. About half the patients die from ischaemic heart disease, and others from cerebral infarction or renal complications.

Lewy body disease

The name refers to the characteristic pathology. It is a progressive dementing illness which can be distinguished from Alzheimer's by its fluctuating course, the occurrence of hallucinations (especially visual), delusions, and signs of parkinsonism. There may be repeated falls and transient disturbances of consciousness.

Other causes of dementia in the elderly

Table 15.5 lists causes of dementia in old age.

The differential diagnosis of dementia in the elderly

General aspects of the diagnosis of dementia are discussed in Chapter 10. In the elderly, dementia must be differentiated from:

1. *Delirium* suggested by impaired and fluctuating consciousness, and by perceptual misinterpretations and visual hallucinations.

2. *Affective disorders* (see Chapter 8).

3. *Paranoid states* (see p. 324).

It is important to *consider treatable causes* of dementia, even though they are rare.

Assessment

The assessment should always include a thorough search for treatable causes of a delirium superimposed upon dementia. About 10% initially considered as having dementia will have a treatable cause (Table 15.6).

The aims of assessment are:

- to identify rare treatable conditions which may present as dementia;
- to diagnose any condition which may exacerbate dementia (e.g. a superimposed delirium);
- differential diagnosis of the cause of dementia;
- to obtain information needed to plan continuing care.

Early diagnosis is important because it enables planning with the patient and with all those involved in care. Information from carers about the impairment caused by the dementia is essential (Table 15.7). Because impairments develop gradually they are often attributed at first to normal ageing. Important clues to dementia are:

- General forgetfulness
- Misplacing items

- Forgetting names of close family members
- Increased anxiety or depression.

Questioning about the patient's functional capacity may reveal defects in self-care, ability to cope with familiar tasks, and emotional changes (Table 15.8).

Examination and investigation

The mental state examination should include a systematic assessment of cognitive functions. A full physical examination and investigation is required in any patients with rapid onset of fluctuating cognitive impairment, for those with unusual patterns of cognitive impairment and clear consciousness, and for all patients with onset under the age of 75 years. Specific investigations are usually not indicated in those with the insidious onset of the typical pattern of dementia over the age of 75.

To determine the cause of dementia, biochemical or other physical investigations may be indicated. According to the diagnostic possibilities, these may include blood count and film, ESR, VDRL serology, thyroid function, urea and electrolytes, liver function, vitamin B_{12}, chest X-ray, skull X-ray, ECG, and EEG. A CT scan is indicated when a localized lesion is suspected.

Treatment of dementia in the elderly

The first step is to treat any treatable physical disorder causing the dementia in the hope of arresting or possibly reversing it to some extent. If the physical disorder has caused an associated delirium, the mental state may improve considerably with treatment of the physical disorder. Even minor medical problems, such as constipation and urinary infection, may worsen the behavioural problems of a demented person (Table 15.10).

In early dementia, all those involved should consider what the patient should be told about the diagnosis. The patient may wish to know and there may be important reasons for early plans for future care, avoidance of unsuitable activities (such as driving), and planning family life and financial matters.

Psychological and social treatment For elderly demented patients psychological and social treatments are similar to those for younger patients.

Whenever feasible, patients should be *cared for at home* especially when family and friends can contribute to their care. If necessary, help can be provided by a community psychiatric nurse or social worker. *Day care* may be needed to help patient and family. *In-patient care* may be needed to tide over a crisis, or to enable the family to have a period of rest or a holiday. If the patient cannot be managed at home, *residential care* may be appropriate in an old people's home. Table 15.11 summarizes the assessment of a number of common practical problems.

In most cases, *long-term care in hospital* is required only when intensive nursing is needed. The role of the primary care team is summarized in Table 15.12.

Drug treatment Medication should be used with care as side effects may be greater than benefits. It is occasionally appropriate to consider sedative drug treatment, such as thioridazine or promazine, for restlessness when it is exhausting both for carers and the patient.

Antipsychotic drugs may be required to control paranoid delusions, and antidepressants may be indicated when depressive symptoms are prominent.

It has been reported that central cholinesterase inhibitors are of specific benefit for the dementia of Alzheimer's disease, delaying deterioration and possibly resulting in some improvement in cognitive function. Their clinical role is

Table 15.7.
History from carer

- Forgetfulness
- Memory lapses
- Personality changes
- Failure to recognize people
- Failure to cope with previous routine tasks
- Lack of self-care and reduction in personal standards
- Giving up previous interests and hobbies
- Emotional changes: anxiety, depression, irritability, lack of care, and concern
- Nocturnal confusion
- Disorientation for time and place
- Difficulty in speech
- Extent to which changes have been gradual or have suddenly worsened

Table 15.8.
Assessment of needs: functional capacity

- Continence
- Dressing
- Self-care
- Cooking ability and nutrition
- Shopping/housework
- Degree of orientation in the home
- Capacity to manage financial affairs
- Formal and informal supports
- Social contacts
- Safety in the home

Table 15.9.

Referral to a hospital consultant

- Early diagnosis of a possible dementia and the cause
- Detection of reversible conditions mimicking dementia
- Specialist advice about management, including advice on drug treatment
- Uncontrollable agitation
- Assessment and management of challenging behaviours
- Access to specialist services

Table 15.10.

Treatment of dementia

- Treat any primary disorder
- Treat the cause of superimposed delirium
- Treat even minor medical problems (see text)
- Involve and support the relatives
- Arrange practical help in the home
- Arrange help for carers (e.g. 'holiday admissions')
- Medication for night- and daytime restlessness
- If home care fails, arrange residential or hospital care

Table 15.11.

Assessment of common problems

Aggression
- Is it verbal or physical?
- To whom is it directed and when—is there a reason?
- What resources are available?
- Should drugs be used?

Incontinence
- What kind and how often?
- Are there contributing medical factors (e.g. drugs)?
- What means of containment are available (e.g. pads or laundry services)?

Wandering
- Frequency?
- What is the degree of danger?

Refusal of services
- How do the risks balance against the choices of the individual?
- What alternative sources of help are available?
- When should the situation be reassessed?

Refusal to accept admission to residential care
- How can risks of wandering and self-neglect be limited?
- Is additional community support available?
- Are compulsory procedures appropriate?
- Can some one be appointed to take on legal powers for financial and other matters?

Table 15.12.

The role of the primary care team

- Investigate exclusion of treatable causes (present in about 10%)
- Exclude coincident condition: especially depression, delirium, paranoid disorder symptoms, and concurrent physical illnesses
- Minimize associated disabilities
- Decide whether to refer to consultant (see Table 15.9)
- Manage and co-ordinate access to other resources
- Help carers. Provide information and advice, especially about the emotional and behavioural changes which have taken place or may do so

limited and their use should only be considered as a part of specialist care. A second generation of drugs is being developed and they can be expected to be available in the next few years.

Depressive disorder

Depressive disorders are common in later life with a prevalence of about 10–15% for those aged 65, of which a quarter are severe. Many of these disorders are in people who have had a depressive disorder at an earlier age; first depressive illnesses decline in incidence after the age of 60, and are rare after the age of 80. The incidence of *suicide* increases steadily with age and is usually associated with depressive disorder.

Clinical features

There are no fundamental differences between depressive disorders in the elderly and those in younger people, but some symptoms are more common in the elderly. Anxiety and hypochondriacal symptoms are frequent, and depressive delusions of poverty and physical illness are more common among severely depressed patients. Hallucinations of an accusing or obscene kind are also more frequent in the elderly.

A few of the retarded depressed patients have conspicuous difficulty in concentrating and remembering but they show no corresponding defect ('*pseudo-dementia*') in clinical tests of memory function. The possibility of a depressive disorder should be considered whenever an elderly patient develops apparent cognitive impairment, or anxiety or hypochondriacal symptoms.

Course

Untreated depressive disorders in the elderly often have a *prolonged course*, some lasting for years. With treatment, most patients improve considerably within a few months, but about 15% do not recover completely even after vigorous treatment. Long-term follow-up of recovered patients shows that relapse is frequent. Suicide is more likely than in younger people.

Factors predicting a better prognosis are:

- onset before the age of 70;
- short duration of illness;
- good previous adjustment;
- no concurrent disabling physical illness;
- good recovery from previous episodes.

Aetiology

In general, the aetiology of depressive disorders in late life resembles that of similar disorders occurring in earlier life (see Chapter 8), except that genetic factors may be less important. Neurological and other physical illnesses seem to be more frequent than among depressed elderly patients than younger ones, and may act as provoking or maintaining factors.

Differential diagnosis

- **from dementia** The most difficult differential diagnosis is between *depressive pseudodementia* and *dementia*, and a specialist opinion is often required (Table 15.13).

Table 15.13.

Dementia and pseudodementia

Dementia	Pseudodementia
Prolonged progressive course	Course of weeks or months
Impaired orientation	Normal orientation
Mood changes secondary	Begins with mood symptoms
Memory impaired, may confabulate	Unwillingness to answer
Progressive course	May be diurnal variation
	May be past history of mood disorder

The distinction (Table 15.13) depends on a detailed history from other informants, and careful observation of the mental state and behaviour. In depressive pseudodementia mood disturbance usually precedes other symptoms, and the depressed patient's lack of interest and unwillingness to answer can usually be distinguished from the demented patient's true failure of memory. In depression, there may be diurnal variation and a past history of mood disorder. The diagnostic problem is made more difficult because dementia and depressive disorder sometimes coexist.

• **from a paranoid disorder** When paranoid ideas are prominent in a depressive disorder, it has to be differentiated from a *paranoid disorder*. In a depressive disorder, the patient usually believes that the supposed persecution is justified by his own wickedness; in paranoid disorder he usually resents it as unjustified. Depressive symptoms usually follow the onset of paranoid disorder, but it is often difficult to be certain of the sequence.

• **from anxiety disorder** Depressive disorder with symptoms of agitation may be mistaken at first for an *anxiety disorder*. It is essential to look for characteristic pessimism and other symptoms of low mood.

Treatment

In most respects the treatment of depressive disorders is the same for the elderly as for people of other ages (see Chapter 8). Suicide risk should be assessed (see p. 244).

Antidepressant drugs are effective in the elderly, but should be used cautiously and adjusted with relation to side effects and response. Tricyclic antidepressants are usually the first choice but SSRIs (specific serotonin reuptake inhibitors) are an alternative. They are particularly useful for those who find the side effects of tricyclic antidepressants intolerable, for those with cardiac arrhythmias or epilepsy, and in those in which the risk of delirium is high (e.g. patients with dementia). To reduce side effects, the starting dose is about half the usual dose for younger patients, and the drug may be given more than once a day. Although it is appropriate to start cautiously, it is important to achieve a full therapeutic dose.

After recovery, antidepressant medication should be reduced slowly and then continued in reduced dose for at least two years. Patients with a history of recurrent depression require long-term continuation treatment.

Electroconvulsive therapy is useful for severe and distressing agitation, life-threatening stupor, or failure to respond to drugs. Special care is needed with the anaesthesia. It may be necessary to space out treatments at longer intervals than in younger patients to reduce the post-treatment memory impairment is not a problem.

Mania

Unlike depressive disorder, mania does not increase in incidence with age. Hence, in old age mania is much less frequent than depressive disorder, accounting for 5–10% of affective disorders. In the elderly, depressive symptoms are often present with the manic symptoms, and the condition is frequently recurrent. Treatment of the acute illness is similar to that for younger patients (Chapter 8), although with special caution about the side effects of drugs. Lithium prophylaxis is valuable but the blood levels should be kept at the lower end of the therapeutic range used for younger patients, and monitored with special care.

Paranoid syndromes

Paranoid syndromes, with persecutory beliefs, delusions or hallucinations, may be due to: (1) dementia; (2) affective disorder; (3) schizophrenia and delusional disorder (sometimes referred to as late paraphrenia); and (4) paranoid personality disorder. The commonest syndromes are those secondary to dementia or affective disorders.

Schizophrenia and delusional disorder may begin in old age or have begun earlier in life and continued into old age. In the elderly, the symptoms are generally less florid, and the behaviour less disturbed than in young patients. Patients with long histories in younger life will require continuing specialist care which takes account of the changing circumstances of old age. The same aetiological factors have been identified as in younger adults, but evidence of previously suspicious personality, social isolation, and deafness seem to be particularly important.

Differential diagnosis In the elderly, *schizophrenia and delusional disorders* are diagnosed by the same criteria as in younger patients. In *dementia* there is cognitive impairment and visual hallucinations may occur. In *affective disorder*, the mood disturbance is more profound than in paranoid states, and the persecutory delusions are usually associated with ideas of guilt. In *paranoid personality disorder* there are lifelong suspiciousness and distrust, with sensitive ideas but no delusions.

Treatment

In general, the treatment of these disorders in the elderly are similar to those for younger people (see Chapter 8). Out-patient treatment may be possible, but admission to hospital is often required for adequate assessment and treatment. Most patients require antipsychotic medication but the dosage is usually less than that needed for younger adults, for example, 2–5 mg of trifluoperazine three times a day or haloperidol 1–10 mg once daily. As with younger patients a depot preparation should be considered. Any sensory deficit, such as deafness or cataract, should be assessed and, if possible, treated. Attendance at a day hospital or day centre may be needed to avoid social isolation, ensure adequate supervision, and prevent relapse. (See *case study*.)

Case study: paranoid symptoms

The son of an 82-year-old widow comes to your surgery to say that he is concerned about his mother. He has noticed, over a period of months, that his mother has complained of increasingly numerous events in which neighbours and other people have apparently shouted abuse from outside her house and persecuted her. She believes that they have stolen objects and that they have moved her furniture around. She thinks that there is a complex conspiracy that involves a number of her neighbours and which is intended to drive her out of her own home. The son has realized that many of the allegations are a fantasy and unbelievable and has tried to persuade his mother to seek help. However, she has maintained that she is perfectly well and that problems lie with her neighbours' behaviour.

You have known the patient for many years and have occasionally visited her to treat minor ailments. You say that you will visit her home and say that you are making one of your regular visits to the older patients in your practice. When you arrive, the patient is initially somewhat suspicious but lets you in and, having offered you a cup of tea, tells you about the way in which she believes she is being persecuted. When you express some doubt, it is clear that she will not be dissuaded from these beliefs.

You feel that it is unlikely that she would agree to a visit from a psychiatrist and that you should try and establish the diagnosis. While your patient is upset about what has been happening, it is also apparent that when she discusses her own family and other issues she is cheerful and retains her usual sense of humour. You conclude she is not suffering from a depressive illness. At the same time, it is apparent that her memory of past events and of previous discussions with you is excellent and that she has a good knowledge of current events. It is clear that she is not suffering from dementia. She is not deaf. You conclude that she is almost certainly suffering from primary paranoid disorder.

You conclude that medication would be appropriate and you are eventually able to persuade your patient that she should try some new tablets to treat the very considerable distress which she reports in association with the persecutory symptoms. You prescribe Stelazine 5 mg a day and arrange to visit her again. When you return to your surgery, you consult the local psychiatrist for the elderly and agree that the present plan is appropriate and that, if necessary and the patient consents, a psychiatric consultation could be arranged at a later stage.

Two weeks later you are pleased to find that the patient is no longer describing the persecutory symptoms which she says have stopped several days previously (although she apparently still believes that they were genuine). She agrees that the medication has been helpful for her distress and is willing to continue for the time being. You suggest that you will check on the medication when you see her for her usual blood pressure review.

Anxiety, minor affective disorder, and personality disorder

Anxiety and minor affective disorder are as common in the elderly as in younger people, but occur rarely for the first time in old age. There is often a predisposing personality disorder. Common precipitating factors are physical illness, retirement, bereavement, and change of accommodation. Among the elderly these syndromes are usually of a non-specific kind, with anxiety, depressive, and hypochondriacal symptoms. Specific obsessional, phobic, and conversion disorders are less common. It is important to identify anxiety which is secondary to depressive disorders in early dementia.

Personality disorder may cause difficulties for elderly patients and their families. Paranoid traits may become accentuated with the social isolation of old age, sometimes to the extent of resembling a paranoid disorder. Personality disorder in the elderly often leads to isolation and to self-neglect, which can be extreme.

The **treatment** of emotional and personality disorders in old age is similar to that in younger adult life. It is essential to treat any physical disorder. Social measures are usually more useful than psychological treatment, but psychotherapy and behavioural treatments should not be ruled out because of age alone.

Abuse of alcohol and drugs

Although excessive drinking declines with increasing age, the problem is still a significant among the elderly. Sometimes the excessive drinking began at a younger age and sometimes in old age, often as a response to loneliness, boredom, or unhappiness. The management of the problem in the elderly is similar to that for younger people (see Chapter 13).

Overuse of prescribed drugs especially hypnotics, analgesics, and laxatives is common and it may be difficult to distinguish between deliberate overuse and that consequent on poor memory for the correct dosage or for the time when the last dose was taken.

Physical abuse of the elderly

Cruelty and physical maltreatment of elderly people may occur by carers at home or in residential care. It is especially likely where there is a long history of disturbed relationships, where carers are ignorant, unsympathetic, or overwhelmed by the behavioural difficulties and, occasionally, for financial exploitation. Doctors need to be aware of the possibility of physical abuse and be prepared to intervene in whatever way will prevent continuing abuse and deal with underlying problems.

Further reading

Jacoby, R. and Oppenheimer, C. (1997). *Psychiatry in the Elderly* (2nd edn). Oxford University Press.
A comprehensive work of reference.

Appendix: Mini Mental State Examination*

(Add points for each corrrect response)		Score	Points
Orientation			
1. What is the	Year?	—	1
	Season?	—	1
	Date?	—	1
	Day?	—	1
	Month?	—	1
2. Where are the	State?	—	1
	Country?	—	1
	Town or City?	—	1
	Hospital?	—	1
	Floor?	—	1

Registration

3. Name three objects taking one second
to say each. Then ask the patient all three
after you have said them.   —   3
Give one point for each correct answer.
Repeat the answers until the patient learns
all three.   —   3

Attention and calculation

4. Serial sevens. Give one point for each correct
answer.
Stop after five answers.
Alternative: Spell 'WORLD' backwards   —   5

Recall

5. Ask for names of three objects learned in Q3
Give one point for each correct answer.   —   3

Language

6. Point to a pencil and a watch. Have the patient
name them as you point.   —   2
7. Have the patient repeat 'No ifs, ands and buts'.   —   1
8. Have the patient follow a three-stage command:
'Take a paper in your right hand. Fold the paper
in half. Put the paper on the floor'.   —   3
9. Have the patient read and obey the following:
'CLOSE YOUR EYES'. (Write it in large letters.)   —   1
10. Have the patient write a sentence of his or her choice.
(These sentence should contain a subject and an
object, and should make sense. Ignore spelling
errors when scoring.)   —   1

11. Enlarge the design printed below to 1.5 cm per side, and have the patient copy it. (Give one point if all sides and angles are preserved and if the intersecting sides form a quadrangle.)

      —   1

      —— = Total 30

* Reprinted from Anthony, J. C., Le Resche, L., Niaz, U., Von Korf, M. R., and Folstein, M. F. (1982). Limits of the 'Mini Mental State' as a screening test for dementia and delirium among hospital patients. *Psychological Medicine*, 12, 397–408.

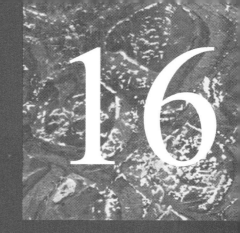

16

Drugs and other physical treatments

- General considerations
- Review of drugs used in psychiatry
- Other physical treatments

Drugs and other physical treatments

This chapter is about the use of drugs and electroconvulsive therapy. Psychological treatment is considered separately in Chapter 17. This is a convenient way of dividing the subject matter of a book, but in practice these *physical treatments are always combined with psychological treatment*, most often supportive or problem-solving counselling, but also one of the specific methods described in Chapter 17.

The account in this chapter is concerned with practical therapeutics rather than basic pharmacology, and it will be assumed that the reader has studied the pharmacology of the principal types of drug used in psychiatric disorders. (Readers who do not have this knowledge should consult a textbook, for example, *The Oxford Textbook of Clinical Pharmacology and Drug Therapy* by D. G. Grahame-Smith and J. K. Aronson.) Nevertheless, a few important points about the actions of psychotropic drugs will be considered, before describing the specific groups of drugs.

New drugs are produced every year. Chapter 4 contains advice about finding a review of evidence about the effectiveness of new drugs.

General considerations

Pharmacokinetics of psychotropic drugs

To be effective, psychotropic drugs must reach the brain in adequate amounts. How far they do this depends on their absorption, metabolism, excretion, and passage across the blood–brain barrier.

Absorption Most psychotropic drugs are absorbed readily from the gut, but absorption can be reduced by intestinal hurry or a malabsorption syndrome.

Metabolism Most psychotropic drugs are metabolized partially in the liver on their way from the gut via the portal system to the systemic circulation. The amount of this so called *first pass metabolism* differs from one person to another, and it is altered by certain drugs, taken at the same time, which induce liver enzymes (e.g. barbiturates) or inhibit them (e.g. monoamine oxidase inhibitors—MAOIs). Although first pass metabolism reduces the amount of the original drug reaching the brain, the metabolites of some drugs have their own therapeutic effects.

Because many psychotropic drugs have active metabolites, the *measurement of plasma concentrations of the parent drug is generally a poor guide to treatment*. Such measurement is *used routinely only with lithium carbonate*, which has no metabolites (see p. 353).

Distribution In plasma, psychotropic drugs are bound largely to protein. Because they are lipophilic, they pass easily into the *brain*. For the same reason they enter into *fat stores* from which they are released slowly, often for many weeks after the patient has ceased to take the drug. They also pass into *breast milk*—an important point when a breast-feeding mother is treated.

Excretion Psychotropic drugs and their metabolites are excreted through the kidneys, so smaller doses should be given when renal function is impaired. Lithium is unique among the psychotropic drugs in being filtered passively in the glomerulus and then partly reabsorbed in the tubules by the mechanism that absorbs sodium. The two ions compete for reabsorption so that when sodium levels fall, lithium absorption rises and lithium concentrations increase—potentially to a toxic level.

Drug interactions

When two drugs are given together one may either interfere with the other, or enhance its therapeutic or unwanted effects. Interactions can take place during absorption, metabolism, or excretion; or at the cellular level. For psychotropic drugs, most pharmacokinetic interactions are at the stage of liver metabolism, the important exception being lithium for which interference is at the stage of renal excretion. An important pharmacodynamic interaction is the antagonism between tricyclics and some antihypertensive drugs (see p. 346). When prescribing a psychotropic and another drug the manufacturer's literature or a work of reference should be consulted to determine whether the drugs interact.

Drug withdrawal

When some drugs are given for a long period, the tissues adjust to their presence and when the drug is withdrawn there is a temporary disturbance of function until a new adjustment is reached. This disturbance appears clinically as a withdrawal syndrome. Among psychotropic drugs, anxiolytics and hypnotics are most likely to induce this effect (see p. 338).

General advice about prescribing psychotropic drugs

Use well-tried drugs When there is a choice of equally effective drugs, it is generally good practice to use the drugs whose side effects and long-term effects are understood better. Also, well-tried drugs are generally less expensive than new ones. Clinicians should become familiar with a few drugs of each of the main types—antidepressants, antipsychotics, and so on. In this way they will become used to adjusting dosage and recognizing side effects.

Change drugs only for a good reason If there is no therapeutic response to an established drug given in adequate dosage, it is unlikely that there will be a better response to another from the same therapeutic group. The main reason for changing medication is that side effects have prevented adequate dosage. It is then appropriate to change to a drug with a different pattern of side effects; for example, from an antidepressant with strong anticholinergic effects to another with weaker ones.

Combine drugs only for special reasons Generally, drug combinations should be avoided (see drug interactions above). However, some drug combinations are of proven value for specific purposes, for example, benzodiazepines and antipsychotics to control acute symptoms of schizophrenia (see p. 175), and lithium and antidepressant for drug-resistant depressive disorder (see p. 144). Usually, drug combinations are initiated by a specialist because the adverse effects of such combinations can be more hazardous than those of a single drug. However, general practitioners may be asked to continue prescribing.

Adjust dosage carefully Dose ranges for some commonly used drugs are indicated later in this chapter, others will be found in the manufacturers' data sheets, or a work of reference. Within these ranges, the correct dose for an individual patient is decided from the severity of the symptoms, the patient's age and weight, and any factors that may affect drug metabolism or excretion.

Plan the interval between doses Less frequent administration has the advantage that patients are more likely to be reliable in taking drugs. The duration of action of most psychotropic drugs is such that they can be taken once or twice a day while maintaining a therapeutic plasma concentration between doses.

Decide the duration of treatment The duration depends on the risk of dependency and the nature of the disorder. In general, anxiolytic and hypnotic drugs should be given for a short time—a few days to two or three weeks—because of the risk of dependency. Antidepressants and antipsychotics are given for a long time—several months—because of the risk of relapse.

Advise patients Before giving a first prescription for a drug, the doctor should explain several points:

1. the likely *initial effects* of the drug (e.g. drowsiness or dry mouth);

2. the *delay* before therapeutic effects appear (about two weeks with antidepressants);

3. the likely *first signs of improvement* (e.g. improved sleep after starting an antidepressant);

4. *common side effects* (e.g. fine tremor with lithium);

5. *any serious effects* that should be reported immediately by the patient (e.g. coarse tremor after taking lithium);

6. any *restrictions* while the drug is taken (e.g. not driving or operating machinery if the drugs reduce alertness);

7. *how long* the patient will need to take the drug: for anxiolytics, the patient is discouraged from taking them for too long; for antidepressants or antipsychotics, the patient is encouraged to continue after symptoms have been controlled.

Compliance with treatment
Many patients do not take the drugs provided for them. Their unused drugs are a danger to children and a potential source of deliberate self-poisoning. Other patients take more than the prescribed dose, especially of hypnotic or anxiolytic drugs. It is important to check that repeat prescriptions are not being requested before the correct day.

To comply with treatment, a patient must be:

1. **Convinced of the need to take the drug.** Schizophrenic or seriously depressed patients may not be convinced that they are ill, or may not wish to recover. Deluded patients may distrust their doctors.

2. **Free from fears about its dangers.** Some patients fear that antidepressant drugs will cause addiction; some fear unpleasant or dangerous side effects.

3. **Able to remember to take it.** Patients with memory impairment may forget to take medication, or take the dose twice.

Time spent at the start of treatment in discussing reasons for drug treatment and the patient's concerns and explaining the beneficial and likely adverse effects of the drugs, increases compliance. Compliance should be checked at subsequent visits and, if necessary, the discussion should be repeated and extended to include any fresh concerns of the patient.

What to do if there is no therapeutic response

The first step is to find out whether the patient has taken the drug in the correct dose. If not, the points described above under 'compliance' should be considered. If the prescribed dose has been taken, the diagnosis should be reviewed: if is confirmed, an increase of dosage should be considered. Only when these steps have been gone through should the original drug be changed.

Box 16.1 Prescribing for special groups

Children

Most childhood psychiatric disorders are treated without medication. The indications for drug treatment are considered in Chapter 19. When drugs are required, care must be taken in selecting the appropriate dose. Usually, medication will have been started by a specialist who will advise about continuing treatment.

Elderly patients

These patients are often sensitive to drug side effects and may have impaired renal or hepatic function, so it is important to start with low doses and increase to about half the adult dose in appropriate cases.

Pregnant women

Psychotropic drugs should be avoided if possible during the first trimester of pregnancy because of the risk of teratogenesis. If medication is needed for a woman who could become pregnant, advice is given about contraception. If the patient is already pregnant and medication is essential the manufacturer's advice should be followed and the risks discussed with the patient. If the patient becomes pregnant while taking a psychotropic drug the risk of relapse should be weighed against the reported teratogenic risk of the drug. In general, it is safer to use long-established drugs for which there has been ample time to accumulate experience about safety. The following points concern the classes of psychotropic drugs.

- *Anxiolytics* are seldom essential in early pregnancy since psychological treatment is usually an effective alternative.
- If *antidepressants* are required, amitriptyline and imipramine have been in long use, without convincing evidence of teratogenic effects.
- *Antipsychotic drugs* It is important to discuss contraception with schizophrenic women, and to re-evaluate the need for antipsychotics if the patient becomes pregnant.
- *Lithium carbonate* should not be started in pregnancy because its use is associated with an increased rate of cardiac abnormality in the fetus (see p. 355). Contraception is especially important for women who may become manic and it is prudent to leave a month between the last dose of lithium and the ending of contraceptive measures. If a patient conceives when taking lithium, there is no absolute indication for termination but the risks should be explained, specialist advice obtained, and the fetus examined by ultrasound. Mothers who are taking lithium at term should if possible stop gradually well before delivery. The drug should not be taken during labour. Serum lithium concentration should be measured frequently during labour and the use of diuretics avoided.

Mothers who are breast-feeding

Psychotropic drugs should be prescribed cautiously to women who are breast-feeding because they pass into breast milk and the possibility is not ruled out that they may affect brain development. Some authorities recommend that women receiving psychotropic medication should not breast-feed. Others continue treatment cautiously with careful monitoring of the baby. Benzodiazepines pass readily into breast milk, causing sedation. Most neuroleptics and antidepressants pass rather less readily into the milk; sulpiride, doxepin, and dothiepin are secreted in larger amounts and should be avoided. Lithium carbonate enters milk freely and breast-feeding should be avoided. The advice of a specialist should be obtained.

Patients with concurrent medical illness

Special care is needed in prescribing for patients with medical illness, especially liver and kidney disorders, which may interfere with metabolism and excretion of drugs. Conversely, medical disorders may be exacerbated by the side effects of some psychotropic drugs. For example, cardiac disorder and epilepsy may be affected adversely by some antidepressant drugs (see pp. 346–7); while drugs with anticholinergic side effects exacerbate glaucoma and may provoke retention of urine.

Review of drugs used in psychiatry

Psychotropic drugs are those which have effects mainly on mental symptoms, they are divided into six groups according to their principal actions. Several have secondary actions used for other purposes. For example, antidepressants are sometimes used to treat anxiety (see Table 16.1):

1. **Anxiolytic** drugs reduce anxiety. Because they have a general calming effect, they are sometimes called *minor tranquillizers* (major tranquillizer is an alter-

Table 16.1.

Psychotropic drugs

Type	Indications	Classes of drug
Anxiolytic	Acute anxiety	Benzodiazepines Azapirones
Hypnotic	Insomnia	Benzodiazepines Cyclopyrrolones Zopiclone
Antipsychotic[a]	Delusion and hallucinations Mania To prevent relapse in schizophrenia	Phenothiazines Butyrophenones Substituted benzamides
Antidepressant	Depressive disorders Chronic anxiety Obsessive-compulsive disorder Nocturnal enuresis	Tricyclics MAOIs[b] SSRIs[c]
Mood stabilizer	To prevent recurrent mood disorder	Lithium Carbamazepine
Psychostimulant	Narcolepsy Hyperkinetic disorder in children	Amphetamine

[a]Antiparkinsonian drugs are used to control side effects of antipsychotics.
[b]MAOIs, monoamine oxidase inhibitors.
[c]SSRIs, specific serotonin reuptake inhibitors.

native name for antipsychotic drugs, see below). In larger doses these drugs produce drowsiness and for this reason are sometimes called *sedatives*.

2. **Hypnotics** promote sleep; many hypnotics are of the same type as drugs used as anxiolytics.

3. **Antipsychotic** drugs control delusions, hallucinations, and psychomotor excitement in psychoses. Sometimes they are called *major tranquillizers* because of their calming effect; or *neuroleptics* because of their parkinsonian and other neurological side effects. (**Antiparkinsonian** agents, are sometimes employed to control parkinsonian side effects.)

4. **Antidepressants** relieve the symptoms of depressive disorders but do not elevate the mood of healthy people. Antidepressant drugs are also used to treat chronic anxiety disorders, obsessive compulsive disorder, and occasionally, nocturnal enuresis.

5. **Mood-stabilizing** drugs are given to prevent recurrence of recurrent affective disorders.

6. **Psychostimulants** elevate mood but are not used for this purpose because they can cause dependence. Their principal use in psychiatry is in the treatment of hyperactivity syndromes in children (see p. 410).

The main groups of drugs will be reviewed in turn. For each group, an account will be given of important points concerning therapeutic effects, the compounds in most frequent use, side effects, toxic effects, and contraindications. General advice will also be given about the use of each group of drugs, but *specific applications to the treatment of individual disorders will be found in the chapters dealing with these conditions*. Drugs with a use limited to the treatment of a single disorder (e.g. disulfiram for alcohol problems), are discussed solely in the chapters dealing with the relevant clinical syndromes.

Anxiolytic drugs

Anxiolytic drugs reduce anxiety, and in larger doses produce drowsiness (they are *sedatives*) and sleep (they are also *hypnotics*). (Hypnotics are discussed on p. 339.) These drugs are prescribed widely, and sometimes unnecessarily for patients who would improve without them. Anxiolytics used most appropriately to reduce severe anxiety. They should be prescribed for a short time usually a few days, seldom for more than 2–3 weeks. Longer courses of treatment may lead to tolerance and dependence.

Buspirone (see below) seems to be an exception to the general rule that anxiolytics produce dependency but its anxiolytic effect develops more slowly and is less intense than that of the benzodiazepines. The drugs called *anxiolytics* are not the only ones that reduce anxiety, antidepressant and antipsychotic drugs also have anxiolytic properties. Since they do not induce dependence, they are sometimes used to treat chronic anxiety. Beta-adrenergic agonists are used to control some of the somatic symptoms of anxiety (see Table 16.2).

Benzodiazepines

Benzodiazepines act on specific receptor sites, linked with GABA (gamma-aminobutyric acid) receptors. They enhance GABA neurotransmission and affect indirectly 5-HT (serotonin or 5-hydroxytrypamine) and noradrenaline systems. As well as anxiolytic, sedative, and hypnotic effects benzodiazepines have muscle relaxant and anticonvulsant properties. Benzodiazepines are rapidly absorbed and metabolized into a large number of compounds many of which have their own therapeutic effects.

Compounds in frequent use The many benzodiazepines are divided into short and long acting drugs. Short acting drugs are useful for their brief clinical effect, free from hangover. Their disadvantage is that they are more likely than long acting drugs to cause dependence. Examples of commonly used drugs of each group are shown for reference in *Additional information*.

Side effects are mainly *drowsiness*, with ataxia at larger doses (especially in the elderly). These effects, which may *impair driving skills* and the operation of machinery, are potentiated by alcohol. Patients should be warned about both these potential hazards. Like alcohol, benzodiazepines can *release aggression* by reducing inhibitions in people with a tendency to this kind of behaviour. This should be remembered, for example, when prescribing for women judged to be at risk of child abuse, or anyone with a history of impulsive aggressive behaviour.

Table 16.2.
Drugs used to treat anxiety

- Primary anxiolytics
  - benzodiazepines
  - buspirone
- Other drugs with anxiolytic properties
  - some antidepressants
  - phenothiazines
  - beta-adrenergic agonists

Additional information **Grouping of benzodiazepines**

Group	Approximate Duration of action	Examples
Short-acting	< 12 hours	Lorazepam Temazepam Oxazepam Triazolam
Long-acting	> 24 hours	Diazepam Nitrazepam Flurazepam Chlordiazepoxide Clobazam Chlorazepate Alprazolam

Toxic effects are few, and most patients recover even from large overdoses. There is no convincing evidence of teratogenic effects; nevertheless, these drugs should be avoided in the first trimester of pregnancy unless there is a strong indication for their use.

Withdrawal effects occur after benzodiazepines have been prescribed for more than a few weeks; they have been reported in up to half the patients taking the drugs for more than six months. The frequency depends on the dose and the type of drug. The withdrawal syndrome is shown in Table 16.3. Seizures occur infrequently after rapid withdrawal from large doses. The obvious similarity between benzodiazepine withdrawal symptoms and those of an anxiety disorder makes it difficult, in practice, to decide whether they arise from withdrawal of the drug, or the continuous presence of the anxiety disorder for which treatment was initiated. A helpful point is that withdrawal symptoms generally begin 2–3 days after withdrawing a short-acting drug, or 7 days after stopping a long-acting one, and diminish again after 3–10 days. Anxiety symptoms often start sooner and persist for longer. Withdrawal symptoms are less likely if the drug is withdrawn gradually over several weeks. (For the treatment of benzodiazepine dependence see p. 285.)

Buspirone

This anxiolytic, which is an azapirone, has no affinity for benzodiazepine receptors but stimulates 5-HT$_{1A}$ receptors and reduces 5-HT transmission. It does not cause sedation but has side effects of headache, nervousness, and light-headedness. It does not appear to lead to tolerance and dependence. Its action is slower than that of benzodiazepines and less powerful. It cannot be used to treat benzodiazepine withdrawal.

Beta-adrenergic antagonists

These drugs do not have general anxiolytic effects but can relieve palpitation and tremor. They are used occasionally when these are the main symptoms of a chronic anxiety disorder. An appropriate drug is *propranolol* in a starting dose of 40 mg

Table 16.3.

Benzodiazepine withdrawal syndrome

- Apprehension and anxiety
- Insomnia
- Tremor
- Heightened sensitivity to stimuli
- Muscle twitching
- Seizures (rarely)

daily increased gradually to 40 mg three times a day. The several **contraindications** limit the use of these drugs. These are: *asthma* or a history of *bronchiospasm*, or *obstructive airways disease*; incipient *cardiac failure* or *heart block*; *systolic blood pressure below 90 mm mercury*; *a pulse rate less than 60 per minute*; metabolic acidosis for example in *diabetes*; and after prolonged fasting as in *anorexia nervosa*. *Other contraindications* and precautions are listed in the manufacturer's literature. There are **interactions** with some drugs that increase the adverse effects of beta-blockers. Before prescribing these drugs, it is important to find out what other drugs the patient is taking, and consult a work of reference about possible interactions.

General advice about use of anxiolytics

- **Use sparingly.** Usually, attention to life problems, an opportunity to talk about feelings, and reassurance are enough to reduce anxiety to tolerable levels.
- **Brief treatment.** Benzodiazepines should be given seldom for more than three weeks.
- **Withdraw drugs gradually** to reduce withdrawal effects. When the drug is stopped, patients should be warned that they may feel more tense for a few days.
- **Short- or long-acting drug.** If anxiety is intermittent, a short-acting compound is used; if anxiety lasts throughout the day a long-acting drug is appropriate.
- **Consider an alternative.** As explained in the section on anxiety disorders (p. 111) some antidepressant and antipsychotic drugs have secondary anxiolytic effects and are useful alternatives to benzodiazepines.

Hypnotics

An ideal hypnotic would increase the length and quality of sleep without changing sleep structure, leave no residual effects on the next day, and cause no dependence and no withdrawal syndrome. No hypnotic drug meets these criteria, and most alter the structure of sleep: rapid eye movement sleep is suppressed while they are being taken and resumes once they have been stopped.

Benzodiazepines are the most frequently used hypnotic drugs: A short-acting drug such as temazepam is suitable for cases of initial insomnia and less likely to cause effects the next day then long-acting compounds such as nitrazepam. These hangover effects can be hazardous for people who drive motor vehicles or operate machines.

Chloral hydrate, chlormethiazole edisylate, and **zopiclone** are used as alternatives to benzodiazepines. (*Barbiturates* although effective hypnotics are dangerous in overdose, causing respiratory depression and should be avoided.)

Patients should be warned that *alcohol potentiates* the effects of hypnotic drugs, sometimes causing dangerous respiratory depression. This effect is particularly likely to occur with chlormethiazole and barbiturates, which should not be prescribed to people taking excessive amounts of alcohol except under careful supervision in the management of withdrawal (see p. 272).

Hypnotic drugs are prescribed too frequently and for too long. Some patients are started on long periods of dependency on hypnotics by the prescribing of night sedation in hospital. These drugs should be prescribed only when there is a real need, and should be stopped before the patient goes home. (The management of insomnia is discussed on p. 237.)

Prescribing for special groups For *children* the prescription of hypnotics is not justified except occasionally for the treatment of night terrors or somnambulism. *For the elderly* hypnotics should be prescribed with particular care since they may become confused and thereby risk injury.

Antipsychotic drugs

These drugs reduce psychomotor excitement, hallucinations, and delusions occurring in schizophrenia, mania, and organic psychoses. Antipsychotic drugs block dopaminergic receptors, and this action may account for their therapeutic effects, and certainly explains their extrapyramidal side effects. They also block noradrenergic and cholinergic receptors and these actions account for some of their many side effects. Extrapyramidal side effects are reduced by anticholinergic drugs. Antipsychotics such as chlorpromazine, which have strong anticholinergic effects, cause fewer extrapyramidal effects than do antipsychotics, such as haloperidol, which have weak anticholinergic effects.

Antipsychotic drugs are well absorbed and partly metabolized in the liver into numerous metabolites, some of which have antipsychotic properties of their own. Because of this metabolism to active compounds, measurements of plasma concentrations of the parent drug are not helpful for the clinician.

Compounds available

There are many antipsychotic drugs, with different chemical structures. For non-specialists, the following simplified grouping is sufficient:

'Typical' antipsychotics bind strongly to post-synaptic dopamine D_2 receptors. This action seems to account for their therapeutic effect but also their propensity to cause movement disorders (see p. 342). Most antipsychotics are in this group.

There are several newer atypical antipsychotics which vary in the extent to which they bind to dopamine D_2/D_4, 5-HT_2, alpha$_1$-adrenergic, and muscarinic receptors. They are less likely to cause movement disorders than the typical antipsychotics and do not cause hyperprolactinaemia. This group of drugs includes **clozapine, olanzapine, riperidone, quetiapine,** and **sertindole.**

Clozapine was the first atypical and it binds only weakly to D_2 receptors and has a higher affinity for D_4 receptors. It also binds to histamine H_1, 5-HT_2, alpha$_1$-adrenergic, and muscarinic receptors. At the time of writing, clozapine is the only antipsychotic which is sometimes effective in patients who are unresponsive to typical antipsychotics. Clozapine does not cause extrapyramidal side effects, but it causes neutropenia in 2–3% of patients which progresses to agranulocytosis in 0.3% of patients. For this reason, it is used only when other drugs have failed and then with regular blood tests, and an explanation of the risks and benefits.

Table 16.4.

Unwanted effects of typical antipsychotic drugs

	Effect	Comments
Antidopaminergic effects	Acute dystonia Akathisia Parkinsonism Tardive dyskinesia	See text
Antiadrenergic effects	Postural hypotension Nasal congestion Inhibition of ejaculation	Hypotension particularly likely after intramuscular ingestion and in the elderly
Anticholinergic effects	Dry mouth Reduced sweating Urinary hesitancy and retention Constipation Blurred vision Precipitation of glaucoma	Retention and glaucoma especially important in elderly
Other effects	Cardiac arrhythmias Weight gain Amenorrhoea Galactorrhoea Hypothermia Worsening of epilepsy (some) Photosensitivity (some) Accumulation of pigment in skin, cornea, lens (some)	Hypothermia especially important in the elderly Chlorpromazine and some other drugs worsen epilepsy. It causes photosensitivity and pigmentation
Neuroleptic malignant syndrome	See Table 16.9	See text

Slow-release depot preparations are given by injection to patients who improve with drugs but cannot be relied on to take them regularly by mouth. These preparations are esters of the antipsychotic drug, usually in an oily medium. Examples include fluphenazine decanoate and flupenthixol decanoate. Their action is much longer than that of the parent drug, usually 2–4 weeks after a single intramuscular dose. Because their action is prolonged, a small test dose is given before the full dose is used.

Side effects The numerous side effects of the typical antipsychotic drugs are related mainly to the antidopaminergic, antiadrenergic, and anticholinergic effects of the drugs (see Table 16.4). Because it is often difficult to achieve a therapeutic effect without troublesome side effects, they are described in some detail. When prescribing, the general account given here should be supplemented with that found in the manufacturer's literature, or in a standard pharmacological work of reference.

Table 16.5.

Extrapyramidal effects of antipsychotic drugs

Effect	Usual interval from starting treatment
Acute dystonia	Days
Akathisia	Days to weeks
Parkinsonism	A few weeks
Tardive dyskinesia	Many years

Table 16.6.

Clinical features of acute dystonia

- Torticollis
- Tongue protrusion
- Grimacing
- Spasm of ocular muscles
- Opisthotonus

Table 16.7.

Clinical features of parkinsonism

- Akinesia
- Expressionless face
- Lack of associated movements when walking
- Stooped posture
- Rigidity of muscles
- Coarse tremor
- Festinant gait (in severe cases)

Table 16.8.

Clinical features of tardive dyskinesia

- Chewing and sucking movements
- Grimacing
- Choreo-athetoid movements
- Akathisia

Antidopaminergic effects give rise to four kinds of **extrapyramidal** symptoms and signs (see Table 16.5). These effects often appear at therapeutic doses.

1. **Acute dystonia** occurs soon after the treatment begins. It is most frequent with butyrophenones and phenothiazines with a piperazine side chain. The clinical features are shown in Table 16.6. The term *oculogyric crisis* is sometimes used to denote the combination of ocular muscle spasm and opisthotonus. The clinical picture is dramatic and sometimes mistaken for histrionic behaviour. Acute dystonia can be controlled by an anticholinergic drug such as biperiden given carefully by intramuscular injection following the manufacturer's advice about dosage.

2. **Akathisia** is an unpleasant feeling of physical restlessness and a need to move, leading to inability to keep still. It starts usually in the first two weeks of treatment but can be delayed for several months. The symptoms are not controlled reliably by antiparkinsonian drugs but generally disappear if the dose is reduced.

3. **Parkinsonian effects** are the most frequent of the extrapyramidal side effects. They are listed in Table 16.7. The syndrome often takes a few weeks to appear. Parkinsonism can sometimes be controlled by lowering the dose. If this cannot be done without losing the therapeutic effect, an antiparkinsonian drug can be prescribed. With continued treatment, parkinsonian effects may diminish even though the dose of the antipsychotic stays the same. It is appropriate to check at intervals that the antiparkinsonian drug is still required since these compounds may increase the risk of tardive dyskinesia.

4. **Tardive dyskinesia** is so called because it is a late complication of antipsychotic treatment. The clinical features are shown in Table 16.8.

The condition may be due to supersensitivity of dopamine receptors resulting from prolonged dopamine blockade. Tardive dyskinesia occurs in about 15% of patients on long-term treatment. Since it does not always recover when the antipsychotic drugs are stopped, and responds poorly to treatment, *prevention* is important. This is attempted by keeping the dose and duration of dosage of antipsychotic drugs to the effective minimum and by limiting the use of antiparkinsonian drugs (see above).

The only agreed *treatment* for tardive dyskinesia is to stop the antipsychotic drug when the state of the mental illness allows this. At first the dyskinesia may worsen, but often it improves after several drug-free months. If the condition does not improve, or if the antipsychotic drug cannot be stopped, an additional drug can be prescribed in an attempt to reduce the dyskinesia. No one drug is uniformly successful and specialist advice should be obtained. (The specialist may try a dopamine receptor antagonist such as sulpiride or a dopamine depleting agent such as tetrabenazine.)

Antipsychotic drugs may cause *depression* but as this symptom is part of the clinical picture of chronic schizophrenia, and it is not certain whether antipsychotic drugs have an independent effect.

Toxic effects Before using any of these drugs it is advisable to study the manufacturer's literature, noting the side effects and toxic effects of the chosen compounds.

The neuroleptic malignant syndrome is a rare but an extremely serious effect of neuroleptic treatment especially with high potency compounds. The cause is unknown. The symptoms which begin suddenly, usually within the first 10 days of treatment, are summarized in Table 16.9 (and listed for reference in *Additional information*).

Treatment is symptomatic. The drug is stopped, the patient cooled, fluid balance maintained, and any infection is treated. There is no drug of proven effectiveness. The condition is serious and about a fifth of patients die. If a patient has had this condition in the past, specialist advice should be obtained before any further antipsychotic treatment is prescribed.

Adverse effects of clozapine About 2–3% of patients taking clozapine develop leucopenia, and this can progress to agranulocytosis. With regular monitoring

Table 16.9.
Neuroleptic malignant syndrome

Principal features
Fluctuating level of consciousness
Hyperthermia
Muscular rigidity
Autonomic disturbance

Additional information Neuroleptic malignant syndrome

Additional features	
Mental symptoms	Fluctuating consciousness
	Stupor
Motor symptoms	Increased muscle tone
	Dysphagia
	Dyspnoea
Autonomic symptoms	Hyperpyrexia
	Unstable blood pressure
	Tachycardia
	Excessive sweating
	Salivation
	Urinary incontinence
Laboratory findings	Raised white cell count
	Raised creatinine
	Phosphokinase (CPK)
Consequent problems	Pneumonia
	Cardiovascular collapse
	Thromboembolism
	Renal failure

leucopenia can be detected early and the drug stopped: usually the white cell count returns to normal. (Monitoring is usually weekly for 18 weeks and twice weekly thereafter.)

Clozapine may also cause excessive salivation, postural hypotension, weight gain, and hyperthermia; and, in high doses, seizures. Clozapine is sedating and respiratory depression has been reported when it has been combined with benzodiazepines.

Teratogenesis Although the drugs have not been shown to be teratogenic, they should be used with caution in early pregnancy.

Contraindications There are few contraindications to the use of antipsychotic drugs. They include myasthenia gravis, Addison's disease, glaucoma, and past or present bone marrow depression. Caution is required when there is liver disease (chlorpromazine should be avoided), renal disease, cardiovascular disorder, parkinsonism, epilepsy, or serious infection. The manufacturer's literature should be consulted for further contraindications to the use of specific drugs.

Choice of drug

Of the many compounds available, the following are among the appropriate choices:

- a more sedating drug—chlorpromazine
- a less sedating drug—trifluoperazine or haloperidol
- a drug with fewer extrapyramidal side effects—sulpiride or risperidone
- an intramuscular preparation for rapid calming—chlorpromazine, or haloperidol
- a depot preparation—fluphenazine decanoate or flupenthixol decanoate
- for patients resistant to other antipsychotics—clozapine (to be initiated by a specialist).

Antiparkinsonian drugs

Although these drugs have no direct therapeutic use in psychiatry, they are used to control the extrapyramidal side effects of antipsychotic drugs. For this purpose the anticholinergic compounds used most commonly are benzhexol, benztropine mesylate, procyclidine, and orphenadrine. An injectable preparation of biperiden is useful for the treatment of acute dystonia (see p. 342).

Although these drugs are used in psychiatry to reduce the side effects of antipsychotic drugs, they have side effects of their own. Their anticholinergic side effects can add to those of the antipsychotic drug to increase constipation, and precipitate glaucoma or retention of urine. Also, they may increase the likelihood of tardive dyskinesia (see p. 342). *Benzhexol, and procyclidine, have euphoriant effects, and are sometimes abused to obtain this action.*

Antidepressants

Antidepressant drugs have therapeutic effects in depressive illness, but do not elevate mood in healthy people (contrast the effects of stimulants like amphetamine). Drugs with antidepressant properties are divided conveniently into: tricyclic antidepressants; modified tricyclic and related drugs; specific serotonin reuptake inhibitors (SSRIs); serotonin (5-HT) and noradrenaline reuptake inhibitors (SNRIs); specific noradrenaline uptake inhibitors; and monoamine oxidase inhibitors (MAOIs). These drugs have not been shown to differ in efficacy or speed of action but only in their side effects.

All antidepressant drugs increase 5-HT function and many increase noradrenaline function. The development of specific 5-HT reuptake inhibitors suggested that the antidepressant effects result from increased 5-HT function. However, specific noradrenaline reuptake inhibitors have been developed and they too are antidepressants. Thus, the mechanism of antidepressant action remains uncertain.

Antidepressants have a long half-life and most can be given once a day. Antidepressants should be withdrawn slowly, because sudden cessation may lead to restlessness, insomnia, anxiety, and nausea. Antidepressant action appears usually 10–14 days after the drug was first taken. The reason for this delay is not known. To avoid relapse the drugs have to be continued for several months after symptoms have been controlled; six months is a usual period.

Tricyclic antidepressants

These drugs, are so named because their chemical structure has three benzene rings. They have many side effects (see below) and toxic effects on the cardiovascular system. Because of these effects tricyclics are being replaced for many purposes by drugs without these side effects. However, they are still important because they are of proven effectiveness in severely depressed patients. Also, they are generally less expensive than other antidepressant drugs.

Side effects Tricyclic antidepressants have many side effects which can be divided conveniently into the groups shown in Table 16.10 Most of the effects are

Table 16.10.
Side effects of tricyclic antidepressants

Anticholinergic effects	Dry mouth
	Constipation
	Impaired visual accommodation
	Difficulty in micturition
	(Worsening of glaucoma)
	Confusion (especially in elderly)
Alpha-adrenoceptor blocking effects	Drowsiness
	Postural hypotension
	Sexual dysfunction
Cardiovascular effects	Tachycardia
	Hypotension
	Cardiac conduction deficits
	Cardiac arrhythmia
Other effects	Seizures
	Weight gain

common and those that are infrequent are important, so the list should be known before prescribing. The following points should be noted:

- Difficulty in micturition may lead to retention of urine in patients with prostatic hypertrophy.

- Cardiac conduction deficits are more frequent in patients with pre-existing heart disease. If it is necessary to prescribe a tricyclic drug to such a patient, a cardiologist's opinion should be sought (it is often possible to choose a drug of another group without this side effect, see below).

- Seizures are infrequent but important. Antidepressant drugs should be avoided if possible in patients with epilepsy; if their use is essential, the dose of anticonvulsant should be adjusted—usually with the advice of the neurologist treating the case.

Toxic effects In overdosage, tricyclic antidepressants can produce serious effects requiring urgent medical treatment. These effects include: ventricular fibrillation, conduction disturbances, and low blood pressure; respiratory depression; agitation, twitching, convulsions; hallucinations, delirium, and coma; retention of urine, and pyrexia.

Teratogenic effects have not been proved but antidepressants should be used cautiously in the first trimester of pregnancy and the manufacturer's literature consulted.

Interactions with other drugs These should be studied before prescribing. They are summarized in *Additional information*.

Contraindications Contraindications include *agranulocytosis*, severe *liver damage*, *glaucoma*, and *prostatic hypertrophy*. The drugs should be used *cautiously in epileptic* patients because they are epileptogenic, in the elderly because they cause hypotension, and after myocardial infarction because of their effects on the heart.

Modified tricyclics and related drugs

The chemical structure of the tricyclics has been modified in various ways to produce drugs with fewer side effects. Of the many drugs, two will be mentioned.

Additional information **Principal interactions between tricyclic antidepressants and other drugs**

> **With antihypertensives** Tricyclic antidepressants interact with adrenergic neurone blockers such as bethanidine, debrisoquine, and guanethidine, and with clonidine. (They do not interfere with beta-adrenoreceptor antagonists or thiazide diuretics.) They can *increase* the hypotensive effect of angiotensin converting enzyme (ACE) inhibitors such as captopril.
>
> **With monoamine oxidase inhibitors** These important interactions are described on p. 351.
>
> **With phenytoin** Because they share a metabolic pathway, tricyclic antidepressants may increase concentrations of phenytoin.
>
> **With pressor amines** Tricyclic antidepressants potentiate the pressor effects of *adrenaline and noradrenaline*, so that there is a potential hazard when a local anaesthetic is used with a pressor amine (e.g. in dentistry).

Table 16.11.
Side effects of SSRIs

Gastrointestinal	Nausea
	Flatulence
	Diarrhoea
Central nervous system	Insomnia
	Restlessness
	Irritability
	Agitation
	Tremor
	Headache
	(Acute dystonia, rarely)
Sexual	Ejaculatory delay
	Anorgasmia

1. **Lofepramine** has less strong anticholinergic side effects than amitriptyline and is less sedating; however it may cause anxiety and insomnia. In overdose it is less cardiotoxic than conventional tricyclics.

2. **Trazodone** also has few anticholinergic effects, but has strong sedating properties.

Specific serotonin reuptake inhibitors (SSRIs)

These drugs selectively inhibit the reuptake of serotonin (5-HT) into pre-synaptic neurones. Examples are fluoxetine, fluvoxamine, paroxetine, and sertraline. Their antidepressant effect is comparable to that of the tricyclic anti-depressant drugs and because they lack anticholinergic side effects they are safer for patients with prostatism or glaucoma, and when taken in overdose. They are not sedating. Their side effects are listed in Table 16.11.

Drug interactions SSRIs with **MAOIs** (monoamine oxidase inhibitors) should be avoided since the combination may produce a 5-HT toxicity syndrome with hyperpyrexia, rigidity, myoclonus, coma, and death. **Lithium** and **trypto-phan** also increase 5-HT function when given with SSRIs. Combinations of lithium and SSRIs are sometimes used cautiously by specialists for depressive disorders resistant to other treatment. Other interactions are listed in the manufacturer's literature.

Toxic effects Overdosage leads to vomiting, tremor, and irritability.

Indications see Table 16.12.

Serotonin and noradrenaline reuptake inhibitors (SNRIs)

Venlafaxine blocks 5-HT and noradrenaline reuptake but does not have the anti-cholinergic effects that characterize tricyclic antidepressants and is not sedative. Side effects resemble those of SSRIs; in full doses it may cause hypotension. At the time of writing, SNRIs have not been evaluated fully in relation to other antide-pressants. (See p. 68 for advice on searching for evidence about the effectiveness of new drugs.)

Table 16.12.
Indications for SSRI treatment for depressive disorder

Concomittant cardiac disease*
Intolerance to anticholinergic side effects
Significant risk of deliberate overdose
Excessive weight gain with previous tricyclic treatment
Sedation undesirable
Obsessive-compulsive disorder with depression

*SSRIs are safer than tricyclics but caution is required.

Specific noradrenaline reuptake inhibitors

Several tricyclic antidepressants are relatively specific noradrenaline reuptake inhibitors (e.g. desimiprimanine and lofepramine). Recently, a non-tricyclic drug has been developed, reboxetine, with a specific action on noradrenaline reuptake. Clinical trials show that it has antidepressant effects greater than placebo and is comparable to other antidepressants. At the time of writing reboxetine has not been evaluated fully. (See p. 68 for advice on searching for evidence about the effectiveness of new drugs.)

Choice of antidepressant

The clinician should become familiar with the use of one drug from each of the following three groups in each of which a possible choice of drugs is shown:

1. A sedating tricyclic—amitriptyline or trazodone.

2. A less sedating tricyclic—imipramine or lofepramine.

3. A drug with few anticholinergic effects—one of the SSRIs.

Since there are no differences between antidepressants in efficacy or speed of action, choice depends on an assessment for each patient of the likely importance of side effects, toxic effects, and interactions with other drugs. Finally, cost should be taken into account.

• **Side effects** Sedating side effects are useful when depression is accompanied by anxiety and insomnia, but may be troublesome for drivers of motor vehicles or other forms of transport, and for operators of machinery. Anticholinergic side effects need to be avoided for patients with prostatism or glaucoma.

• **Toxic effects** Cardiotoxic effects should be considered especially when there is an increased risk that the patient may take a deliberate overdose, or there is cardiac disease.

• **Epilepsy** All antidepressants have the potential of provoking seizures and so that the dose of antiepileptic drugs may have to be increased in patients with epilepsy.

• **Interaction with other drugs used to treat medical disorders** A work of reference should be consulted if the patient is taking or is likely to commence medication for another condition, and a choice made to prevent drug interactions.

• **Cost** It is appropriate to choose the least expensive drug within the group that is clinically appropriate.

Advice to patients Before prescribing, the following points should be explained and discussed with the patient:

Delayed response The therapeutic effect is likely to be delayed for up to two or three weeks but side effects will appear sooner.

Side effects The common effects should be described including drowsiness, and a warning given of the dangers of driving a motor vehicle or using machinery even when only slightly drowsy. With tricyclics, dry mouth and accommodation difficulties are common side effects. Patients taking 5-HT reuptake blockers may feel irritable or restless.

Effects of alcohol The effects of alcohol are increased when antidepressants are taken.

Older patients Older patients should be warned about the effects of postural hypotension and told how to minimize these (e.g. by rising slowly from bed). Effects of tricyclics on bladder function should be explained. Reassurance can be given that most of these effects are likely to decrease with time.

Starting treatment When tricyclics are prescribed, the starting dose should be moderate; for example, amitriptyline 75–100 mg per day increased after 3–7 days to 125–150 mg per day according to the urgency. The dose may be increased further if there is no response, after the extent of the side effects has been observed.

Drugs with sedative side effects can be given in a single dose at night, so that sedative effects help the patient to sleep and the peak of other side effects occurs during sleep. SSRIs and other drugs that cause insomnia should be given in the first half of the day, usually in a single dose.

Doses should be reduced for elderly patients, those with cardiac disease, or prostatism, or other conditions that may be exacerbated by the drugs, and those with disease of the liver or kidneys. If agitation, as a symptom of depressive disorder, is not controlled by a sedative antidepressant, a phenothiazine can be added.

Since patients feel the side effects of the drug before experiencing its benefits, they should be seen again after a week, or earlier if the disorder is severe. At this interview, the severity of depression is reassessed, side effects are discussed, and encouragement given to continue taking the medication until the therapeutic response occurs.

Non-response The management of depressed patients who fail to respond to antidepressant medication is discussed on p. 152.

Monamine oxidase inhibitors

Monoamine oxidase inhibitors (MAOIs) are seldom used as the first antidepressant treatment because of their side effects and hazardous interactions with other drugs and foodstuffs (described below). They are started usually by a specialist but since general practitioners and hospital doctors may treat patients who are taking MAOIs, their hazardous interactions should be known.

Monoamine oxidase inhibitors inactivate enzymes that metabolize noradrenaline and 5-hydroxytryptamine (5-HT) and this action probably accounts for their therapeutic effects. They also interfere with the metabolism of tyramine, and certain other pressor amines taken medicinally. MAOIs also interfere with the metabolism in the liver of barbiturates, tricyclic antidepressants, phenytoin, and antiparkinsonian drugs. When the drug is stopped, these inhibitory effects on enzymes disappear slowly, usually over about two weeks, so that the *potential for food and drug interactions outlasts the taking of the MAOI*. Recently, MAOIs with more rapidly **reversible actions** have been produced. Reversible MAOIs are less likely to give rise to serious interactions with foodstuffs and drugs.

The various MAOIs differ little in their therapeutic effects. Commonly used drugs include **phenelzine**, **isocarboxazid**, and **tranylcypromine**. The latter has an amphetamine-like stimulating effect in addition to its property of inhibiting monoamine oxidase. This additional effect improves

Table 16.13.

Side effects of MAOIs

Autonomic	Dry mouth
	Dizziness
	Constipation
	Difficulty in micturition
	Postural hypotension
Central nervous system	Headache
	Tremor
	Paraesthesia
Other	Ankle oedema
	Hepatotoxicity (hydrazines)

mood in the short term but can cause dependency. **Moclobemide** is a *reversible* MAOI.

Side effects The side effects of MAOIs are listed in Table 16.13.

Interactions with foodstuffs and drugs **With tyramine in food and drinks** Some food and drinks contain tyramine, a substance that is normally inactivated in the body by monoamine oxidases. When these enzymes are inhibited by MAOIs, tyramine is not broken down and exerts its effect of releasing noradrenaline, with a consequent pressor effect. (As noted above, with most MAOIs the inhibition lasts for about two weeks after the drug has been stopped. With the 'reversible' MAOI, meclobemide, inhibition lasts for a shorter time, usually about 24 hours.) If large amounts of tyramine are ingested, blood pressure rises substantially with a so-called *hypertensive crisis* and, occasionally, a cerebral haemorrhage. An important early symptom of such a crisis is a severe, usually throbbing, headache.

The main tyramine-containing food and drinks to be avoided are listed for reference in *Additional information*. About four-fifths of reported interactions between foodstuffs and MAOIs, and nearly all deaths, have followed the consumption of *cheese*. It is important to consult this list and the manufacturer's literature before prescribing MAOIs. Patients should be given a list of foodstuffs and other substances to be avoided (available usually from the manufacturer).

Drugs. Patients taking monoamine oxidase inhibitors should not be given drugs metabolized by enzymes inhibited by MAOIs or those which enhance 5-HT functions. The former fall into three groups.

1. *Drugs metabolized by amine oxidases and with pressor effects*. Of these ephedrine is a constituent of some 'cold cures', and adrenaline is used with local anaesthetics.

2. *Drugs metabolized by other enzymes affected by MAOIs*. The most important of these drugs are listed for reference in *Additional information*. Sensitivity to oral antidiabetic drugs is increased leading to the risk of hypoglycaemia.

3. *Drugs that potentiate brain 5-HT function—see Additional information*. Combinations of the drug with MAOI may produce a **5-HT syndrome** with:

Additional information Interactions of MAOIs with drugs and food

---

Due to inactivation of monoamine oxidase

- *Foods and drinks with high tyramine content*
  Most cheeses
  Extracts of meat and yeast
  Smoked or pickled fish
  Hung poultry or game
  Some red wines

- *Drugs with pressor effects*
  Adrenaline, noradrenaline
  Amphetamine, ephedrine
  Fenfluramine
  Phenylpropanolamine
  L-Dopa, dopamine

Due to effects on other enzymes

  Morphine, pethidine
  Procaine, cocaine
  Alcohol
  Barbiturates
  Insulin and oral hypoglycaemics

Drugs that promote brain 5-HT function

  SSRIs
  Clomipramine
  Imipramine
  Fenfluramine
  L-Tryptophan
  Buspirone

- Hyperpyrexia
- Restlessness, muscle twitching, and rigidity
- Convulsions and coma.

Combinations of MAOIs and tricyclics In specialist practice, combinations of MAOIs and tricyclic antidepressants are sometimes used for resistant depression. Other doctors are unlikely to start this treatment but they may treat patients already taking the combination. Key points about the combined treatment are summarized in Box 16.2.

Treatment of hypertensive crises Hypertensive crises are treated by parenteral administration of phentolamine or to block alpha-adrenoceptors, if this drug is not available, by intramuscular chlorpromazine. Blood pressure should be followed carefully.

Treatment of the 5-HT syndrome All medication should be stopped and supportive measures given. Drugs with 5-HT antagonists properties may be tried but their benefits have not been proved: propranolol and cypropeptadine are possible choices.

Contraindications to MAOIs These include liver disease, phaeochromocytoma, congestive cardiac failure, and conditions which require the patient to take any of the drugs that react with MAOIs.

Box 16.2 **Combinations of MAOIs and tricyclics**

To avoid a 5-HT syndrome, combinations of MAOI with imipramine or clomipramine should be avoided. (Also, MAOIs and SSRIs should not be combined, see p. 347). When an MAOI and a suitable tricyclic are combined they should be started together, both at low dosage; or MAOI is added to previously prescribed tricyclic. *Tricyclics should not be added to MAOI* since this sequence is more likely to provoke a 5-HT syndrome. Since the effects of MAOIs (except moclobemide) continue for at least two weeks after the drugs have been stopped, tricyclics should not be given for this period after stopping an MAOI. (If tricyclics are given first no drug-free interval is required.) The value of this combined therapy has not been evaluated fully and generally it should be started by a specialist.

Box 16.3 **Monoamine oxidase inbibitors (MAOIs). Treatment card**

Treatment card

Carry this card with you at all times. Show it to any doctor who may treat you other than the doctor who prescribed this medicine, and to your dentist if you require dental treatment.

Instructions to patients

Please read carefully

While taking this medicine and for 14 days after your treatment finishes you must observe the following simple instructions:

1. Do not eat CHEESE, PICKLED HERRING, or BROAD BEAN PODS.
2. Do not eat or drink BOVRIL, OXO, MARMITE, or ANY SIMILAR MEAT or YEAST EXTRACT.
3. EAT ONLY FRESH foods and avoid food that you suspect could be stale or 'going off'. This is especially important with meat, fish, poultry, or offal. Avoid game.
4. Do not take any other MEDICINES (including tablets, capsules, nose drops, inhalations, or suppositories) whether purchased by you or previously prescribed by your doctor, without first consulting your doctor or your pharmacist.

   NB Treatment for coughs and colds, pain relievers, tonics, and laxatives are medicines.
5. Drink ALCOHOL only in moderation and avoid CHIANTI WINE completely.

Keep a careful note of any food or drink that disagrees with you, avoid it and tell your doctor.

Report any severe symptoms to your doctor and follow any other advice given by him.

Prepared by the Royal Pharmaceutical Society and the British Medical Association on behalf of the Health Departments of the United Kingdom (revised September 1998). Reproduced from the *British National Formulary* (copyright BNF).

Management Because the drugs have so many interactions, MAOIs should not be prescribed as the first drug for the treatment of depressive disorders, and usually specialist advice should be obtained when they appear to be indicated.

Information for patients The dangers of interactions with foods and other drugs should be explained carefully, and a warning card provided (see Box 16.3). Patients should be told to show this card to any doctor or dentist who is treating them. They should be warned not to buy any proprietary drugs except from a qualified pharmacist, to whom the card should always be shown.

Choice of drug Phenelzine is a suitable choice, starting with 15 mg twice daily and increasing cautiously to 15 mg four times a day. Tranylcypromine which has amphetamine-like effects as well as MAOI properties, is often effective but as noted above some patients become dependent on its stimulant action.

Changing drugs As noted above, if an MAOI is not effective, *at least two weeks* must pass between ceasing the MAOI and starting another kind of antidepressant. As MAOIs should be discontinued slowly, the time for changeover is even longer. These periods are shorter for the reversible MAOI, moclobemide (see above).

Mood-stabilizing drugs

Three drugs are effective in preventing the recurrence of affective disorder: (1) lithium, (2) carbamazepine, and (3) sodium valproate. Lithium is also used to treat acute mania and, in special cases, to augment the effects of tricyclic antidepressants.

Lithium

Pharmacology It is not known which of lithium's many pharmacological actions explains its therapeutic effects, but its effect in increasing brain 5-HT function may be relevant.

Lithium is absorbed and excreted by the kidneys where, like sodium, it is filtered and partly reabsorbed. Lithium concentrations rise, sometimes to dangerous levels in three circumstances:

(1) *dehydration*: when the proximal trubule absorbs more water, more lithium is reabsorbed;

(2) *sodium depletion*: lithium is carried by the mechanism that carries sodium, and more lithium is transported when there is less sodium;

(3) *thiazide therapy*: thiazide diuretics increase the excretion of sodium but not of lithium and plasma lithium rises.

Dosage and plasma concentrations General practitioners are often asked to supervise continuing treatment with lithium started by specialists, and hospital doctors treat these patients for other conditions. Because the therapeutic and toxic doses are close together, it is essential to measure plasma concentrations of lithium regularly during treatment. Measurement is made first after 4–7 days; then weekly for 3 weeks; and then, provided that a satisfactory steady state has been achieved, once every 6 weeks.

The *timing of the measurement* is important. After an oral dose, plasma lithium levels rise by a factor of two or three within about four hours and then fall to the steady state level. Since the steady state level is important in therapeutics,

Table 16.14.
Side effects of lithium

1. *Early effects*
   Diuresis
   Tremor
   Dry mouth
   Metallic taste
   Weakness and fatigue

2. *Later effects*
   Fine tremor[a]
   Polyuria and polydipsia
   Thyroid enlargement
   Hypothyroidism
   Impaired memory (see text)
   ECG changes[b]

3. *Long-term effects on the kidney*
   See text

[a] Coarse tremor is a sign of toxicity.
[b] T wave flattening; QRS widening (reversible when drug is stopped).

concentrations are normally measured *12 hours after the last dose*, usually just before the morning dose which can be delayed if necessary for an hour or two. It is the steady state level 12 hours after the last dose, not to the 'peak' which is the level referred to when discussing the concentrations aimed at in treatment and prophylaxis. If an unexpectedly high concentration is found the first step is to find out whether the patient has inadvertently taken the morning dose before the blood sample was taken.

The required plasma concentrations are:

* for prophylaxis: 0.4–0.8 mmol/litre—increased occasionally to a maximum of 1.2 mmol/litre;

* for treatment of acute mania: 0.9–1.2 mmol/litre.

Toxic effects begin to appear over 1.5 mmol/litre and may be serious over 2.0 mmol/litre.

Although the therapeutic effects is related to the steady state concentration of lithium, any renal effects caused by the drug (see below) may relate to the peak concentrations. For this reason, the drug is often given twice a day. Delayed release tablets have been introduced for the same reason but the time-course of plasma levels resulting from these tablets is not substantially different from that of standard preparations.

Unwanted effects These effects are listed in Table 16.14; the following points should be noted.

* **Polyuria** can lead to dehydration with the risk of lithium intoxication. Patients should be advised to drink enough water to compensate for the fluid loss.

* **Tremor** Fine tremor occurs frequently. Most patients adapt to this; for those who do not, propranolol 10 mg three times daily often reduces the symptom. *Coarse tremor is a sign of toxicity.*

* **Enlargement of the thyroid** occurs in about 5% of patients taking lithium. The thyroid shrinks again if thyroxine is given while lithium is continued; and it returns to normal a month or two after lithium has been stopped.

* **Hypothyroidism** occurs commonly (up to 20% of women patients) with a compensatory rise in thyroid stimulating hormone. Tests of thyroid function should be performed every six months, and a continuous watch kept for suggestive clinical signs particularly lethargy and substantial weight gain. If hypothyroidism develops and lithium treatment is still necessary, thyroxine treatment should be added.

* **Impaired memory** Usually this takes the form of everyday lapses such as forgetting well-known names. The cause is not known.

* **Long-term effects on the kidney** 10% of patients develop a persistent impairment of concentrating ability. A few patients develop nephrogenic diabetes insipidus due to interference with the effect of antidiuretic hormone. This syndrome does not respond to antidiuretic treatments but usually recovers when the drug is stopped. Provided doses are kept below 1.2 mmol/litre, renal damage is rare in patients whose renal function is normal at the start. Nevertheless, it is usual to test renal function every six months.

Toxic effects The toxic effects of lithium (see Table 16.15) constitute a serious medical emergency for they can progress through coma and fits to death. If these symptoms appear, lithium should be stopped at once and a high intake of fluid provided, with extra sodium chloride to stimulate an osmotic diuresis. Lithium is cleared rapidly if renal function is normal but in severe cases renal dialysis may be needed. Most patients recover completely, some die, and a few survive with permanent neurological damage.

Teratogenesis Lithium crosses the placenta and, there are reports of increased rates of **fetal abnormalities** most affecting the heart. Therefore, the drug should be avoided in the first trimester of pregnancy. If possible, lithium should be stopped a week before delivery or otherwise reduced by half and stopped during labour to be restarted afterwards. However, lithium is **secreted into breast milk** to the extent that plasma lithium concentrations of breast-fed infants can be half or more of that in the maternal blood. Therefore, bottle-feeding is usually advisable.

Drug interactions There are several important interactions between lithium and other drugs. The manufacturer's literature or a book of reference should be consulted whenever lithium treatment is started and a second drug is prescribed for a patient taking lithium. The principal interactions are listed for reference in Box 16.4.

Contraindications These include *renal failure* or *recent renal disease*, *cardiac failure* or *recent myocardial infarction*, and *chronic diarrhoea* sufficient to alter electrolytes It is advisable not to use lithium for *children* or, as explained above, in *early pregnancy*. The

Table 16.15.
Toxic effects of lithium

- Nausea, vomiting
- Diarrhoea
- Coarse tremor
- Ataxia, dysarthria
- Muscle twitching, hyper-reflexia
- Confusion, coma
- Convulsions
- Renal failure
- Cardiovascular collapse

Box 16.4 **Principal interactions between lithium and other drugs**

1. Lithium concentrations may be increased by several drugs, including:
   - Haloperidol.
   - Thiazide diuretics (potassium sparing and loop diuretics seem less likely to increase lithium levels but should be used cautiously).
   - Muscle relaxants: when a patient on lithium is to have an operation the anaesthetist should be informed in advance because the effect of muscle relaxants may be potentiated. If possible, lithium should be stopped 48–72 hours before the operation.
   - Non-steroidal antiinflammatory agents (NSAIDs).
   - Some antibiotics—metronidazole and spectinomycin.
   - Some antihypertensives—angiotensin converting enzyme inhibitors and methyldopa.
2. Interaction with antipsychotics:
   - Potentiation of extrapyramidal symptoms.
   - Occasionally, confusion and delirium.
3. Interaction with specific serotonin reuptake inhibitors (SSRIs):
   - 5-HT syndrome (see p. 351).
4. Later action with ECT may cause a reaction similar to a 5-HT syndrome.

Additional information **The management of patients on lithium**

Treatment with lithium is usually started by a specialist but other doctors are often involved in continuing it.

A careful routine of management is essential because of the effects of therapeutic doses of lithium on the thyroid and kidneys, and the toxic effects of excessive dosage. The following routine is one of several that have been proposed.

Before starting lithium, a note should be made of any other medication taken by the patient and a *physical examination* should be carried out. *Laboratory tests* of renal and thyroid function are carried out, usually the estimation in blood of electrolytes, and creatinine, and T4 as a screening test, followed by thyroid stimulating hormone and other tests if indicated. Haemoglobin, ESR, and a full blood count are often done as well. *If indicated, ECG, and pregnancy tests*, should be done. If these tests show no contraindication to lithium treatment, the doctor should consult the manufacturer's data sheets about interactions and avoid especially thiazide diuretics.

Advice to the patient The doctor should explain:

(1) the common side effects;

(2) early toxic effects which would indicate an unduly high blood level of lithium;

(3) the need to keep strictly to the dosage prescribed;

(4) the arrangements for monitoring blood levels of lithium;

(5) the circumstances in which unduly high levels are most likely to arise—low salt diet, unaccustomed severe exercise, gastroenteritis, renal infection, or dehydration secondary to fever; and

(6) the need to stop the drug and seek medical advice if these conditions arise.

If the patient consents, it is usually appropriate to include another member of the family in these discussions. An explanatory leaflet should be provided, repeating the same points for reference.

Starting lithium prophylaxis Lithium carbonate may be given in a single dose or in two doses 12 hours apart. The starting dose is 750–1000 mg per day, adjusted on the basis of weekly blood level estimations of lithium until an appropriate concentration is achieved. For prophylaxis, a lithium level of 0.4–0.8 mmol/litre (in a sample taken 12 hours after the last dose) is usually aimed for; if this is not effective, a higher range of 0.7–1.2 mmol/litre may be recommended by a specialist. In judging response, it should be remembered that it may take several months before lithium achieves its full effect.

As treatment continues lithium estimations should be carried out every six weeks, with thyroid and renal function tests every six months. It is important to have a way of reminding the doctor about the times for the next repeat investigation. If two consecutive thyroid function tests a month apart show hypothyroidism, lithium should be stopped or L-thyroxine prescribed. Mild but troublesome polyuria is a reason for attempting a reduction in dose, whereas severe persistent polyuria is an indication for specialist renal investigation. A persistent leucocytosis is not uncommon and is apparently harmless; it reverses soon after the drug is stopped.

While lithium is continued, the doctor must keep in mind the possibility of interactions if new drugs are required by the patient.

precautions needed during delivery and lactation are referred to on p. 355. Lithium should not be prescribed if the patient is judged unlikely to observe the precautions required for its safe use.

Management

Details of management are shown for reference in *Additional information*. Lithium is usually **continued for at least two years**, and often for much longer. The need for the drug should be reviewed once a year, taking into account any persistence of mild mood fluctuations which suggest the possibility of relapse if treatment is stopped. Continuing medication is more likely to be needed if the patient has previously had several episodes of affective disorder within a short time, or if previous affective disorders were so severe·that even a small risk of recurrence should be avoided. There should be compelling reasons for continuing treatment for more than five years although patients have taken lithium safely for longer periods.

Lithium should be withdrawn gradually over a few weeks; sudden withdrawal may cause irritability, emotional lability and, occasionally, relapse (more often into mania than depression).

Carbamazepine

Carbamazepine was introduced as an anticonvulsant. Later it was found to prevent the recurrence of affective disorder. It is effective in some patients unresponsive to lithium, and for some with rapidly recurring manic-depressive disorder. Dosage is similar to that for epilepsy. Side effects, which may be troublesome if plasma levels are high, include drowsiness, dizziness, nausea, double vision, and skin rash. *A rare but serious side effect is agranulocytosis.* Carbamazepine can accelerate the metabolism some other drugs and of the hormones in the contraceptive pill, reducing its effectiveness. It is advisable therefore to consider another form of contraception. Drug interactions should be checked in a reference source before prescribing other drugs to a patient taking carbamazepine. The long-term prophylactic effects of carbamezapine are less certain than those of lithium, and some patients require treatment with both drugs.

Sodium valproate

Like carbamezepine, sodium valproate was introduced as an anticonvulsant. Later it was found to control acute mania. The evidence is less strong that it prevents recurrence of bipolar disorder, but it is sometimes tried for patients who do not respond to or cannot tolerate lithium or lithium with carbamazepine. Common side effects include sedation, tiredness, tremor, and gastrointestinal disturbance. Sodium valproate may cause thrombocytopenia and has other unwanted effects that should be studied in a reference source before a patient is treated.

Drugs for Alzheimer's disease

Drugs claimed to improve memory in Alzheimer's disease are considered on p. 319.

Other physical treatments

Electroconvulsive therapy (ECT)

ECT is given by psychiatrists. The general reader requires only a general knowledge of its use: those requiring further information should consult the *Oxford Textbook of Psychiatry* or another specialist text.

In ECT, an electric current is applied to the skull of an anaesthetized patient to produce seizure activity while the consequent motor effects are prevented with a muscle relaxant. The electrodes which deliver the current can be placed with one on each side of the head (bilateral ECT) or with both on the same side (unilateral ECT). Unilateral placement on the *non-dominant side* results in less memory impairment but may be less effective than bilateral ECT. Bilateral placement is therefore preferred when a rapid response is essential, or when unilateral ECT has not been effective.

The beneficial effect, which depends on the cerebral seizure, not on the motor component, is thought to result from neurotransmitter changes probably involving 5-HT and noradrenaline transmission. ECT acts more quickly than antidepressant drugs, although the outcome after three months is similar.

Indications

The main indications for ECT are:

1. **The need for an urgent response**
   - when life is threatened in a severe depressive disorder by refusal to drink or eat or very intense suicidal ideation;
   - in puerperal psychiatric disorders when it is important that the mother should resume the care of her baby as quickly as possible.

2. **For a resistant depressive disorder**, following failure to respond to thorough treatment with antidepressant medication.

3. **For two uncommon syndromes:**
   (i)   catatonic schizophrenia
   (ii) depressive stupor

Side effects of ECT

ECT has few side effects; some patients have a brief period of headache after the treatment. There are occasional effects from the anaesthetic procedure: the teeth, tongue, or lips may be injured while the airway is introduced and, rarely, muscle relaxants cause prolonged apnoea.

Memory problems Some patients fear long-lasting impairment of memory following ECT but memory tests have not confirmed this. The few patients who complain of lasting poor memory after ECT generally have persistent depressive symptoms, suggesting that the poor memory is related to the depressive disorder and not to the ECT.

Mortality of ECT The death rate from ECT is about 4 per 100 000 treatments, closely similar to that of an anaesthetic given for any minor procedure to a similar group of patients. Mortality is greater in patients with cardiovascular disease, and due usually to ventricular fibrillation or myocardial infarction

Contraindications

The contraindications are those for any anaesthetic procedure and any condition made worse by the changes in blood pressure and cardiac rhythm that occur even in a well-modified fit: serious heart disease, cerebral aneurysm, and raised intra-cranial pressure.

Extra care is required with diabetic patients who take insulin and for patients with sickle cell trait. Although risks rise somewhat in old age, so do the risks of untreated depressive disorder and of drug treatment.

Consent to ECT

Before ECT, a full explanation is given of the procedure and its risks and benefits, before asking for consent. If a patient refuses consent or is unable to give it; for example, because he is in a stupor, and if the procedure is essential, the psychiatrist seeks a second opinion and discusses the situation with relatives (although they cannot consent on behalf of the patient). In the UK and many other countries there are procedures for authorizing ECT when the patient refuses but it is essential (these are set out in the Mental Health Act or corresponding legislation). Patients treated under these provisions seldom question the need for treatment once they have recovered.

The technique

ECT is administered by a psychiatrist, who applies the current, and anaesthetist, and a nurse. The procedure is described in specialist textbooks. ECT is usually given twice a week with a total of 6–12 treatments, according to progress. Response begins usually after 2 or 3 treatments; if there has been no response after 6–8 treatments, it is unlikely that more ECT will produce useful change.

As some patients relapse after ECT, antidepressants are usually started towards the end of the course to reduce the risk of relapse.

Treatment with bright light

This treatment is sometimes used for seasonal affective disorder (SAD) (see p. 131). Not all patients respond; when a therapeutic effect appears it is rapid, but relapse is common. Light is administered usually at 6–8 am using a commercially available light box. The intensity of the light is usually about that of a bright spring day. The mode of action is uncertain; the light may correct circadian rhythms which seem to be phase-delayed in seasonal affective disorder.

Psychosurgery

Psychosurgery refers to the use of neurological procedures to modify the symptoms of psychiatric illness by operating either on the nuclei of the brain or on the white matter. The treatment had a period of wide use after its introduction in 1936 and until the development of effective psychotropic drugs in the 1960s. Nowadays, it is used rarely and then only in a few special centres, mainly for a very small minority of patients with obsessional or prolonged depressive disorders which have failed to respond to vigorous and prolonged pharmacological and behavioural treatment.

Modern surgery involves small lesions placed by stereotaxic methods usually to interrupt the frontolimbic connections. With these restricted lesions, side effects are unusual; when they occur they include apathy, weight gain, disinhibition, and epilepsy.

There have been no randomized controlled trials to test the value of the operation, and its use is diminishing even further as pharmacological and behavioural treatments continue to improve.

Further reading

Lader, M. and Herrington, R. (1990). *Biological Treatments in Psychiatry*. Oxford University Press.
A comprehensive survey of drug treatments and ECT.

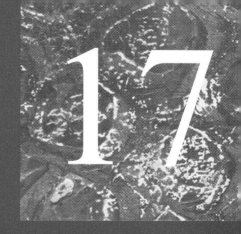

Psychological treatment

- Basic procedures

- Supportive treatment

- Problem-solving techniques

- Cognitive-behaviour therapies

- Dynamic psychotherapy

- Treatment involving more than one patient

Psychological treatment

There are many kinds of psychological treatment but only a few are of direct concern to non-specialists. All doctors need to be able to employ basic psychological procedures in their everyday practice. They also need to know enough about the commonly used special methods of psychological treatment to be able to decide when to refer patients appropriately. In this chapter, psychological treatments will be described under five headings:

1. **Basic procedures** common to every form of therapy and relevant also to all interactions between doctor and patient

2. **Supportive treatment** which is a part of all clinical practice

3. **Problem-solving techniques** useful for patients with adjustment disorders and similar conditions

4. **Behavioural and cognitive treatments** which are used to alter patterns of behaviour and thinking that prevent recovery from certain psychiatric disorders

5. **Psychodynamic methods** that enable patients to recognize unconscious determinants of their behaviour and thereby gain more control over it.

Most patients are treated individually but methods are available for treating couples, families, and small groups of unrelated people who share a common problem. These methods will be described briefly in the last section of this chapter.

Two terms may cause confusion because each is used with more than one meaning. *Psychotherapy* is sometimes used to mean all forms of psychological treatment, often with an additional qualifying term; for example, behavioural psychotherapy. In the second usage, the term refers solely to psychodynamic methods. *Counselling* is used to refer to a wide range of the less technically complicated psychological treatments ranging from the giving of advice, through sympathetic listening, to structured ways of encouraging problem solving. By itself, the term does not have a precise meaning and should usually be qualified to indicate what procedures are being employed (e.g. problem-solving counselling) or what problem is being addressed (e.g. bereavement counselling).

Basic procedures

Certain basic procedures are involved in all forms of psychological treatment whatever additional techniques are employed. These procedures also form part of all therapeutic relationships including those involved in prescribing drugs or supporting patients for whom there is no effective specific treatment. The processes can be summarized as follows:

1. **Use of the doctor–patient relationship** to gain patients' confidence, improve their compliance with more specific methods, and sustain them through

periods of distress. Although helpful in these ways, the doctor–patient relationship can become too intense and impede progress (this problem is discussed below). Patients should feel that the doctor is concerned about them but understand that the relationship is professional, clearly distinct from a friendship, and one that the doctor maintains with other patients.

2. **Listening** to patients' concerns. Patients feel helped when they can describe their problems to a sympathetic person, and many complain that doctors do not spend enough time listening to their concerns before giving advice. Adequate time needs to be provided for listening and patients should feel that they have the doctor's undivided attention and have been understood. Non-verbal signs of attention and occasional rephrasing of what has been said help to achieve this.

3. **The expression of emotion** to relieve distress. It is everyday experience that the expression of strong emotion is followed by a sense of relief. Some patients feel ashamed to reveal their feelings to a doctor and need to be assured that the process is not a sign of personal weakness. Sometimes the process has to be gone through more than once but frequently repeated outpourings of emotion are not generally helpful unless accompanied by constructive efforts to improve the situation that is giving rise to distress.

4. **Information, explanation, and advice** should of course be accurate and relevant to the patient's physical and mental condition. It should correct any misunderstandings about the nature of the condition or the likely outcome. Such misunderstandings are common and often arise because patients were so anxious when the information was first given that they could not concentrate on it. Explanations of the cause of symptoms should be clear, free from jargon, and positive. It is not enough, for example, to explain that no organic cause has been found for symptoms, a convincing account should be given of their psychological origin.

5. **Improving morale** Patients who have prolonged or recurrent medical or social problems may understandably give up hope of improvement. Low morale undermines efforts at treatment and rehabilitation. Even if the doctor cannot offer hope of recovery, it is usually possible to improve morale; for example, by describing ways of reducing pain and distress, or discussing with a disabled patients how remaining abilities could be developed.

6. **Encourage self-help** Patients should be helped to achieve an appropriate balance between compliance with treatment, and determination to be self-sufficient. It is usually possible to achieve this important aim even with the most handicapped patients provided a dependent relationship is not allowed to develop.

The problem of excessive dependency It is important that the relationship between patient and doctor does not become too dependent. This problem is most likely to arise during psychological treatment but it can occur whenever time is spent in talking with patients about their problems.

Signs that the *relationship is becoming too intense* include questions from the patient about the doctor's personal life, and efforts to prolong interviews beyond the agreed time or to contact the doctor for unwarranted reasons. At the same time, patients become dependent and do not make appropriate efforts to help themselves. If the doctor does not respond to patients' demands for increased attention, they may become anxious or angry. If such signs appear, the doctor should discuss them and explain why too intense a relationship is unhelpful.

An intense relationship between patient and doctor is called a **transference**. The term is used because in such a relationship the patient transfers to the doctor feelings and thoughts that originated in another close relationship—often with one or other parent. When the transferred feelings are positive, there is said to be a *positive transference*; when the transferred feelings are negative, there is said to be a *negative transference*. Not only may patients transfer to their doctors feelings that properly belong elsewhere, doctors may do the same with their patients, feeling strongly about them because they remind them, consciously or unconsciously, of an aspect of a parent or another close figure in their lives. These feelings of the therapist toward the patient are called **counter-transference** and referred to as positive or negative as explained under transference. If counter-transference is not recognized in its early stages and corrected, it may impair the doctor's ability to provide impartial advice for that patient and to maintain an appropriate professional relationship.

Supportive treatment

The basic processes described above enter into all doctor–patient relationships. Sometimes they are used to assist patients for whom no other treatment is necessary or possible. When this is done, the procedure is called *supportive therapy* (Table 17.1). It is used to relieve distress during a short episode of illness or personal misfortune, or in the early stages of treatment before specific measures have had time to act (e.g. while waiting for the effect of an antidepressant drug). Supportive therapy is used also to sustain a patient who has a medical or psychiatric condition that cannot be treated, or stressful life problems that cannot be resolved completely (e.g. the problems of caring for a handicapped child). Before choosing supportive therapy, the question should always be asked whether a more active form of psychological or other treatment could bring about change.

Sessions of supportive therapy generally last for about 15 minutes though the first session of treatment is often rather longer to allow adequate time for listening and emotional release. Sessions are often weekly until the major problems have been discussed; thereafter they can then be less frequent. The length, frequency, and number of sessions should be agreed with the patient at the start.

Problem-solving techniques

The aim of these treatments is to help patients to solve stressful problems and to make changes in their lives. These methods are used as the main treatment for acute reactions to stress and for adjustment disorders; and they are used as an addition to other treatments for psychiatric disorders in which associated life problems need to be resolved.

Problem solving is used for problems requiring a *decision*; for example, whether a pregnancy is to be terminated, or an unhappy marriage brought to an end. It is

Table 17.1.

Basic procedures of supportive treatment

- Develop a therapeutic relationship
- Listen to the patient's concerns
- Give information, explanation, and advice
- Encourage the expression of emotion
- Improve morale
- Review and develop intact assets
- Encourage self-help

Table 17.2.
Problem-solving counselling

Basic techniques of supportive therapy, plus:

1. Define and list the problems
2. Choose a problem for action
3. List alternative courses of action
4. Evaluate the courses of action and choose the best
5. Try the selected course of action
6. Evaluate the results

Repeat until the important problems have been resolved

also used for problems requiring *adjustment* to new circumstances such as bereavement or the discovery of terminal illness, or a move to an unfamiliar environment (e.g. by a student starting university life). Problem solving is used also to help a person to *change*, giving up an unsatisfactory way of life and adopting a more healthy one; for example, as part of treatment for dependence on alcohol or drugs.

Problem solving begins with the basic processes described above (Table 17.1). To these are added the following six steps (Table 17.2):

1. A **list of problems** is drawn up by the patient with help from the therapist who helps the former to define the problem and separate its various aspects.

2. The **patient chooses** one of these problems to work on.

3. The patient is helped to **list alternative courses of action** that could solve or reduce the problem. Written problem lists greatly help in arriving at courses of action that are practical and likely to succeed. All problems in the list are eventually considered in the same way, taking one at a time. The courses of action should be specific, indicating what is to be done, and how success will be judged.

4. The **patient considers the pros and cons** of each action plan and chooses the most promising.

5. The patient **attempts** the chosen **course of action** for the selected problem.

6. The **results** of the trial are **evaluated.** If it has been successful, another problem is chosen for action. If the plan has not succeeded, the attempt is reviewed constructively by the patient and therapist to decide how to increase the chance of success on the next occasion. Lack of success is not viewed as a personal failure but as an opportunity to learn more.

Throughout treatment, patients are encouraged to take the lead in identifying problems and solutions so that they learn not only a way of resolving present difficulties but also a strategy for dealing with future problems. Sessions of this kind take about 30 minutes. Four to eight sessions are usual according to the complexity of the problems.

Crisis intervention

When patients are overwhelmed by stressful events or adverse circumstances they are said to be in crisis and help for them is often called *crisis intervention*. People in crisis include those who have harmed themselves (see Chapter 12), victims of physical or sexual assault, and people involved in man-made or natural disasters. Such patients are highly aroused and usually require some additional help to reduce this arousal before they can concentrate effectively on problem solving.

The *additional steps for patients in crisis* are:

• **Lower anxiety and promote sleep** by encouraging the distressed person to talk and express feelings. Although this is one of the basic steps in psychological treatment and therefore part of problem solving, it is particularly important for patients in crisis and is therefore listed first for emphasis. It may be necessary to prescribe an anxiolytic or hypnotic drug (usually a benzodiazepine) for a few days to calm the patient and ensure sleep.

- **Recall traumatic events** It is thought that avoidance of memories of the traumatic experience prolongs the stress reaction. For this reason patients in crisis are often encouraged to remember and relive that experience, even if this induces severe emotion. Although this step reduces distress in the short term, it has not been shown to reduce the frequency of long-term effects of the stressful experience

These steps are additional to the problem-solving techniques described above and to the basic processes of psychological treatment (p. 364).

Cognitive-behaviour therapies

Behaviour therapy is used to treat symptoms and abnormal behaviours that are persisting because of certain actions taken by the patient or of other people, usually to relieve immediate distress. **Cognitive therapy** is used to treat symptoms and abnormal behaviours which persist because of the way that patients think about them. Because such thoughts and actions often occur together, both behavioural and cognitive techniques are often required for the same patient and it is usual to speak of *cognitive-behaviour therapy* to emphasize the close relation between the two.

The actions that help to maintain a disorder in the longer term often produce an initial relief of distress and this is one reason why these maladaptive ways of thinking and behaving are often hard to change. An example of an action that reduces distress but prolongs symptoms is avoidance of situations that provoke anxiety. An example of an action by another person that has the same effect is paying more attention to the patient when behaving abnormally than when behaving normally. In contrast, abnormal ways of thinking usually increase anxiety in both the short and long term; for example, thoughts that palpitations, occurring in fact as part of the anxiety response, are evidence of an impending heart attack (see p. 118).

Most cognitive-behaviour therapies require special training and are carried out by specialists. However, some less complex procedures can be used by non-specialists; these are *relaxation*, *exposure*, and *anxiety management*.

Principles of cognitive-behaviour therapy

The *general approach* to cognitive-behaviour therapy is that the therapist helps patients first to become aware of and then to modify their maladaptive thinking and behaviour. Because patients have to practise new ways of thinking and behaving between the sessions of treatment, it is particularly important that they understand the procedures clearly and are well motivated to carry them out. Written instructions are often used to supplement the explanations given by the therapist during treatment sessions. Other features common to all forms of cognitive-behaviour therapy are:

- **Behavioural analysis** Symptoms, cognitions, and behaviour are monitored by recording them in a diary in which are noted the occurrence of symptoms, and of the thoughts and events that precede and possibly provoke them, and the thoughts and events that follow and possibly reinforce them (Table 17.3). This detailed examination of thoughts, behaviour, and provoking events is called *behavioural analysis*.

Table 17.3.

Examples of behaviour diaries

A. A diary to record anxiety

Date/Time	The situation in which you felt anxious	Symptoms	Rating of anxiety 0–10	What you were thinking	What you did
12/6/98 4 pm	In a queue at the supermarket	Palpitations and dizziness	8	I am going to die	Ran away from the queue
13/6/98 10 am	In town centre	Palpitations and sweating	5	I must relax	Stood still tried to relax

B. A diary to record an eating disorder

Date/Time	The problem	The situation at the time		What were you thinking	What you did
18/7/98 7 pm	Ate a whole loaf of bread with butter and jam	Feeling despondent after being criticised at work		Ev erything I do goes wrong	Made myself vomit
19/7/98 1 pm	Bought 3 bars of chocolate and a cake	Angry with my friend		No one r espects me	Sat alone and ate it all

- **Graduated approach** Treatment takes the form of a graduated series of tasks and activities such that patients gain confidence in dealing with less severe problems before attempting more severe ones.

- **Experimental format** Tasks and activities are presented as experiments in which the achievement of a goal is a success, while non-achievement is not a failure but an opportunity to learn more by analysing constructively what went wrong. This format helps to avoid discouragement and maintain motivation.

Techniques of behaviour therapy (Table 17.4)

Relaxation training

This treatment is used to reduce anxiety by lowering muscle tone and autonomic arousal. Relaxation training is useful in the treatment of some physical conditions that are made worse by stressful events (e.g. some cases of mild hypertension). Used alone, relaxation is not effective for severe anxiety disorders but it is a component of anxiety management training (see below) which is often effective in these conditions.

The essential procedures are: relaxing the muscles one by one; breathing slowly as in sleep; and clearing the mind of worrying thoughts by concentrating on an image of; for example, a tranquil scene. These techniques can be combined in a variety of ways but the results of the resulting methods are similar.

In one method of relaxation training the patient goes through the following steps:

- *Distinguish between tension and relaxation* by first tensing a group of muscles and then letting go.

- *Breathe slowly* and regularly as in sleep.

- *Imagine* a *restful scene* such as a quiet beach on a warm cloudless day.

- *Relax a single muscle group* (e.g. the muscles of the left forearm). Follow this by relaxing other groups in a sequence such as: whole left arm, right arm, neck and shoulders, face, abdomen, back, left leg, right leg.

- *Relax more extensively* (e.g. all the muscles of a limb together) so that complete relaxation is achieved more rapidly.

- At the end, *become active gradually* as in waking from sleep.

The first relaxation session may last up to 30 minutes while each subsequent session usually lasts about 15 minutes. Throughout the sessions the person continues to breathe slowly and imagine restful scenes. After about six sessions, most people can relax rapidly. At this stage it is useful to associate relaxation with a keyword that can be used to promote relaxation rapidly at times of stress. It is useful to provide a tape recording of the instructions for relaxation to be used at home in quiet surroundings at a time when disturbance is unlikely.

Exposure

Exposure is used mainly for phobic disorders. The basic procedure is to persuade patients to enter, repeatedly, situations that they have avoided previously or, if this is not practicable to imagine doing so. When re-entry to feared situations is

Table 17.4.

Some techniques of behaviour therapy

- Relaxation training
- Exposure
- Response prevention
- Thought stopping
- Assertiveness training
- Self-control
- Contingency management
- (Aversion therapy)

gradual the term *desensitization* is used. When the re-entry to feared situations is rapid, the term *flooding* is used.

The **stages of treatment** are:

- Determine in detail which *situations* are *avoided*.

- Arrange these situations in order of the amount of anxiety that each provokes (the resulting list is called a *hierarchy*). The items in the hierarchy are chosen so that the difference in the amount of anxiety induced by each one and the next is about the same throughout the list. A list might include items such as the local shop when there are no other customers; the local shop when it is crowded; a supermarket when there are no queues at the checkouts; a supermarket with long queues.

- *Teach relaxation training* which is then used to reduce anxiety during exposure.

- Persuade the patient *to enter a situation* at the bottom of the hierarchy and stay until anxiety has declined. The procedure is repeated with the next situation on the hierarchy and then with next until the top of the hierarchy is reached. Anxiety should have subsided before the patient leaves the situation otherwise no benefit will follow.

This sequence brings about a reduction in the anxiety experienced in the situation and generalization to the next situation in the hierarchy so that less anxiety is experienced when this is entered. If repeated and adequately prolonged exposure does not cause a reduction in anxiety, a new situation is chosen lower on the hierarchy. When one stage has been accomplished, the patient enters the next situation on the list, and so on through the hierarchy. Patients should practise exposure for about an hour every day. To ensure this it is often helpful to enlist a relative or friend who can encourage practice, praise success, and sustain motivation if there are setbacks.

Other behavioural methods

Response prevention

Response prevention is used to treat obsessional rituals. It is based on the observation that rituals diminish in frequency and intensity after patients have made repeated and determined efforts to suppress them for a time. To be effective, the ritual must be suppressed until the associated anxiety has waned, and this may take up to an hour. Since the immediate effect of response prevention is an increase in anxiety, patients require much support if they are to suppress the rituals for long enough. When response prevention has been achieved, patients are encouraged to do the same in situations known to provoke the rituals. As the procedures are repeated there is a gradual decline not only in the rituals but also in any intensity of associated obsessional thoughts.

Thought stopping

Thought stopping is used to treat obsessional thoughts occurring without obsessional rituals (and therefore not treatable by response prevention). An intense stimulus is used to interrupt the thoughts; for example, the mildly painful effect of snapping an elastic band worn around the wrist. By repeating this action, some patients gradually become more able to interrupt the thoughts on their own, without the distracting stimulus.

Assertiveness training

Assertiveness training is used for people who are abnormally shy or socially awkward. Direct but socially acceptable expression of thoughts and feelings is encouraged as follows: *analysis* of the social behaviour in terms of facial expression, eye contact, posture, and tone of voice, and what is said; *enactment* of the social encounters which cause difficulty for the patient while the therapist demonstrates an appropriate response and helps patients to copy it. Sometimes therapist and patient *exchange roles* to help the patient understand the viewpoint of the other person in the situation. Finally, patients *practise* appropriate social behaviour in everyday life, and keep a diary record of the outcome of this practice.

Self-control

Self-control techniques are used to increase control over behaviours such as excessive eating or smoking. The treatment has two stages: self-monitoring and self-reinforcement. *Self-monitoring* is the keeping of daily records of the problem behaviour and of the circumstances in which it occurs. Thus, a patient who overeats may record what is eaten, when it is eaten, and any associations between eating and stressful events or moods. The keeping of such records is itself a powerful aid to self-control, because many patients have previously avoided facing the true extent of their problems. *Self-reinforcement* is rewarding oneself when a goal has been achieved successfully. For example, a woman might buy herself a new pair of shoes when she reaches a target. Simple rewards of this kind help to maintain motivation.

Contingency management

Contingency management is used when abnormal behaviour is being reinforced unwittingly by other people; for example, by parents who attend more to a child during temper tantrums than at other times. The *treatment* has two aims: first, to identify and reduce the reinforcers of abnormal behaviour; and second, to find ways of rewarding desirable behaviour. Praise and encouragement are the usual rewards but they may be added to with material rewards such as points or stars that will earn a child a desired toy or treat.

Contingency management has four stages:

1. The *behaviour* to be changed is *recorded* by the patient or another person (e.g. a parent might count the frequency of a child's temper tantrums).

2. Events that immediately follow the behaviour and appear to be *reinforcers are identified*; usually these involve extra attention given to the child, when behaving badly.

3. *Alternative rewarding consequences* are *devised* to reinforce appropriate behaviour (e.g. the parent would attend more to the child when behaving well).

4. The *undesirable behaviour* is *ignored* as far as this is practicable.

Parents *monitor progress* by recording the frequency of each kind of behaviour. Although this treatment is concerned mainly with factors that follow and reinforce behaviour, attention is also given to events that precede and seem to provoke the behaviour. For example, the child's temper tantrums may occur after the mother pays attention to a younger sibling. The approach may seem mechanistic, but in practice the procedures can be carried out in a caring way.

Aversion therapy

In this method, undesirable behaviour is linked to a negative reinforcement such as a mild electric shock. Aversion therapy has fallen out of use because of the ethical problems in giving repeated painful stimuli as treatment, and its lack of long-term effectiveness.

Outline of cognitive therapy

Cognitive therapy proceeds through four stages:

1. *Identify maladaptive thinking* by asking patients to keep a daily record of the thoughts that precede and accompany their symptoms or abnormal behaviour. The thoughts are recorded as soon as possible after they have occurred.

2. *The maladaptive thinking is challenged* by correcting misunderstandings with accurate information, and pointing out illogical ways of reasoning.

3. *Alternative ways of thinking* are worked out with the patient.

4. *These alternative explanations* are tested in behavioural experiments.

Until maladaptive thinking has been changed, use is made of *distraction*, brought about by:

- *Refocusing attention* from the thoughts to some external object (e.g. patients may count blue cars in the street or look intently at an object in the room).

- *Carrying out mental exercises*, such as mental arithmetic, that require full attention.

The examples that follow illustrate how these principles are put into practice in treating common disorders.

Cognitive therapy for anxiety management

Anxiety management reduces anxiety directly by relaxation and indirectly by changing two kinds of maintaining factor: (1) anxiety-provoking cognitions; and (2) avoidance. The procedures are listed in Box 17.1. The following points should be noted.

The first step is to assess the intensity of the anxiety response, the pattern of symptoms, the situation in which anxiety occurs, any anxiety-provoking situations, and the use of avoidance as a way of coping with anxiety. This assessment guides the choice of subsequent procedures.

Relaxation training is given in all cases. Patients are told about the normal anxiety response and the harmless natures of the symptoms of anxiety. This information is discussed in relation to the particular symptoms and concerns of the patient revealed in the initial assessment; for example, that rapid heart action could cause damage to the heart.

The therapist explains how fear of the effects of anxiety ('fear of fear') produces a vicious circle; for example, fear that anxiety will lead to fainting, or fear that other people will observe tremor and think unfavourably of the patient.

Box 17.1 **Anxiety management**

- **Use a behaviour diary** (see Table 17.3) to assess:
  - prominent symptoms
  - severity of symptoms
  - situations in which anxiety occurs
  - avoidance
- Teach **relaxation** (see p. 369)
- Give **information** to correct misunderstanding about the cause of symptoms
- **Explain** the vicious circle of anxiety ('fear of fear') and the effects of avoidance
- Teach **exposure** (see p. 369) when anxiety-provoking situations are avoided
- Teach **distraction** from anxious thoughts (see p. 372)

For further information see Kennerley, H. (1995). *Managing anxiety* (2nd edn). Oxford University Press.

Most anxiety patients avoid situations that provoke anxiety and this avoidance maintains anxiety. Training in exposure (p. 369) is an important component of anxiety management whenever the assessment reveals avoidance.

Although explanation of the nature of anxiety reduces anxiety-provoking thoughts, it does not remove them. Distraction (see above) is useful in all cases to deflect attention from these thoughts when anxiety is beginning to develop.

Cognitive therapy for panic disorder

Patients with panic disorder believe that physical symptoms of anxiety are evidence of serious physical illness (e.g. that palpitations are evidence of an impending heart attack). Such ideas are sometimes called catastrophic cognitions. These convictions cause further anxiety and a cycle of mounting anxiety is set up (see p. 118). The four stages of cognitive therapy are used, with the following special features:

1. Patients who find it difficult to identify the cognitions associated with panic may be helped if panic is induced in the treatment session by voluntary hyperventilation or exercise.

2. The link between cognitions and anxiety may be demonstrated by asking patients to dwell on the catastrophic cognitions—which increases anxiety—and to distract attention from them—which reduces anxiety.

3. The therapist explains how physical symptoms occur as part of the normal response to stress, and how a vicious circle model of mounting anxiety is set up when patients fear the consequences of physical symptoms of anxiety (see p. 117).

4. Patients are encouraged to think in the new way when they experience symptoms in situations outside the clinic, and to observe the effect of this on the severity of their anxiety.

Cognitive therapy for depressive disorder

The cognitive disorder in depressive disorder is particularly complex, and cognitive treatment is correspondingly more elaborate than that for anxiety disorder. There are three kinds of cognitive abnormality. The *first* are **intrusive thoughts**, usually of a self-depreciating kind (e.g. 'I am a failure'). When they are weak such thoughts can be counteracted by distraction, using the methods described above, but when they are strong they are difficult to control.

The *second kind* of depressive thinking is the making of **logical errors** that distort the interpretation of experience and help to maintain the intrusive thoughts. These errors are known as: exaggeration, catastrophizing, overgeneralization, and ignoring the positive.

Exaggeration is magnifying small mistakes and thinking of them as major failures.

Catastrophizing is expecting serious consequences from minor problems (e.g. thinking that a relative who is late home has been involved in an accident).

Overgeneralizing is thinking that the bad outcome of a particular event will be repeated in every similar event in future (e.g. that having lost one partner, the person will never find a lasting relationship).

Ignoring the positive is to dwell on personal shortcomings or on the unfavourable aspects of a situation while overlooking favourable aspects.

The therapist helps the patient recognize these and other errors and adopt more reasonable ways of thinking.

The *third kind* of depressive thinking involves **maladaptive assumptions** often about social acceptability; for example, the assumption that a person is liked only if good looking and successful. These assumptions are seldom revealed directly but can be discovered by questioning patients about their reasons for feeling depressed. Repeated questioning of this kind is a characteristic feature of cognitive therapy.

Cognitive therapy for depression focuses on identifying and then challenging these three kinds of cognition by asking why patients hold their beliefs, and examining the consequences of thinking as they do. As in other forms of cognitive therapy, the therapist also helps patients to consider the consequences of thinking as they do, and in new ways. The therapist also suggests activities to overcome the depressed patient's tendency to withdraw and to be inactive ('activity scheduling'). This last procedure is especially important for severely depressed patients.

Cognitive-behaviour therapy for bulimia nervosa

This treatment begins with behavioural self-control methods (see p. 371) which are used to re-establish normal patterns of eating (three meals a day and no snacks between meals) before cognitive techniques are introduced. Patients keep records of what and when they eat, and what events and emotions precede a binge. They

Box 17.2 Self-help for bulimia nervosa

• Monitoring	• a daily record of eating, binges, and vomiting
	• weighing once a week
• Regular planned meals	• three normal sized meals a day with three small between-meal snacks
• Stop binges	• eat only the planned amount
	• keep other food out of sight
	• keep limited stocks
	• take just enough money when buying food
• Control vomiting	• urge to vomit declines as binges stop
• Control purging and use of diruetics	• reduce laxatives/diuretics, if necessary, in stages
• Find alternatives to binge-eating	• list distracting activities
	• try them out
• Reduce life problems	• see problem-solving counselling (Table 17.2)

For further information see Fairburn, C. G. (1995). *Overcoming binge eating*. Guilford Press, New York and London.

also record vomiting and laxative abuse. The self-control procedures reduce binge-ing, vomiting, and laxative abuse but to avoid relapse cognitive procedures have to be added. The four basic stages of cognitive therapy are used. Abnormal cognitions are identified using daily records; the logical basis of these cognitions is challenged; alternative views are formulated; and the effect of thinking in new ways is tested. A simplified account of a self-help programme for bulimia nervosa is shown in Box 17.2.

The cognitive approach in everyday practice

Although cognitive therapies are complex procedures requiring special training, several features of the cognitive approach are useful in everyday clinical practice. It is particularly useful to ask patients to keep daily records to: (1) find out what they are thinking before and while they experience symptoms; (2) record abnormal behaviours and their attempts to control them, and (3) evaluate progress.

Dynamic psychotherapy

Brief psychodynamic therapy

In this treatment, patients are helped to obtain a greater understanding of aspects of their disorder of which they were unaware (unconscious aspects) as a means to gaining more control over their symptoms and abnormal behaviour, and of dealing better with situations and relationships that have been difficult. The treatment may be brief and focused on a small number of specific problems, or long-term and dealing with a broader range of problems. Brief dynamic therapy is sometimes called *focal psychotherapy*. Doctors other than psychiatrists are unlikely to use dynamic psychotherapy but they may need to refer patients for treatment and for this they need a basic understanding of its indications and techniques.

The main **indications** for brief dynamic therapy are problems of low self-esteem and difficulties in making relationships either of which may be accompanied by emotional disorders, eating disorders, or sexual disorders. Patients referred for dynamic psychotherapy need to be insightful and willing to consider links between their present difficulties and problems at earlier stages of their lives.

The **techniques** of brief psychotherapy (see Table 17.5) can be summarized as follows:

1. Patient and therapist *agree on the problems* that will be the focus of treatment.

2. Patients *discuss recent and past experiences* of the problem. To encourage this self-revelation the therapist speaks infrequently and responds more to the emotional than the factual content of what is said; for example, instead of asking for more factual detail he may say 'you seem angry when you talk about that experience'.

3. Patients are encouraged to *review their own part in problems* that they ascribe to other people, and *identify common themes* in what they are describing; for example, fear of being rejected by other people.

4. Patients are helped to *recall similar problems* at an earlier stage of life. They are encouraged to consider whether the present maladaptive behaviour may have originated as a way of coping that was adaptive at that time but has continued as a self-defeating pattern of response. For example, failure to trust others following the experience of sexual abuse in childhood.

5. To help patients *make connections between past and present* behaviour, or between different aspects of their present behaviour, the therapist makes **interpretations**. These are suggestions about these connections which should be framed as hypotheses to be considered by the patient, rather than truths to be accepted.

6. The patient is encouraged to consider *alternative ways of thinking and relating* and to try these out first with the therapist and then in everyday life.

In this kind of psychotherapy the relationship with the therapist becomes particularly intense. In this treatment, transference can be put to good use since it reflects the patient's relationship with the parents. The ways in which the transference is expressed is therefore an indirect indication of the way the patient related to the parents earlier in life and this may suggest how the present problems developed. Explanations of this kind are called **transference interpretations**. Although transference can be useful in this way, it is important to reduce the intensity in the later stages of treatment otherwise the patient is left in a dependent state and it is difficult to end treatment at the planned time.

Table 17.5.

Techniques of brief psychodynamic therapy

- Agree problems to be discussed
- Discuss recent and past experiences of the problem
- Review patients' part in problems they ascribe to others
- Identify common themes
- Link present with past behaviour (interpretations)
- Examine relationship with the therapist (transference interpretations)
- Consider alternative ways of thinking and relating

Long-term dynamic psychotherapy

This is the most ambitious kind of psychological treatment but its value is disputed. The aim is to modify longstanding patterns of thinking and behaviour that contribute to personal and relationship problems which may be associated with psychiatric disorder or problems in themselves. These forms of psychotherapy originate directly or indirectly from Freud's method of psychoanalysis The basic techniques resemble those of the shorter forms of dynamic psychotherapy (described above) but with additional procedures intended to uncover more deeply hidden aspects of the problems.

Most of the special techniques are intended to access memories of events which occurred early in life and have been strongly repressed. These methods (see Table 17.6) are:

- **free association** (i.e. encouraging patients to allow their thoughts to wander freely and illogically from a starting point of relevance to the problem);
- **recall of dreams** and discussion of their meaning;
- **intense transference** which causes behaviour in the interview that reflects behaviour with the parents in earlier years.

Intense transference is achieved by seeing the patient frequently (three or more times a week), and by the therapist saying little and revealing little of himself. This intense transference may lead also to strong emotional reactions in the sessions with the opportunity to discover ways of controlling these, and similar feelings experienced outside the sessions. As transference becomes more intense, so does counter-transference; for this reason therapists who use this kind of treatment are required to seek greater self-understanding by undergoing a period of dynamic therapy themselves.

The problems of reducing the intensity of the transference, discussed under *brief dynamic therapy*, are even greater with reconstructive methods and it is a disadvantage of this treatment that it sometimes lasts well beyond the planned date of termination. No randomized controlled trials have demonstrated that this intensive form of psychotherapy is more effective than brief dynamic treatment or cognitive-behaviour methods.

Treatment involving more than one patient

Group therapy

When several patients are treated together, certain psychological processes develop which do not occur in individual therapy. These processes are useful both in psychiatric treatment and in the general practice of medicine where groups may be used to support patients or their relatives. These additional factors (Table 17.7) are:

1. **Group support** which can help the members through difficult periods in treatment or in their lives outside.

2. **Learning from others** (e.g. how others in the group have overcome problems similar to the patient's own).

Table 17.6.

Techniques of long-term dynamic therapy

- Free association
- Recall of dreams
- Intensify transference
  - frequent sessions
  - passive therapist

Table 17.7.

Additional therapeutic influences in group therapy

- Group support
- Learning from one another
- Testing opinions against those of others
- Practising social behaviour

3. **Testing** opinions against those of others. (This procedure is often more effective in changing beliefs and attitudes than advice from a doctor.)

4. **Practising social behaviour** especially for those who are shy or socially awkward.

In group therapy, close relationships develop between patients as well as between each patient and the therapist. An important task of the therapist is to ensure that these relationships do not become too intense, and particularly that they do not continue outside the group meetings.

Group therapy can be used for the purposes for which individual therapy is used that is for support, problem solving, behavioural treatment, and dynamic psychotherapy. The length of treatment, the intensity of involvement of patients, and the techniques vary according to the purpose, as they do with individual therapy.

Special forms of group

There are several kinds of special group treatment, of which only two will be mentioned. In **psychodrama** problems are enacted (as in a play) rather than merely talked about. In **encounter groups** a confrontational style of questioning and interpretation is used in the hope that it will hasten change. There is no research evidence that confrontational methods produce additional benefit and in some patients they may provoke a temporary increase in symptoms. For these reasons confrontational methods should be used only after special training and then with patients selected to have enough inner strength.

Large-group treatment

In some psychiatric wards, patients meet regularly in a group containing 20 or more people. The usual purpose is supportive, enabling patients to talk about the problems of living together in the ward, and thereby to prevent any increase in these problems. **A therapeutic community** uses group methods not just for support but in any attempt to modify personality. Patients reside usually for many months, living and working together, and attending small and large groups in which they discuss problems in relationships and try to help each other to recognize and resolve their problems. This kind of treatment has been used mainly for patients with personality disorders characterized by antisocial or aggressive behaviour. The value of these methods is uncertain and the approach is limited to a few special centres.

Self-help groups

These groups are organized by people with a shared problem, such as obesity, alcoholism, postnatal depression, or the rearing of a child with a congenital disorder. The groups meet without a professional therapist and are often led by a person who has overcome the problem. Alcoholics Anonymous (see p. 274) is an example of such a group, Weight Watchers is another. When well run by informed persons these groups are valuable sources of support.

Psychotherapy with couples and families

Marital therapy

Marital therapy (otherwise called **couple therapy**) is used to help couples who have problems in relationships. In medical practice this therapy is used when relationship problems are maintaining a psychiatric disorder (e.g. a depressive disorder) in one or both partners. Treatment focuses on the ways in which the couple interact rather than on their individual problems. The aim is to promote concern by each partner for the welfare of the other, tolerance of differences, and an agreed balance of decision making and dominance. To avoid imposing the therapist's own values, it is usual to start by helping the couple to identify the difficulties they wish to put right, before helping them to understand each other's point of view. The therapist remains neutral, and is careful not to take sides with either partner. Common problems of communication include failure to express wishes directly, failure to listen to the other's point of view, 'mind reading' (A knows better than B, what is in B's mind) and making positive comments followed by criticism (the sting in the tail).

Marital therapy can be carried out in several ways. It can use simple **problem-solving methods** (see p. 365). It can use a **behavioural approach** which focuses on the ways that each person reinforces, or fails to reinforce, the behaviour of the other. It can use **transactional methods** in which attention is given to the private rules that govern the couple's behaviour towards each other; and to the question of who makes these rules (e.g. who decides which person's work has priority). **Dynamic** methods are used to uncover hitherto unconscious aspects of the couple's interaction; for example, the possibility that a husband repeatedly criticizes his wife because she fails to show the self-reliance that he lacks himself. Depending on the nature of the marital problem, and on the couple's capacity for psychological insight, each approach can be of value.

Family therapy

Family therapy is usually employed when a child or adolescent has an emotional or conduct disorder. In addition to the young person, the parents are involved together with any other family members (such as siblings or grandparents) who are involved closely with the young person. The aim of treatment is to reduce the problem rather than to produce some ideal state of family life.

Problems-solving methods, transactional methods, and *dynamic approaches,* can be used as in marital therapy. Specific forms of family therapy have been devised to deal with factors thought to lead to relapse in eating disorders and schizophrenia.

Further reading

Bloch, S. (ed.) (1966). *An Introduction to the Psychotherapies* (3rd edn). Oxford University Press.
Outlines methods used in each of the commonly used forms of psychotherapy.

Hawton, K., Salkovskis, P. M., Kirk, J., and Clark, D. M. (1989). *Cognitive Behaviour Therapy for Psychiatric Problems: A Practical Guide.* Oxford University Press.
A comprehensive account with examples of the use of cognitive-behaviour therapy in a range of psychiatric disorders.

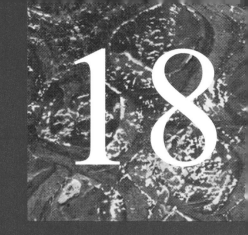

18

Mental health care for a community

- Psychiatric disorder in the community
- The provision of mental health services

Mental health care for a community

This chapter is concerned with the provision and organization of services for people with psychiatric disorder. It is not concerned with the treatment of individuals, but with the provision of mental health services for a population. It deals mainly with the services needed for people between the ages of 18 and 65 (services for children are discussed on pp. 400–2, and services for the elderly on p. 312). It does not deal with services for people with mental retardation (these services are described on pp. 438–41).

The way mental services are organized differs from country to country. This chapter describes mainly the provision of services in Britain but the principles apply much more widely.

The chapter begins by describing the overall epidemiology of mental disorder. This gives a measure of the need for services. It then goes on to describe the principles of providing services and current models of service provision.

Psychiatric disorder in the community

Prevalence

To understand what range of psychiatric services are required for a community it is necessary to know:

(1)   the frequency of mental disorders in the population; and

(2)   how patients with these disorders come into contact with the health services.

The local prevalence of mental disorders will vary from place to place, but approximate estimates can be obtained from national surveys. Table 18.1 shows prevalence estimates from a large population surveys in Britain. From this table it can be seen that mental disorders are common. From this and other studies, it appears that between 1 in 4 and 1 in 5 of the population at risk experience such disorders in the course of a year.

Higher rates of neurotic disorder are found in people who are:

* divorced/separated
* single parents
* unemployed
* city or town dwellers.

Higher rates of psychotic illness are found in:

* homeless people
* inner cities.

Table 18.1.

Approximate prevalence of psychiatric disorder in the community (1-week prevalence per 1000 population; Age: 16–65 years)

	Women	Men
Any non-psychotic mental disorder	200	125
Non-specific neurotic disorder	100	50
Generalized anxiety disorder	50	40
Depressive episode	30	20
Obsessive-compulsive disorder	20	10
Panic disorder	10	10
Functional psychosis*	5	5
Alcohol dependence*	20	75
Drug dependence*	15	30

*1-year prevalence per 1000 population.

Figures based on: Jenkins, R., Lewis, G., Bebbington, P., Brugha, T., Farrell, M., Gill, B., and Meltzer, H. (1997). The National Psychiatric Morbidity Surveys of Great Britain—initial findings from the Household Survey. *Psychological Medicine*, 27, 775–89.

Psychiatric disorders in different health care settings

The prevalence of psychiatric disorder also varies in different health care settings. This information can be used as an estimate of *need* for mental health services as well as describing where the majority of mental disorders are treated.

The relationship between primary and secondary care

A commonly used model of the proportion of mental illness that is seen at different levels of service is that of Goldberg and Huxley, who described a *pathway to psychiatric care* (Table 18.2).

Less severe conditions such as anxiety and depressive disorder are very common in primary care. It has been estimated that about 5% of general practice attenders suffer from a significant depressive disorder. In specialist psychiatric care, more severe disorders such as schizophrenia are more common.

Psychiatric disorders in general hospital settings

The prevalence of psychiatric disorder is also high in general hospitals, both in patients with physical illness and in patients with somatoform disorders. This subject is dealt with fully in Chapter 11.

The provision of mental health services

The basic principles of the provision of mental health services are the same as for any other health service. They should be:

1. Accessible to all users

2. Relevant to the need of the whole community

Table 18.2.

Pathway to psychiatric care and the approximate prevalence of mental disorders in the population and health care settings

Level 1. Mental disorder in the community
200 per 1000 population aged 16–65
Filter 1. The decision to consult a doctor

Level 2. Mental disorders in all primary care patients
180–200 per 1000 population aged 16–65
Filter 2. The detection of mental disorder in primary care

Level 3. Mental disorders diagnosed in primary care patients
100 per 1000 population aged 16–65
Filter 3. Referral to secondary mental health services

Level 4. All mental disorders in secondary care patients
20 per 1000 population aged 16–65
Filter 4. Admission to psychiatric hospitals

Level 5. Patients in psychiatric hospital
< 5 per 1000 population aged 16–65

From Goldberg, D. and Huxley, P. (1980). *Mental Illness in the Community*. Tavistock, London.

3. Effective

4. Equitable (fair)

5. Socially acceptable

6. Efficient and economical.

In this section, we will describe the different kinds of services available for people suffering from mental disorders.

What makes mentally ill people seek help?

Not everyone with a psychiatric disorder seeks medical advice. Some people with minor emotional reactions to stress obtain help from their family, friends, the Church, or non-medical counselling agencies (see Chapter 6). Many people with problems of substance abuse do not seek help of any kind. Nevertheless, in Britain, about 9 in 10 of people with mental disorder attend a general practitioner, although many do not complain directly of psychological symptoms (see below). Whether a person with **clinically significant** psychiatric disorder consults a general practitioner depends on several factors (see Box 18.1). There is a great deal of misunderstanding and stigma about mental disorders among the general population. For example, that majority of people believe that depression is wholly due to adverse life events, the best treatment is counselling, and that antidepressants are addictive. There have been recent efforts to improve the general population's knowledge although the effectiveness of such campaigns remains unknown.

Box 18.1 **Factors influencing a person's decision to seek medical advice**

- the *severity and duration* of the disorder;
- the *person's attitude* to psychiatric disorder—some people feel ashamed of the disorder and embarrassed to ask for help;
- the *attitudes* and knowledge of *family and friends*; if these people are unsympathetic the affected person may be less likely to admit the problem or seek help for it;
- the person's *knowledge* about possible help; if he does not know that help can be provided, or if he has false expectations about the likely treatment he may not seek help;
- the person's *perception of the doctor's attitude* to psychiatric disorder; if the doctor is viewed as unsympathetic, the person is less likely to ask for help.

Psychiatric disorder in primary care

Detection of psychiatric disorder

Most people with psychiatric disorder who seek help from a general practitioner have symptoms of anxiety or depression. Not all these patients tell the doctor about these psychiatric symptoms; many describe physical symptoms. These physical symptoms may be of an associated minor physical illness, or may be somatic symptoms of anxiety (e.g. palpitations), or of depression (e.g. tiredness). Patients present physical rather than psychological symptoms for two reasons. Some patients are aware of the emotional symptoms as well as the physical ones but are uncertain whether the doctor will respond sympathetically to a request for help with psychological symptoms; they hope he will discover them for himself. Other patients are unaware that their physical symptoms may have a psychological cause. Up to a third of people who consult a general practitioner present in the above two ways. General practitioners vary in their ability to detect these undeclared psychiatric disorders. The general practitioner's success in detection of psychiatric disorder depends on two factors:

1. Always consider the **possibility of mental disorder** in consultations.

2. **Interviewing skills** (see pp. 21–3). This is the ability to gain the patient's confidence (and so enable him to disclose any psychiatric symptoms) and to identify any psychological factors that are contributing to physical symptoms.

General practitioners can improve their ability to detect common psychiatric disorders, such as depression, by using screening questions or questionnaires and by improving their interviewing skills (see Chapter 2).

The treatment of psychiatric disorder in primary care

The majority of identified psychiatric disorder is treated by general practitioners themselves. Thus, they deal with nearly all adjustment disorders, the majority of the anxiety and depressive disorders, and many problems of alcohol abuse. They refer to psychiatrists about 5–10% of the patients identified as having psychiatric disorders selecting particularly those with severe depressive disorders, schizophrenia, dementia, and other disorders when severe and persistent.

For depressive disorders, drug treatment is usually indicated. There is evidence that depressive disorders are undertreated in primary care—both in terms of dose and duration of treatment. It has been shown that if depressive disorders in primary care are optimally treated, the outcome is much improved. The undertreatment is often related to under-recognition of depressive disorders—and to an erroneous belief that antidepressants are ineffective if low mood is related to adverse life events and, therefore, understandable. Problem-solving therapy (pp. 365–6) may also be effective in mild and moderate depressive disorders, and this is an alternative if the patient prefers a psychological treatment and if it is available.

For most adjustment and anxiety disorders, psychological treatments are more important than drugs (p. 110). Most general practitioners do not have the time to provide psychological treatments for all who need it. Unless there is another way to obtain treatment, it may be necessary to prescribe anxiolytic drugs to suppress symptoms in the short term (p. 337). An alternative is for the primary care team to include other people who can provide brief psychological therapies for patients. Many primary care teams now include a counsellor, who may be providing one of the specific brief psychological therapies, but more often will be providing non-specific counselling.

Patients who do not respond to treatment, have severe illnesses, or need treatments not available in primary care need to be referred to the specialist psychiatric services. The decision to refer to a psychiatrist is determined by several factors (see Box 18.2).

The psychiatrist working in general practice
A way of increasing the number of patients with psychiatric disorders who can be managed in primary care is to arrange visits to the health centre by a psychiatrist.

Box 18.2 Factors influencing a general practitioner's decision to refer to the specialist psychiatric services

- Uncertainty about diagnosis
- Severity of the condition: the most severely ill patients may need admission to hospital
- Serious suicidal ideas
- The need for treatment which is unavailable in primary care
- Willingness of the patient to see a psychiatrist
- Accessibility of psychiatric services, how far the patient has to travel, and how promptly patients are seen by the psychiatrist

There are two main ways in which a psychiatrist can work:

1. **'Consultation–liaison' model** in which the psychiatrist advises the general practitioner about the assessment or management of patients whom the latter continues to treat: the psychiatrist may advise about drug dosage, or the conduct of brief psychological treatment. The psychiatrist can assess patients when the general practitioner is uncertain about diagnosis or about the advisability of specialist treatment.

2. **'Shifted out-patient' model** The psychiatrist transfers most of his out-patient work from the hospital to primary care, spending a large part of his time there.

In general, a combination of the two is preferred because it permits more patients to receive the benefit of psychiatric expertise and at the same time strengthens the clinical skills of the general practitioner. However, the precise details of the arrangement chosen depends on several local factors including the needs of the general practitioners, the accessibility of out-patient clinics to patients, and the number of psychiatrists available to provide services for the population. Other members of the psychiatric team may also develop links to general practices.

Specialist psychiatric services

The patients reaching psychiatric services are a selected group of the population of people with mental disorder. The number and type of patient referred depends on the general practitioner's confidence, ability, and willingness to treat psychiatric problems, and on the resources at his disposal. The principles which apply to the provision of psychiatric services are:

- to treat patients outside hospital whenever feasible;
- to provide services close to patients' homes;
- to prevent the occurrence and recurrence of mental disorder;
- to involve families and voluntary organizations in the planning and provision of care.

All psychiatric services must provide for patients with serious disorders such as severe and chronic anxiety disorders, severe affective disorder, schizophrenia, dementia, and people who are suicidal or dangerous to others by reason of mental disorder. Specialist adult psychiatric services consist of a range of services including:

- community mental health teams (CMHTs);
- out-patient clinics;
- day hospitals;
- hospital beds;
- rehabilitation resources.

Community mental health teams (CMHTs)

These have been developed in order to avoid unnecessary admission to hospital, to provide services as close as possible to a patient's home, and to provide continuity of care for patients with chronic psychiatric disorders. They are usually **multidisciplinary**, including several other clinical disciplines as well as psychiatry (Table 18.3). In a well-functioning CMHT, the members will work flexibly as well as performing their own specific tasks.

Table 18.3.

Mental health professionals in a community mental health team (CMHTs)

Profession	Role
Psychiatrist	The clinical leader of the team and responsible for psychiatric assessments. Initiates and supervises drug treatments and provides brief psychological interventions. Supervises out-patients, in-patients, and day patients.
Community mental health nurse	The core members of the team who usually work exclusively in the CMHT. Act as **key workers** for patients with chronic mental disorders, monitor medication and side effects, and provide psychological treatments.
Clinical psychologist	Performs psychological assessments and provides a full range of psychological treatments.
Occupational therapist	Performs functional assessments, provides social skills training, psychological treatments, and assists the patient in finding occupation.
Social worker	Performs social and Mental Health Act assessments and assists the patient in meeting accommodation and financial needs. May also provide some psychological treatments.

There are two main models of community care. In the first, **case management,** a *key worker* is identified. The key worker is often a mental health nurse and is reponsible for making sure that the patient's needs and clinical status are regularly assessed. This assessment often takes place at a multidisciplinary meeting. Other members of the team are involved as required to fulfil specific functions. For example, if the patient's clinical state deteriorates, a psychiatrist will be involved and if the patient needs help with housing, the social worker will be involved. In the alternative model, **assertive community treatment**, only a limited number of the the most severely ill patients are treated by the CMHT. Unlike case management, the clinical responsibility for each patient is shared by the team. Another difference is that each member of the assertive community treatment team will need to be involved with each patient. The focus of treatment is on ensuring compliance with treatment and avoiding the need for hospital admission.

In the UK, ease management is the main model used. Whichever model of community care is used, several elements are required to make sure that a CMHT is able to work effectively with patients suffering from severe mental illness, such as schizophrenia.

1. *Regular reassessment of the patient's clinical status and needs*
This should be performed systematically on a regular basis. It may be necessary to arrange a **multidisciplinary needs assessment** in which CMHT members with specific skills (see Table 18.3) assess the patient's functioning and decide which interventions are likely to help.

2. *Effective collaboration between those involved in care*

Team members should meet regularly and communicate effectively about patients between meetings with the patients themselves, relatives or carers, and others involved in the patient's care including social services and the general practitioner. A written **care plan** should be made for each patient and circulated to everyone who needs to know about the arrangements. Care planning meetings are particularly important before a patient is discharged from hospital.

3. *Adequate support for carers*

Family and friends are the main carers of most patients living outside hospital. They encourage suitable behaviours such as getting up and eating at appropriate times; maintaining personal hygiene; and using time constructively. They provide psychological support and encourage compliance with treatment. They have to tolerate unusual behaviour or social withdrawal. Prolonged involvement in care can be stressful and carers may need counselling as well as periods of respite.

Voluntary carers play a significant part in community care. Trained volunteers may provide counselling and practical support for patients and families. Charitable organizations provide some professional carers and hostel staff. Voluntary carers need training, supervision, and adequate access to mental health professionals.

4. *Provision of suitable accommodation*

Many patients live with their families, and some can care for themselves in rented accommodation. Others need more help, which can be provided in two main ways.

(i) **Group homes** Some patients are able to live in group homes which are houses in which 4 or 5 patients live together. These houses are often owned by voluntary organization charities. Patients perform the essential tasks of running the house together, even though separately they could not do so. They receive support and supervision, usually from a community nurse who ensures that arrangements are continuing to work well.

(ii) **Staffed hostels** More handicapped patients can live in hostels where members of staff are present throughout the day and often at night, ensuring greater supervision and assistance than in a group home.

Difficulties finding suitable accommodation can often delay a patient's discharge from hospital.

5. *Provision of appropriate occupation*

Some patients with chronic psychiatric disorder can take normal employment or, if beyond retirement age, can take part in the same activities as healthy people of similar age. Other patients require specially arranged *sheltered work*, in which they can work productively, but more slowly than would be possible elsewhere. Often such work includes the making of craft items or horticulture. If patients who are too handicapped to undertake sheltered work, they need *occupational therapy* to avoid boredom, understimulation, and lack of social contacts.

6. *Arrangements to ensure the patient's collaboration with treatment*

This is one of the main challenges of community care. Several methods have been tried, ranging from providing the patient with good quality information about their treatment to using compulsory treatment orders (see pp. 451–3). The most promising approaches are currently using family interventions (p. 379) and 'insight therapy', a hybrid of cognitive therapy and motivational interviewing.

Out-patient clinics

Out-patient clinics are an efficient way of providing psychiatric assessment and treatment. Most of the treatment could be provided in general practice or the community by a visiting psychiatrist or other mental health clinician, but central clinics have three advantages, they:

(1) employ the time of the professional staff effectively because they do not spend time travelling;

(2) ensure that a senior person is available immediately to give advice to less experienced staff;

(3) provide facilities for physical examination and investigations which may not be so readily available in the community.

Their disadvantages are that patients may have to travel long distances and that it may be more difficult for family members to attend when this necessary.

Day services

There are two main functions of day services:

1. **Day hospitals** provide assessment and treatment for patients who need intensive treatment but can sleep safely at home or in a hostel. Day hospitals provide supervised drug treatment, occupational therapy and rehabilitation, and a range of psychological treatments. Such hospitals are suitable for patients with moderately severe depressive disorder, chronic schizophrenia, and severe and chronic neuroses. Day hospitals can shorten the length of in-patient stay and avoid admission altogether for some patients.

2. **Day centres** provide long-term support for patients suffering from chronic mental illness, but do not offer an alternative to hospital admission. Occupational therapy and rehabilitation may be provided, but medical and nursing services are not. Voluntary organizations often provide day centres or 'drop-in centres'.

In-patient facilities

Every specialist pscyhiatric service requires an in-patient unit, capable of treating patients with severe mental disorder, and able to admit patients promptly in an emergency.

Admission to hospital is needed when patients:

• need a level of assessment which cannot be provided elsewhere;

• need a treatment which cannot be provided in any other setting;

• have insufficient social support;

• put themselves or other people at risk;

• when arrangements for care outside hospital break down and a comprehensive care plan needs to be put in place.

Psychiatric in-patient units serving a large area used to be grouped together in a single psychiatric hospital; now they are often smaller, dispersed, and accommodated in general hospitals serving smaller areas. Units in specialist hospitals have the advantage that a wider range of treatments can be made available (e.g. specialized occupational and rehabilitation facilities); units in a general hospital have the advantages of reduced stigma, early liaison with other specialties, and usually, closeness to the patient's home.

In the past, patients often remained in in-patient units long after the acute stage of illness had passed; when recovery was incomplete some patients remained for many years. Now patients with residual problems are usually discharged from hospital and given continuing treatment. The advantage of remaining in hospital ('asylum') is easier provision of accommodation, treatment, rehabilitation, and protection; the disadvantage of a prolonged stay in hospital can be institutionalism that adds to the handicap produced by the disorder. This institutionalism is the result of lack of social stimulation, idleness, and boredom. A monotonous routine with lack of responsibility for personal decisions. If community care can meet the patients' needs it is generally better than prolonged in-patient care and preferred by patients and their carers. However, when patients are discharged from hospital without adequate provision for their needs for accommodation and treatment, community care can be worse for the patient than long-term care in hospital.

A range of specialist residential provision is required to provide adequate services for a population. Approximate estimates of the number of places required in each type of accommodation for a population are shown in Table 18.4. The actual provision required will depend on local factors such as the amount of social deprivation and unemployment (high rates of social deprivation increase the need for residential services).

Table 18.4.

Estimated need for specialist residential provision per 250 000 population

Type of accommodation	Estimate (range)
Acute and crisis care	100 (50–150)
Intensive care unit	10 (5–15)
Secure unit	4 (1–10)
Hostel wards	50 (25–75)
24-hour staffed hostels	75 (40–110)
Day staffed hostels	50 (25–75)
Group homes (visited)	45 (20–70)

From Wing, J. (1992). Epidemiologically based needs assessment In A.Steven and J. Raftery *Epidemiologically based needs assessment*. NHS Executive, London.

Further reading

Goldberg, D. and Huxley, P. (1992). *Common Mental Disorders: A Bio-social Approach.* Routledge, London.
Describes the reasons that lead people with psychiatric disorders to present to doctors, the factors which lead to referral to the specialist psychiatric services.

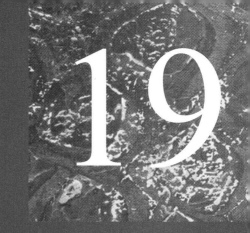

19

Child and adolescent psychiatry

- General issues

- Types of psychiatric disorder in childhood

- A review of childhood psychiatric disorders

- Appendix: A comprehensive scheme for history taking and examination in child psychiatry

Child and adolescent psychiatry

Problems of emotion and behaviour are common among children of all ages, and doctors are often asked for advice about them by parents. It is estimated that about 1 in 5 children have a significant problem in any one year. Many of these children come to the notice of general practitioners but only about 1 in 10 needs the help of a specialist. To help these children and their families the doctor needs a basic knowledge of normal child development and of the behaviour disorders of this time of life, and the skills needed to talk with the child, assess the problem, and manage it.

Common problems among pre-school children concern sleeping, eating, elimination, and rebelliousness. Among school-age children 90% of problems concern anxiety or disordered conduct. Adolescents experience both the problems of late childhood, and the early onset of those of adult life. At all ages, developmental delays are common including those affecting reading. Common problems among adolescents include mood disorders, eating disorders, and conduct disorders. All these problems are likely to be reported by parents but at times, doctors will be involved in cases in which the child is the victim of abuse or neglect by the parents. The last group of problems is considered at the end of the chapter.

After reading this chapter, the reader should know:

(1)   how to interview a child;

(2)   how to assess whether behaviour is abnormal;

(3)   how to assess the child's family;

(4)   the principal features of the common childhood psychiatric disorders;

(5)   the principles of management in general practice;

(6)   the indications for referral for specialist care.

The plan of this chapter is shown in Table 19.1, and starts with a brief account of some relevant aspects of normal development.

General issues

Normal development

Detailed accounts of child development are provided in textbooks of paediatrics. The following account summarizes points which are particularly relevant to the study of childhood emotional and behavioural disorders. It is important to remember that there are wide variations in the speed of development of healthy children.

The first year of life

This is a period of rapid intellectual and motor development. The child learns the basic features of common objects, spatial relationships, and simple links between

Table 19.1.

Organization of the chapter

General issues	Normal development
	Assessment in child psychiatry
	Causes of child psychiatric disorder
	Principal methods of treatment
Problems of pre-school children	Aetiology
	Assessment
	Common problems (Table 19.5)
Disorders of older children	Emotional disorders (Table 19.6)
	Disorders of sleep
	Disorders of elimination
	Hyperkinetic disorder
	Conduct disorder
	Other problem behaviours
Disorders of development	Specific developmental disorders
	Childhood autism
	Other disorders affecting speech
	Gender identity disorders
Psychological disorders of physically ill children	
Disorders of adolescence	see p. 419
Disorders of parent–child relationships	Physical abuse
	Sexual abuse
	Emotional abuse
	Neglect
	Munchausen syndrome by proxy

cause and effect. By about 7 months most children can sit without support, and by about 14 months most can take a few steps unaided. In the first year, the child develops a regular pattern of feeding and sleeping. The child forms a strong, secure emotional bond especially with the mother but also with the father, siblings, and others closely involved. By about 8 months the child shows signs of distress when separated from the mother, and in the presence of strangers.

The second year

The child begins to walk, explores the environment, and learns that this exploration has to be limited at times by the parents (e.g. to avoid danger). The parents demand more of the child as they encourage bowel and bladder training. For a time, the child resists these constraints and demands, and shows frustration, sometimes with displays of temper. Although these tantrums may at first be alarming to the parents, provided they are dealt with consistently and lovingly they gradually resolve, although infrequent tempers may continue into the next year.

Language develops during the second year and by the age of 20 months most children have learnt the words 'dada', 'mama', and three others. As language comprehension increases, it becomes easier for the parents to understand their children's wishes and feelings and to guide their behaviour.

Ages 2–5 years

In this period there is rapid development of language and intellectual functions and children ask many questions. Motor skills are refined and continence is achieved. Children become less self-centred and more sociable and they learn to share in the life of the family. Gender roles become established, the parents' values are absorbed, and a sense of conscience develops. During this period children are capable of vivid fantasy, expressed in imaginative games. Play also helps children learn how to relate to other children and adults, explore objects, and increase their motor skills.

Later childhood

When children start school, they learn about social relationships with other children and with adults other than the parents. Skills and knowledge increase. Ideas of right and wrong develop further at this age as the influence of the school is added to that of the family. Children develop a feeling of self-worth, while learning that they are less successful in some activities than are their peers. A loving family and good teachers help with these developments.

Adolescence

Considerable changes, physical, psychosexual, and social, take place in adolescence and they are usually accompanied by some emotional turmoil. Generally, the latter does not last long and it may go unnoticed by adults. Among older adolescents rebellious behaviour is common, especially during the last years of compulsory attendance at school. Other common behaviours are problems in relationships, sexual difficulties, delinquent behaviour, excessive drinking of alcohol, and abuse of drugs and solvents. These behaviours and the associated emotional turmoil may be difficult to distinguish from psychiatric disorder.

Assessment of a psychiatric problem in childhood

Three special points should be considered when assessing the emotional or behavioural problems of a child or adolescent:

1. It is usually *the parents* and not the child, who *seek help*. For this reason, whether such a disorder becomes known to the family doctor depends not only on its nature and severity but also on the attitudes and tolerance of the parents. Some healthy children are brought to the doctor by over-anxious parents for advice about behaviour that is usual for the child's age; other children with serious problems are not brought to the attention of the medical services.

2. Psychiatric disturbance in a child may *result from problems in other members of the family*, usually the parents; for example, the child may be distressed because the parents quarrel frequently. For this reason assessments in child psychiatry are, even more than in adult psychiatry, concerned with the whole family and not just with the patient.

3. Whether a behaviour is abnormal depends in part on *the child's stage of development*. For example, repeated bed-wetting is clearly normal in a child aged 18

months but clearly abnormal in a child aged 7 years. At intervening ages its significance has to be assessed carefully.

General points

The *aims of assessment* are to:

- obtain a clear account of the presenting problems and make a diagnosis;
- relate these problems to the child's temperament, development, and physical condition;
- relate the problems to the influences of the family, school, and wider social environment;
- make a management plan.

Although the *general approach* to the psychiatric assessment of children resembles that of adults, there are two important differences. First, when the child is young, the parents supply most of the information, nevertheless, the child should usually be seen without the parents at some stage. This arrangement is especially important when child abuse is suspected. Second, when interviewing a child it is often difficult to follow a set routine and a flexible approach to interviewing is required. However, the data should be recorded in a standard order to assist others who may use the case record.

Interviewing the parents (Table 19.2)

The interviewer should put the parents at ease and make them feel that the interview is intended to help them and not to undermine their confidence. They should feel that they are part of the solution to the child's difficulties rather than part of the problem. The interviewer should encourage parents to talk spontaneously about the child's problem before systematic questions are asked. The interviewer then proceeds using the general interview techniques described in Chapter 2. The main items for assessment are shown in Table 19.2 (a more complete list is provided for reference in the Appendix to this chapter, p. 424). Throughout the interview the doctor should be alert to feelings and attitudes as well as to facts.

In assessing more severe problems, it is often helpful for the doctor, a nurse or a social worker to *visit the home*. This visit provides useful information not only about the material circumstances of the home, but also about the relationships between family members and the pattern of their life together.

Interviewing and observing the child

Starting the interview Children are usually brought to the doctor by their parents; few have chosen to come. It is important therefore to establish a friendly atmosphere and win the child's confidence before asking about the problems. With younger children an indirect and gradual approach is needed; for example, by talking first about general topics that may engage the child's interest such as pets, games, or birthdays, before asking about the problems. With older children and adolescents it may be possible to follow an approach similar to that for adults.

Continuing the interview Older children may respond to direct questions about their presenting problem and their circumstances but with young children it is often useful to ask about their likes and dislikes, and what they would request if

---

Table 19.2.

Interviewing parents: the main items*

The presenting problem
Nature, severity, and frequency
Situations in which it occurs
Factors that make it worse or better

Other current problems concerning
Mood and energy level
Activity, concentration
Physical symptoms
Eating, sleeping, elimination
Relationships with parents and siblings
Relationships with other children
Antisocial behaviour
School performance

Family history
Separations from and illness of parents
Quality of relations with parents and siblings

Personal history of the child
Problems in pregnancy and delivery
Previous and current levels of development
Past illness and injury; hospital stays
Attendance and attainments at school

*See Appendix (p. 424) for details.

given three wishes. Children who have difficulty in expressing their problems and feelings directly in words, may do so during imaginative play, or when asked to make a drawing or painting and then to talk about it.

Observing behaviour While trying to engage a child in these ways, the interviewer observes how he interacts with himself and with the parents when they are present. Specific items of the child's behaviour and mental state should be recorded. The main points are listed in Table 19.3 and a more complete list is given in the Appendix to this chapter (p. 424). A general assessment should be made of the child's development relative to other children of the same age.

Physical examination Any relevant physical examination should be performed with particular attention to the central nervous system.

Interviewing other informants

The most important additional informants other than the family are the child's *teachers*. They can describe classroom behaviour, educational achievements, and relationships with other children. They may also make useful comments about the family and home circumstances.

Types of psychiatric disorder in childhood

The psychiatric problems of childhood can be divided into four groups:

1. Behaviour problems of pre-school children.

2. Problems of behaviour and emotion among older children.

3. Disorders of development.

4. Abuse of children by parents or other adults.

The individual disorders within these groups are described in a later section. First, some general issues are discussed concerning the aetiology and treatment of childhood psychiatric disorders.

General causes of childhood psychiatric disorder (Table 19.4)

Although there are causes specific to each disorder, many others are general. The causes of childhood psychiatric disorders are multiple; as in adult psychiatry, they fall into three groups of interacting factors: *heredity, physical disease,* and *environment*. Of these, environmental factors are particularly important.

Heredity

For most conditions genetic factors are thought to exert their effects indirectly through the control of temperament and intelligence, which in turn predispose to some psychiatric disorder. The principal exception is infantile autism in which specific genetic factors are important.

Physical disease

In childhood, any serious physical disease can lead to psychological problems, but brain disorders are particularly likely to have this effect. Serious damage to the brain (usually from birth injury) certainly predisposes to psychiatric disorder. It

Table 19.3.
Principal observations of a child's behaviour and emotional state

- Rapport with the interviewer
- Relationship with parents
- Appearance
- Activity level
- Ability to concentrate
- Mood
- Habits, mannerisms
- Stage of development
- Physical examination

Table 19.4.
Causes of childhood psychiatric disorder

Heredity

Physical disease

Environment

Famil factors:
Separation
Illness of a parent
Parental discord
Personality deviance of parent
Large family size
Child abuse and neglect

Social and cultural factors:
Influences at school
Peer group behaviours
Poor social amenities and overcrowding
Lack of community involvement

has been suggested that minor damage to the brain may be a cause of some otherwise unexplained psychiatric disorders such as conduct disorder. However, evidence for this latter idea is unconvincing.

Environmental factors

These factors are important in most of the psychiatric disorders of childhood. They concern both the family and factors outside the family.

The family To progress successfully from complete dependence on the parents to independence, children need a stable and secure family environment in which they are loved, accepted, and provided with consistent discipline. Lack of any of these elements can predispose to psychiatric disorder.

Prolonged absence or loss of a parent can predispose to both emotional and conduct disorders in the child. How children react to separation depends on their age at the time of separation, their previous relationship with the parents, the reason for the separation (for example, separation due to divorce of the parents may follow a long period of quarrelling which itself affects the child), and how the separation is managed by those remaining with the child. When separation leads to institutional care, this may itself predispose to psychiatric disorder.

Other family factors strongly associated with psychiatric disorder in the child include: *discordant family relationships*, the *illness of a parent*, *personality deviance of a parent*, and *large family size*. (Variations in child-rearing practices might be expected to affect the child, but such variations have not been found to be clearly related to psychiatric disorder, except for grossly abnormal patterns of rearing involving child abuse, neglect, or rejection.)

Social factors outside the family Wider social influences become increasingly significant as the child grows older, spends more time outside the family and is influenced by the attitudes and behaviour of other children, teachers, and older people in the neighbourhood. Such influences are particularly important in the aetiology of conduct disorder.

The importance of social factors is reflected in the finding that rates of childhood psychiatric disorder are higher in areas of social disadvantage, such as deprived inner city areas with overcrowded living conditions, lack of play space for younger children, inadequate social amenities for teenagers, and lack of community involvement.

Principal methods of treatment

General issues

Although treatment necessarily differs according to the type of disorder, there are many common features. For most childhood disorders, treatment need not be complex. The essential steps which can often be carried out by the general practitioner are shown in Table 19.5. It is often enough to reassure the child, discuss the problem with the parents, and give them and the child information about the nature and causes of the disorder and the likely outcome. Discussion with the parents and child does not stop with the giving of information; the parents' concerns should be explored and any misperceptions identified and corrected. Any stressors

Table 19.5.

General treatment plan for childhood psychiatric problems

Engage and reassure the child

Discuss problems with parents:
- nature
- causes
- probable outcome

Reduce stressors on the child:
- at home
- at school
- elsewhere

Assess and if necessary change the response to the problem of parents or others.

Avoid medication except for specific indications (see text).

on the child should be reduced if possible. To achieve this, it may be necessary to talk with other family members or teachers. Simple behavioural principles are often useful, particularly to reduce behaviour that is being inadvertently reinforced by the parents or other members of the family. Drug treatment is seldom required.

Since many childhood problems affect conduct at school and may lead to educational difficulties, the child's teachers often need advice about the best way to respond to disturbed behaviour and may need to be involved in the whole plan. Remedial teaching may be needed, or a change in the child's school timetable. Occasionally, a change of school is indicated.

The role of specialist services Generally, the primary care team can treat the child. A child psychiatry clinic has the additional resource of a team consisting usually of a psychiatrist, social worker, psychologist, and nurses. Usually one of these people is chosen as the 'key worker' to whom the child relates, while the other team members take on specific tasks, such as liaison with parents or teachers, or behavioural treatment. The family is involved closely in treatment, and so is any agency concerned with the child and his family such as social or educational psychology services.

Nearly all children referred for specialist psychiatric treatment are treated as out-patients although a few are day patients. **In-patient care** is seldom necessary. It is chosen for one of three reasons:

1. *To treat a severe behaviour disorder* that cannot be managed in another way (e.g. some cases of childhood autism).

2. *For observation* when the diagnosis is uncertain (e.g. to decide whether an epileptic child's behaviour problems are related to the epilepsy, or to emotional and social factors).

3. *To separate the child* temporarily from a severely disturbing home environment (e.g. when there has been physical abuse).

Sometimes, the *mother is admitted* to hospital with the child to allow observation and modification of the ways in which she responds to the child, most often in cases of child abuse.

Specific techniques of treatment

Problem-solving counselling (see p. 365) for parents and child is part of the treatment of all the problems considered in this chapter.

Family therapy Families are always involved in some way in the treatment of children. Family therapy refers to a specific psychological treatment in which the child's symptoms are considered as an expression of difficulties in the functioning of the family. Members of the family meet to discuss the difficulties that appear related to the child's disorder, while the therapist helps them to find ways of overcoming the problems.

Behaviour therapy Behavioural principles are used in the management of many kinds of childhood psychiatric problem. Often, the aim is to reduce the attention given to a child when a problem behaviour occurs, and increase the attention given to appropriate behaviour. As well as these general approaches, specific techniques of behaviour therapy are used for phobias (see p. 405) and enuresis (see p. 409).

Dynamic psychotherapy for children As noted above, all treatment of childhood psychiatric disorder involves counselling for the child. Some psychiatrists also use dynamic psychotherapy. The techniques used with adults (see p. 375) cannot be used with younger children who cannot easily express themselves in words. Therefore, play is used as an alternative means of expression for these children, and the therapist interprets this play as he would interpret the words and behaviour of an adult patient. Dynamic psychotherapy has not been evaluated adequately in controlled trials with children and is now used infrequently in most health care systems.

Special education Some children benefit from special education to remedy associated problems of backwardness in writing, reading, or arithmetic which often accompany psychiatric disorders especially conduct disorder and hyperkinetic disorder.

Substitute care This term refers to the placement of a child in a foster home, a children's home, or a boarding school. Such placements are sometimes necessary when the family is very unstable, but should be considered only after every practicable effort has been made to improve the home environment.

Drug treatment Medication is considered last because it has little place in the treatment of childhood psychiatric disorders. Although *anxiolytic and hypnotic* drugs are sometimes prescribed occasionally, most anxiety and sleeping problems can be treated better in other ways (see pp. 405 and 407). *Antidepressant drugs* are indicated in the more severe depressive disorders of childhood and adolescence but usually only after psychological and social measures have failed. Antidepressant drugs also have a limited place in the treatment of enuresis (p. 410). *Stimulant drugs* have a beneficial effect in severe hyperkinetic disorder (see p. 410). *Antipsychotic drugs are not indicated* for children.

A review of childhood psychiatric disorders

Problems of pre-school children (Table 19.6)

Common problems at this age are attention-seeking, disobedience, and temper tantrums, and problems of sleeping and feeding. Most problems are short lived and whether they are reported to doctors depends on the attitudes of the parents as well as on the severity of the disorder.

Aetiology

Psychological disorders at this age are related to the child's general stage of development, to temperament, and to influences in the family.

Development As noted earlier, there are wide individual variations in rates of development, seen most obviously in relation to sphincter control and language acquisition.

Table 19.6.
Disorders of pre-school children

Temper tantrums

Breath-holding

Sleep problems
- insomnia
- nightmares and night terrors

Feeding problems
- food fads and food refusal
- pica

Temperament Differences in temperament are evident from soon after birth when some babies are more active and responsive than others. Such early characteristics may affect the parents' response to the child (e.g. how often they pick up the child) and these parental responses may affect the child's subsequent development.

Family problems Many behaviour problems at this age are associated with differences within the family such as inadequate parenting skills, maternal depression, marital disharmony, and rivalry between siblings.

Assessment

In assessing the problems of pre-school children, the doctor has to rely mainly on information from the parents. As mentioned above, it is important to distinguish between abnormal behaviour in the child, and inappropriate concern of parents about behaviour within the normal range. It is important also to find out whether the behavioural problem is part of a wider delay in development suggesting mental retardation (see Chapter 20) or a pervasive developmental disorder (p. 414). Finally, the functioning of the whole family should be assessed since, as explained above, the child's disorder may be a reflection of wider family problems.

Common problems

Temper tantrums Most toddlers have occasional mild temper tantrums, and only frequent or severe tantrums are abnormal. Tantrums are often provoked by inconsistent discipline and reinforced unintentionally by excessive attention to the child when they take place. Parents should be informed about the nature and causes of the problem. Temper tantrums usually improve in response to setting consistent limits to the child's behaviour, enforcing these with kind but firm discipline and to reducing in the attention given to the child during the tantrums. It is important to discover why the parents have been unable to achieve consistent discipline (e.g. there may be marital problems) as well as to give common sense advice on setting and enforcing limits.

Breath-holding Periods of breath-holding are not uncommon in pre-school children. Like temper tantrums, they are often related to frustration leading to a state of rage followed by the breath-holding. The behaviour can be alarming for parents, especially if the child becomes cyanosed before breathing resumes. The parents should be given an explanation of the nature of the attacks, helped to respond calmly, and to avoid reinforcing the behaviour with undue indulgence. In this way, the behaviour disappears with time.

Insomnia Among children between 1 and 2 years of age, about a fifth take at least an hour to settle down to sleep or are repeatedly wakeful for long periods during the night, thus disturbing their parents. Most of these problems resolve within a few months. When wakefulness is an isolated problem and not severe, the only requirement is to reassure parents that it will pass and to help them not to overreact to it. If the sleep problem is more severe or persistent, the parents' response to the problem should be studied. Often, the parents are inadvertently maintaining the problem by responding as soon as the child cries, spending long periods at the child's bedside, allowing the child to return to the living room, or taking the child into their own bed. Parents should be given an explanation of the nature and causes of the condition. Improvement can usually be achieved if they:

- establish a regular bedtime routine;
- do not reinforce the problem behaviour;
- make the child's bedroom a pleasant place.

Hypnotic medication should be used seldom and then only briefly in conjunction with the above measures. At first, it may be difficult to persuade the parents to keep to the new rules, and continued support may be needed from the doctor or a nurse. When this simple approach fails, there may be a wider problem in the child or the family and specialist assessment may be required.

Nightmares and night terrors (see p. 407) are quite common among healthy toddlers but seldom persist for long. Usually all that is needed is to advise the parents to calm the child on waking and help him to return to sleep. If this is not successful, there may be a wider problem, requiring specialist assessment.

Feeding problems *Food fads* and *food refusal* are common in pre-school children. In a minority, the behaviour is severe or persistent. When this happens it is often because the parents are unintentionally reinforcing behaviour that would otherwise be transient. Some parents offer alternative (and sometimes unsuitable) food, or engage in elaborate behaviours to persuade the child to eat. Parents should be helped to understand the causes of the problem and then advised how to manage it differently. They are encouraged to ignore the feeding problem as far as possible, to refrain from offering the child alternatives when he does not eat what is first offered and to stop using other special ways to persuade him to eat.

Pica is the eating of items which are not foods (e.g. soil, paint, and paper). Pica is often associated with other behaviour problems, and sometimes with mental retardation. Parents should be reassured that the problem is a recognized disorder which usually improves. They should take common sense measures to keep the child away from the abnormal items of diet. Any stressful circumstances should be modified if possible. With this approach the problem usually disappears; if it does not there may be a wider problem requiring specialist assessment. Even in these more severe cases the problem usually diminishes as the child grows older.

Disorders of older children

The disorders of older children are grouped as shown in Table 19.7. The age range is between about 5 years and the early years of puberty. This section includes, in addition, an account of three patterns of behaviour which, although not psychiatric disorders, are commonly associated with them: truancy, school refusal, and delinquency.

Emotional disorders (Table 19.8)

The term *emotional disorder* refers to childhood disorders characterized by anxiety or depression, or physical symptoms that are an expression of anxiety or depression ('somatization'), or repetitive and compulsive behaviours. Emotional disorders are common (only conduct disorders are more frequent) but most improve

Table 19.7.
Disorders of older children

- Emotional disorders
- Disorders of sleeping
- Disorders of elimination
- Hyperkinetic disorder
- Conduct disorder

Table 19.8.
Emotional disorders of children

- Anxiety disorder
- Phobic disorder
- Separation anxiety
- Unexplained physical symptoms (somatization)
- Repetitive behaviours and obsessive-compulsive symptoms
- Depressive disorder

with time leaving no residual symptoms. When these disorders continue into adult life, it is usually as an anxiety or affective disorder.

Anxiety disorder The symptoms of childhood anxiety disorder are listed in Table 19.9. Anxiety is common in childhood and there is no clear dividing line between normal and abnormal: the diagnostic criteria is that there should be significant problems in social functioning resulting from the anxiety.

The nature of normal childhood anxiety changes as the child grows older. Infants pass through a stage of fear of strangers; pre-school children fear separation from their parents, and fears of animals and darkness are common; older children fear social situations. Anxiety disorders in childhood follow the same sequence: separation anxiety and phobic disorder start in early childhood, social anxiety starts later.

Aetiology The causes of anxiety disorder are mainly environmental, described on p. 400.

Treatment Attention should be paid to any stressful events, or family problems or other aetiological factors. The child is helped to talk about the worries and reassured appropriately. The parents are informed about the nature and causes of the problem and about ways of helping the child to gain confidence and overcome fears. Anxiolytic drugs should be used only when anxiety is extremely severe, and then only for a few days at a time.

Separation anxiety disorder Children with separation anxiety cling to their parents and are extremely distressed when parted from them. They may worry that an accident or illness may befall the parents. The condition may be initiated by a frightening experience such as admission to hospital, or by insecurity in the family; for example, when the parents are contemplating divorce. Separation anxiety is often maintained by overprotective attitudes of the parents and treatment is directed to changing these attitudes and reassuring the child (see also school refusal, p. 412).

Phobic disorder Phobic symptoms are common in childhood. Most concern animals, insects, darkness, or death. Some children fear going to school so that phobic disorder is a cause of school refusal (see p. 412). Most childhood phobias improve without treatment provided that the parents adopt a firm and reassuring approach. When phobias do not improve with these measures, behavioural treatment is usually effective. The child is helped to return gradually to the feared situations repeating each stage until it can be completed without anxiety, before moving on to the next.

Social anxiety disorder in childhood Younger children with this disorder are abnormally anxious in the presence of strangers, and avoid them. Older children have fears similar to those described as social phobia in adults (see p. 113).

Unexplained physical symptoms Children often complain of somatic symptoms for which no physical cause can be found. The symptoms are usually associated with stressful circumstances which cause anxiety in the child, and by parental anxiety. Common examples are abdominal pain, headache, limb pains, and sickness; abdominal pain is particularly frequent. The term *somatization* is often used for this type of disorder, but the phrase *unexplained physical symptoms* seems preferable for non-specialists.

Table 19.9.

Symptoms of childhood anxiety disorder

Fearfulness and phobia

Timidity

Excessive worrying

Poor concentration

Poor sleep

Physical symptoms
- – headache
- – nausea, vomiting
- – abdominal pain
- – bowel disturbance

Overdependence

Separation anxiety

Treatment The doctor explains to the child and parents that the physical symptoms are undoubtedly real but the causes are psychological. If possible, stressful circumstances are reduced and the child is encouraged to talk about the symptoms, situations in which the symptoms are worse or better, and any related problems. When the symptom is pain, the child and parents are helped to find ways of reducing it without taking analgesics, usually with distracting activities for the child. The parents are helped to convey sympathy but not to focus attention on the pain.

Repetitive behaviours and obsessive-compulsive disorder Many children engage in *repetitive behaviours* such as counting or the repeatedly handling, touching, or avoiding certain objects. These behaviours do not fulfil all the criteria used to define compulsive behaviours in adults (see p. 120) because the child does not struggle against them. In other ways, however, they are similar to obsessive-compulsive symptoms observed in adults.

Obsessional and compulsive symptoms of the adult type are uncommon in childhood. When they occur it is usually as part of an anxiety or depressive disorder.

Treatment Repetitive behaviours usually disappear without treatment. The child and parents should be reassured about recovery, any stressful circumstances should be changed if possible. Since obsessional and compulsive symptoms are usually part of a primary anxiety or depressive disorder, the primary disorder should be treated. In other cases, any stressors should be reduced if this is possible and the child and parents should be supported. Obsessive-compulsive symptoms have a less favourable prognosis than repetitive behaviours.

Depressive disorder In childhood, depression is a normal response to distressing circumstances such as the serious illness of a parent, the death of a close family member, or parental disharmony. The child is sad and tearful and may eat poorly and sleep badly. As well as these normal responses to adversity, older children may develop *depressive disorders*. These disorders seem related to those of adult life because there is an increased rate of depressive disorder among the first degree relatives of the affected children, and there are continuities between depressive disorder in childhood and adult life. The clinical picture of these disorders is generally similar to that in adults with *low mood, loss of interest and pleasure* in usual activities, *self-blame, hopelessness,* and *disturbance of appetite and sleep*. Sometimes *physical symptoms* take the place of obvious low mood. Extreme guilt is less common among children than adults. Depressive disorder is infrequent in childhood, and bipolar disorder does not seem to occur before puberty.

Treatment The parents are informed about the nature of the problem and helped to support the child. Any stressful circumstances are reduced if possible and the child is helped to talk about the feelings of depression. Usually these steps lead to improvement. If they do not, or if the disorder is particularly severe when treatment is started, antidepressant drug treatment can be considered. If used, they should be reserved for older children with definite evidence of a severe depressive disorder. Such children should, if possible, be assessed by a specialist before antidepressant drugs are prescribed.

Prognosis After 9 months, about 50% are still depressed. Poor outcome is related to intensity of initial low mood and family and social difficulties.

Suicide in childhood is considered on p. 244.

Disorders of sleeping

The commonly encountered disorders of sleeping are nightmares, night terrors, and sleep walking (sleep problems of younger children are considered on pp. 403–4).

A **nightmare** is *an awakening from REM (rapid eye movement) sleep* to full consciousness with recall of an unpleasant dream. Nightmares are common in children, especially around the ages of 5 or 6 years. Often, they are provoked by frightening experiences during the day, and frequent nightmares may be accompanied by daytime anxiety.

Treatment The parents should be informed about the nature of the disorder and reassured that it is likely to improve. The child is given information appropriate to his age and any stressful circumstances discussed and reduced if possible.

Night terrors are less common than nightmares. A few hours after going to sleep the child sits up and appears terrified and confused and may scream. Night terrors occur during stages 3 and 4 of non-REM sleep. After a few minutes, the child settles slowly and returns to normal calm sleep.

There is no specific **treatment** The parents should be informed about the nature of the problem. It is sometimes helpful to wake children shortly before the usual time of their night terror. Night terrors rarely persist into adult life.

Sleep-walking In this condition children walk around in a mechanical manner while still asleep. The eyes are usually open and the child avoids familiar objects. Sleep-walking occurs during *deep non-REM sleep*, usually in the early part of the night. The child may appear agitated, and does not respond to questions. They are difficult to wake, although they can usually be led back to bed. Some children do not walk, but sit up and make repetitive movements. Episodes last usually for only a few minutes, though rarely they may continue for as long as an hour. Sleep-walking is most common between the ages of 5 and 12 years, occurring at least once in 15% of children in this age group. Occasionally, the disorder persists into adult life.

There is no specific **treatment** Parents should be told what is known about the condition, and that it usually resolves. Meanwhile, as sleep-walkers occasionally harm themselves, they should protect the child from injury by fastening doors and windows securely, barring stairs, and removing dangerous objects.

Disorders of elimination

Functional enuresis Functional enuresis is the repeated involuntary voiding of urine occurring after an age at which continence is usual, and in the absence of any identified physical disorder. The condition may be **nocturnal** (bed-wetting) or **diurnal** (occurring during waking hours), or both. Nocturnal enuresis is referred to as **primary** if there has been no preceding period of urinary continence for at least one year. It is called **secondary** if there has been a preceding period of urinary continence for this period. Nocturnal enuresis can cause great unhappiness and distress, particularly if the parents blame or punish the child, and if the condition restricts staying with friends or going on holiday.

Most children achieve regular daytime and night-time continence by 3 or 4 years of age, and *5 years is generally taken as the youngest age for the diagnosis.* Nocturnal enuresis occurs in about 10% of children at 5 years of age, 4% at 8 years, and 1% at 14 years. The condition is more frequent in boys. Daytime enuresis has a lower prevalence and is more frequent in girls.

Aetiology *Primary nocturnal enuresis* seems usually to result from delay in maturation of the nervous control of the bladder. Rarely, there is an anatomical or functional abnormality of the bladder itself. Most children are free from psychiatric disorder (although psychiatric disorder is more frequent than that among non-enuretic children). Factors that may contribute to aetiology in some cases include abnormal toilet training, whether unduly lax or unduly rigid, and anxiety due to stressful events. *Secondary cases* are often related to stressful events in the home or at school.

Assessment There are six stages of assessment:

1. *Exclude a primary physical cause,* particularly urinary infection, diabetes or epilepsy.

2. *Exclude a primary psychiatric cause* (i.e. mental retardation or psychiatric disorder).

3. *Identify any stressful circumstances* in the family, at school, or elsewhere.

4. *Identify the child's concerns* about the bed-wetting and any other problems.

5. *Identify the attitudes* of the parents and any siblings to the bed-wetting.

6. *Find out how the parents have tried to help* the child already.

Treatment (Table 19.10) If the enuresis is caused by a physical disorder, this should of course be treated. When enuresis is associated with a serious emotional disorder, the child should be referred to a child psychiatrist. Most mild cases can be treated successfully in general practice. If the enuresis is *primary*, it should be explained to the parents and the child that the condition is common and that the child is not to blame. It should be explained to the parents that punishment and disapproval are inappropriate and ineffective. The parents should be encouraged to reward success (e.g. with star charts), and not to focus attention on failure. If stressors have been found, they should be reduced if possible. Many younger enuretic children improve spontaneously soon after advice of this kind, but those over 6 years of age are likely to need more than advice. The next procedures are *restriction of fluid* intake before bedtime and waking the child to pass urine once during the night.

If children over the age of 6 years do not improve with these simple measures, treatment with an *enuresis alarm* may be given (see Box 19.1). About 70% of children improve within a month of this treatment, but a third relapse within a year.

Treatment with a *tricyclic antidepressant*, usually imipramine or amitriptyline, can reduce bed-wetting. The drug is given in a dose of 25–50 mg at night depending on the age of the child, usually for 4–6 weeks (appropriate dosage should be decided after consulting the manufacturer's literature). Most bed-

Table 19.10.

Treatment of nocturnal enuresis

- Treat any physical disorder
- Treat any psychiatric disorder
- Advice to parents and child
  - avoid disapproval and punishment
  - praise success (star charts)
- Modify stressors if possible
- Restrict fluids before bedtime
- Wake during the night

For persistent cases

- Enuresis alarm (see Box 19.1)
- Tricyclic antidepressants for temporary relief

Box 19.1 **The enuresis alarm**

In its original form (the 'pad and bell'), the alarm consisted of two perforated metal plates, separated by a sheet of cotton, and incorporated in a low voltage circuit including a battery, a switch, and a bell or buzzer. The resistance of the dry cotton prevents current from flowing in the circuit. When the bed is made, the plates are placed where the child's pelvis will rest. As soon as the child begins to pass urine in the bed, the sheet of cotton becomes wet, the circuit is completed, and the bell or buzzer sounds. The child turns off the switch, and rises to complete the emptying of the bladder. The bed is remade and a dry sheet of cotton is put between the metal plates before the child returns.

In the modern version a sensor to detect urine is attached to the child's pyjama trousers and a miniature alarm is carried in the pocket or on the wrist.

wetters improve on the drug, about a third obtaining complete relief. Most relapse, however, when the drug is stopped. Because of this high relapse rate, as well as the side effects of tricyclics and the potential danger of accidental overdose, the use of drugs is limited mainly to enabling the child to be dry over a short but important period such as a school journey.

Functional encopresis Functional encopresis is an uncommon disorder in which there is repeated passing of faeces into inappropriate places after the age at which bowel control is usual. The age at which control is reached is variable but at the age of 3 years 94% of children have control, and 6% are still incontinent of faeces once a week or more. The disorder may be present continuously from the time when bowel control is normally acquired (*primary encopresis*), or it may start after a period of continence (*secondary encopresis*). The condition is more common in boys than girls.

Aetiology *Primary encopresis* may be associated with mental retardation but otherwise the causes are not known. Sometimes, parents have adopted either an excessively strict, or in other cases an inconsistent, approach to bowel training but this is unlikely to be the sole cause because other children reared in these ways develop bowel control. Emotional disorder is common among children with encopresis, but it may be the result rather than the cause of the condition. Sometimes soiling begins after an upsetting event, or during a period of rebellion with the parents. *Secondary encopresis* may occur as a consequence of chronic constipation due to conditions causing pain on defecation (e.g. anal fissure) or of Hirschsprung's disease.

Assessment This is similar to that for enuresis (see above): (1) seek a primary physical or psychiatric cause; (2) identify any stressful conditions, assess the attitudes of the parents and any siblings; and (3) explore the child's concerns about the problem. Finally, the parents are asked how they have tried to help the child already.

Treatment The plan of treatment resembles that for enuresis (see above):

• Treat any primary physical or psychiatric disorder.

• Reassure the parents that the problem occurs in other children and will improve in time.

- Encourage the parents to reward success and not to dwell on failure.
- Modify any stressful circumstances if possible.
- Encourage the child to sit on the toilet for 10 minutes after each meal and try to encourage more normal bowel habits.

Occasionally, admission to hospital is needed to establish a new routine. Untreated encopresis seldom persists beyond the middle teenage years. When treated it usually improves within a year.

Hyperkinetic disorder

About a third of children are described by their parents as overactive, and up to a fifth of schoolchildren are so described by their teachers. These reports encompass behaviour varying from normal high spirits to a severe and persistent disorder. The boundary between normal overactivity and the persistent disorder has to be drawn in an arbitrary way, and there are disputes whether the criterion for disorder should be set high (excluding with certainty, all normal overactivity) or low (making sure no abnormal behaviour is missed). In the USA, a lower cut-off is used than in the UK and many other countries. Hyperkinetic children have a short span of attention. This feature is given prominence in the American classification (DSM-IV), which uses the term **Attention deficit-hyperactivity disorder**. The term used in the International Classification of Diseases (ICD-I0) is **hyperkinetic disorder**.

Clinical features The features of the syndrome are listed in Table 19.11. The overactivity usually becomes evident when the child starts to walk, although sometimes it is seen before that time. The child is constantly on the move and interferes with objects. Attention cannot be sustained, with a consequent difficulty in learning. A child with the fully developed syndrome is impulsive, reckless, and prone to accidents. Mood fluctuates, but depressive mood is common. Minor forms of antisocial behaviour are common, particularly disobedience, temper tantrums, and aggression. These behaviours exhaust the parents.

Aetiology The cause of hyperkinetic disorder is not known. Genetic investigations have been inconclusive. Neurodevelopmental delay has been suggested but again the evidence is not conclusive. Any innate tendency to hyperactivity may be increased by social factors, since overactivity is more frequent among children living in poor social conditions. However, social factors are unlikely to be the sole cause of hyperkinetic disorder. Lead intoxication and food additives have been suggested as causes, but the evidence is not convincing.

Prognosis As the child grows older, the overactivity generally lessens, especially when it is mild and not present in every situation. Usually it ceases by puberty. Associated learning difficulties are less likely to improve, and antisocial behaviour has the worst prognosis. When the overactivity is severe, or accompanied by major learning difficulties, or associated with low intelligence, it may persist into adult life.

Treatment **Help for parents and teachers**   The nature of the condition should be explained and they should be supported in their efforts to contain and live with the overactivity.

Medication For unknown reasons, *stimulant drugs*, such as methylphenidate, sometimes have the paradoxical effect of reducing the overactivity. Parents often ask

Table 19.11.
Hyperkinetic disorder: clinical features

Extreme restlessness
Sustained overactivity

Poor attention
Learning difficulty

Impulsiveness
Recklessness
Accident proneness

Disobedience
Temper tantrums
Aggression

about this treatment but it is generally reserved for severe cases because there may be side effects of irritability, depression, poor appetite, and insomnia and, in some cases, slowing of growth. For this reason a specialist opinion should be obtained before prescribing. Hyperactive children treated in this way do not appear to become addicted to the stimulant drug. About two-thirds of children improve in the short term, but the long-term benefits of the treatment are uncertain.

Remedial teaching is needed if there are significant learning difficulties.

Conduct disorder

This disorder is characterized by severe and persistent antisocial behaviour clearly greater than ordinary mischievousness and rebellion. Extreme cases are easy to define but the dividing line between normal and abnormal conduct is sometimes difficult to draw. It is the most common type of psychiatric disorder among older children and adolescents.

Clinical features *In the pre-school period* the disorder usually manifests as aggressive behaviour to other children, and rebelliousness with the parents, often accompanied by overactivity.

The clinical features in *later childhood* are listed in Table 19.12. It should be noted that: (a) repeated stealing is less significant in young children than at older ages because children below about 7 years do not usually have a full appreciation of what constitutes the ownership of property by other people; and (b) disapproved sexual behaviour in younger children includes frequent masturbation and intrusive sexual curiosity. Alcohol and drug abuse may occur in older children and adolescents.

Aetiology *Environmental factors* are important. Conduct disorder is more frequent among children from unstable, insecure, and rejecting families living in deprived areas. It is more frequent also among children from broken homes, and those who have been in residential care in early childhood. Conduct disorder is related also to adverse factors in the wider social environment, such as overcrowding and high crime rates.

Constitutional factors It is not certain how much these add to effects of environmental factors. Adoption studies suggest that genetic factors are not of great general importance although they may play a part in the aetiology of aggressive behaviour. The association of conduct disorder with speech and reading disorder could reflect a common constitutional cause related to the maturation of the nervous system.

Prognosis Mild conduct disorders generally improve but more severe ones usually run a prolonged course in childhood and adolescence, and some persist into adult life. There are no good indicators of outcome for the individual child, except that the behaviour is more likely to persist when it is severe and when the quality of personal relationships is poor.

Treatment This is directed to the family as well as the child although some families are difficult to help. Mild disorders often recover with time and can be managed by the general practitioner with advice to the parents on consistently setting limits to the child's behaviour. More severe disorders generally require specialist management which includes:

- *Reduction of stressful circumstances*, if this is possible.

- *Behavioural programmes* with parents to reduce reinforcement of undesirable behaviour and increase positive responses to normal behaviour.

Table 19.12.
Conduct disorder: clinical features

Disobedience
Lying
Aggressive behaviour
Problems at school
Truanting
Stealing
Vandalism and fire-setting
Disapproved sexual behaviour
Alcohol and drug abuse

- *Remedial teaching* if there are reading or other educational difficulties.
- *Residential placement* in a foster home, residential home, or special school. This course is taken only with severe and intractable disorders and after discussion between all those involved with the child.
- *Medication has no place* in treatment.

Although these measures may reduce the immediate difficulties, there is no convincing evidence that any treatment affects the long-term course of conduct disorder. However, when adverse social and family factors improve for any reason, the disorder may improve.

Other problem behaviours of older children

In this section, we consider two patterns of behaviour associated with psychiatric disorder but with other causes as well: repeated absence from school and juvenile delinquency.

Repeated absence from school Repeated and prolonged absence from school has four causes:

1. Repeated or prolonged physical illness.

2. Parents who keep the child at home to help with domestic or other work.

3. *Truancy*. The child rebels against going to school.

4. *School refusal*. A physically healthy child wishes to go to school—and the parents support this—but he is unable to do so because of emotional problems.

Of these four causes, *truancy* requires brief discussion and *school refusal* a longer account.

Truancy Truancy is a form of rebellion and requires a direct and energetic approach agreed by the parents and teachers. Strong pressure should be brought to bear on the child to return to school, while an attempt should be made to resolve any educational or other problems at school. If these steps fail, legal proceedings may be initiated by the educational authorities.

School refusal The child shows mounting signs of unhappiness and anxiety when it is time to go to school and is reluctant to leave home. The child may complain of feeling ill, and especially of unexplained somatic physical symptoms of such as headache, abdominal pain, diarrhoea, or sickness. These complaints occur on school days but not at other times. Some children leave home to go to school but become increasingly distressed as they approach it. The final refusal to go to school can arise:

- *gradually* after a period of increasing difficulty of the kind just described;
- *after an enforced absence*, usually due to minor physical illness;
- *after an upsetting event* either *at school* such as bullying, or failure *in the family*, such as discord between the parents, or illness in a parent or grandparent.

Whatever the final sequence of events, these children are extremely resistant to efforts to return them to school, and their evident distress makes it hard for the parents to insist that they go.

Associated disorder In younger children *separation anxiety* is important. In older children there may be a *phobic or depressive disorder*. In the remaining cases there is no disorder and the refusal is an understandable but exaggerated *response to problems at school or at home* of the kind noted above.

Outcome Most younger children eventually return to school. A few severely affected adolescents cannot be returned to school before the age at which compulsory school attendance ends.

Management (see Table 19.13). General practitioners are often asked for help with these problems. They can usually assist all but the severe cases and early intervention can prevent worsening of the condition. The first step is to exclude a primary psychiatric disorder. Then any stressful circumstances are sought and if possible modified. The doctor should explain sympathetically but firmly to the parents and the child the nature of the condition and the need to achieve an early return to school. The arrangements for this need to be agreed with both parents, with the teachers, and if possible with the child. The doctor's role is to support the parents in carrying out the plan. If the parents find it difficult to adopt a firm approach, a nurse or social worker may accompany the child to school on the first few occasions.

If these simple measures fail, referral to a child psychiatrist is appropriate. The psychiatrist will look again for a possible primary psychiatric disorder, explore the causes for the child's distress in more detail, and employ the greater resources of the psychiatric team to help the child overcome the fear of going to school. Occasionally, admission to hospital is arranged to separate the child from particularly stressful circumstances at home or provide intensive treatment for anxiety or depression. Sometimes, a change of school is needed before the child will resume attendance.

Table 19.13.

Management of school refusal

Exclude a primary disorder:		Separation anxiety Other anxiety disorders Depressive disorders
Identify stressors:	*At home*:	marital problems, threats of separation, illness of family member
	At school:	criticism, failure, bullying
Modify stressors if possible:		Advice for parents Discussion with teachers
Return to school:		Firm approach Sympathetic support
Psychiatric opinion if the above fail		

Juvenile delinquency: children who break the law Delinquency is the failure of a young person to obey the law. It is not a psychiatric disorder but its causes include psychiatric disorder, usually conduct disorder. Also, parents often ask for advice from doctors about their delinquent children. Delinquency is most common at the age of 15–16 years. It is much more common in boys than girls. When asked about their own conduct, most adolescent boys admit having broken the law at some time, often with minor acts of shoplifting. Up to a fifth of adolescent boys are found to have carried out an offence, usually a trivial one. Of these only a few continue to offend in adult life. Parents can usually be reassured that a single act, especially if carried out with a group of others, is not of serious significance.

Causes Delinquency is related to low *social class*, *poverty*, *poor housing*, *and poor education,* so that rates are greater in areas of social deprivation. Delinquency is more frequent in children from *broken homes, families with discord, and very large families.* Among boys with *criminal fathers* about half are convicted for an offence, as against a fifth of those whose fathers who have not been convicted. The reasons for this association include poor parenting and shared attitudes to the law.

Management Delinquency is dealt with by the courts. Enquiries are made about problems in the family and educational progress, before deciding on punishment. Usually, the main emphasis is on:

- attempting to improve the family environment;
- helping the offender to develop better skills for solving problems;
- improving educational and vocational accomplishments;
- if possible, reducing harmful peer group influences.

These steps are helpful for the majority but a minority offend repeatedly despite all these forms of help.

Medical reports for the court Such reports are prepared usually by a child psychiatrist. When another doctor is asked to provide a report, the general guidelines about the writing of reports on adult offenders should be followed (see p. 456).

Disorders of development

Disorders of development are divided into specific disorders in which only a single function is involved and pervasive disorders in which a wide range of aspects of psychological development are affected. Autism is the least rare of pervasive development and the only one discussed here. The others are discussed in Chapter 20 of the *Oxford Textbook of Psychiatry*.

Disorders of development do not affect intellectual function; when this is present the condition is mental retardation, see Chapter 20. Specific disorders are more common and family doctors are more often asked for advice about them. Although rare, pervasive disorders are more serious and it is particularly important to them at an early stage and arrange specialist assessment.

Specific developmental disorders

These circumscribed developmental delays are of the four kinds shown in Table 19.14. The disorders do not involve general intellectual development

Table 19.14.

Specific developmental disorders

1. Reading disorder
2. Arithmetic disorder
3. Motor disorder
4. Language disorder

(which occurs in mental retardation) or general social development (which occurs in autism).

Specific reading disorder (dyslexia) This is also known as *developmental reading disorder*. The child's reading age is significantly (two standard deviations) below the level expected from age and IQ and this is not due solely to inadequate education. Writing and spelling are also impaired, but other aspects of development are not. The child's conduct is often disordered, possibly as a reaction to frustrating experiences at school. Compared with children with general backwardness at school, those with specific reading disorder are more often boys and are more likely to have minor neurological abnormalities; they are less likely to come from disadvantaged families.

Aetiology Several kinds of delay in psychological development can interfere with the complex processes of reading, but the causal mechanisms are still unknown.

Prognosis When the disorder is mild, about a quarter of the children read normally by adolescence. When the disorder is severe, most children still have severe problems in adolescence and later.

Management Special education in reading is required, the important first step being to reawaken the interest of the child after what has often been a long experience of failure. For this reason early detection is important.

Specific arithmetic disorder The condition parallels specific reading disorder in its clinical picture, unknown aetiology, and treatment by special education.

Specific motor disorder Children with this disorder have delayed motor development and poor co-ordination without general intellectual impairment or a specific neurological cause. They are late in developing the skills of feeding, walking, and dressing. They are clumsy, tending to break things, and are not good at games. Some have difficulty in writing and drawing.

Aetiology is unknown.

Prognosis Usually there is some improvement with time.

Management There is no specific treatment although special training may improve the child's confidence.

Specific developmental language disorder Children with this disorder have delayed speech development in the absence of general mental retardation or another cause such as deafness, cerebral palsy, or autism. On starting school, 5% of children have difficulty in making themselves understood by strangers and 1% are seriously retarded in speech. Serious delays in the production or understanding of speech has obvious consequences for education and social development and may be associated with behavioural problems.

Aetiology is not known.

Prognosis Mild cases usually improve, severe ones have a varied outcome.

Management is with speech therapy and remedial teaching. Early detection is important.

Table 19.15.
Childhood autism: clinical features

- Inability to relate and gaze avoidance
- Speech and language disorder
- Impaired non-verbal communication
- Resistance to change
- Odd behaviour and mannerisms
- Emotional lability, overactivity, poor concentration
- Seizures

Childhood autism

Although rare, autism is important because it is a serious disorder. All doctors should be able to recognize the possibility that it is present, although positive diagnosis requires a specialist opinion. The abnormal behaviour starts in early childhood after a brief period of normal development. Autism occurs in about 30–40 per 100 000 children, and is four times more common in boys than in girls.

Clinical features The clinical features are listed in Table 19.15. The following additional points should be noted.

• **Inability to relate** Autistic children do not respond to their parents' affectionate behaviour by smiling or cuddling, and are no more responsive to their parents than to strangers. Often, there is no clear difference between their behaviour to people and to inanimate objects. Autistic children avoid eye contact ('gaze avoidance').

• **Speech and language disorder** Speech may develop normally and then decline, or develop late. There may also be specific linguistic deficits. Occasionally, speech never develops.

• **Impaired non-verbal communication** adds to the problems caused by speech and language disorder.

• **Resistance to change** Autistic children are distressed by changes in their daily routine. They prefer the same food, insist on wearing the same clothes, or engage in the same repetitive games.

• **Odd behaviour and mannerisms** are common.

• **Seizures** About a quarter of autistic children develop epileptic seizures, usually about the time of adolescence.

• **Other features** Autistic children may be *emotionally labile*, suddenly becoming angry or fearful without apparent reason. They may be *overactive* and *distractible*. They may *sleep badly*; and they may *wet or soil* themselves.

Aetiology Twin studies indicate that genetic factors are of major importance, but it is not known how these factors lead to autism. The occurrence of seizures in some patients at the time of adolescence (see above) suggests an organic brain disorder. Of the various functional abnormalities, the basic one seems to be cognitive, affecting particularly symbolic thinking and language. One of the deficits in symbolic thinking is inability to judge correctly what other people are thinking.

Abnormal parenting has *not* been shown to be a cause. This is an important point for families to understand since many blame themselves for the child's problems.

Prognosis As autistic children grow up, about half acquire some useful speech, although serious impairments usually remain. Those who improve may continue to show emotional coldness and odd behaviour. As mentioned already, a substantial minority develop epilepsy in adolescence. Between 10% and 20% of children with childhood autism are eventually able to attend an ordinary school and later obtain work. A further 10–20% cannot work but can live at home and attend a training centre. The remainder are unable to lead an independent life.

Differential diagnosis This usually requires the advice of a specialist. Childhood autism has to be distinguished from several other disorders, notably:

- **deafness**, excluded by appropriate tests of hearing;
- **specific developmental language disorder** (see p. 415) in which the child usually responds normally to people;
- **mental retardation** in which there is general intellectual retardation with relatively less language impairment and a more normal response to other people.

Treatment The advice of a specialist should be obtained. There is no specific treatment and management has three aspects:

1. **Management of abnormal behaviour** A behavioural approach is used. Factors are identified that appear to be reinforcing the behaviour; often the parents attend more to the child when behaviour is abnormal than at other times. The reinforcing factors are reduced if possible and the child's response is monitored. These procedures lead to short-term improvement in some cases but have not been shown to produce lasting benefit.

2. **Special schooling** Most autistic children require special schooling to help them achieve their remaining potential for development. Residential schooling may be needed.

3. **Help for the family** The general practitioner has an important role in explaining the nature of the disorder, supporting the parents, and helping them to establish as normal a life as possible for the child and the rest of the family. Day care may be needed. Many parents find it helpful to join a support group of other parents of autistic children where they can discuss common problems.

Other disorders affecting speech

At this point, having considered specific language disorder and autism, it is convenient to consider two other disorders in which speech is affected without general intellectual retardation or autism. These are *stammering* and *elective mutism*.

Stammering This is a disturbance of the rhythm and fluency of speech. It may take the form of repetitions of syllables or words, or of pauses in the production of speech. Stammering is four times more frequent in boys than girls. It is usually a brief disorder in the early stages of language development, but 1% of children suffer from stammering after starting school. Stammering is not usually associated with a psychiatric disorder although it can cause distress and embarrassment.

The **aetiology** of stammering is not known. **Prognosis** Most children improve with time but a minority persist into adult life. **Treatment** is by speech therapy; this may help in the short term but its long-term value is uncertain.

Elective mutism In this rare condition, a child refuses to speak in some circumstances but speaks normally in others. Usually, speech is lacking at school and normal at home. There is no defect of speech or language, only a refusal to speak in certain situations. Often, there is other negative behaviour such as refusing to sit down or to play when asked to do so. The condition usually begins in children between 3 and 5 years of age, after normal speech has been acquired. The **cause** is unknown. **Prognosis** About half improve after five years; the course after that is uncertain.

Treatment There is no specific treatment of proven effectiveness. Parents should be told what is known about the problem. Any stressful circumstances at home or at school should be modified if possible.

Gender identity disorders

Some boys prefer to play at girls' games and dress in girls' clothes, and prefer the company of girls. Some of these boys also have an effeminate manner and say they want to be girls; they have a disorder of gender identity. Some girls show corresponding masculine behaviour. The **cause** of this disorder is unknown. It has been suggested that there may be an innate disorder which is reinforced by the parents' encouragement of feminine behaviour in boys and by a lack of male companions (with the corresponding factors important for girls).

Prognosis Some children with gender identity problems grow up normally, others continue to have problems in adult life.

Management When the behaviour is not extreme parents should be reassured and helped to encourage behaviours appropriate to the child's gender role. When the behaviour is extreme, the child should be assessed by a child psychiatrist who may offer counselling to the parents and child, and use behavioural measures in an attempt to reinforce behaviour more appropriate to the child's gender. It is not known whether such treatment alters the long-term outcome.

Psychological disorders of physically ill children

Psychological problems of physically ill adults are discussed on p. 208. Most of the points made there also apply to children, so only a few special issues will be considered in this section.

Most children adapt well to the experience of physical illness.

Reactions of children

Acute physical illness is more likely to cause delirium in children than in adults. A familiar example is delirium caused by febrile illness. *Chronic physical illness* and its treatment can affect self-esteem, and social development. These problems are particularly common with neurological disorders including epilepsy, leukaemia, and other conditions requiring intensive chemotherapy.

Reactions of parents

Although all parents are distressed when their child develops a chronic physical illness, some experience a more severe immediate reaction similar to bereavement. Some parents *deny* the seriousness of the condition, some *reject* the child, and some are *overprotective*. With time, most parents regain a satisfactory, loving relationship with their ill child, and cope successfully with the difficulties. The family doctor can help parents to achieve a satisfactory adjustment.

Reactions of siblings

The brothers and sisters of children with serious physical illness or handicap generally manage well, and some even acquire increased abilities to cope with stress. However, some siblings develop emotional or behavioural disturbances, feel neglected, or resent having to spend time helping to care for ill or handicapped child. The family doctor should always consider the needs of the siblings as well as those of the affected child and the parents.

Admission to hospital

This has important psychological effects for a child, who may become anxious or depressed, or may regress in behaviour. Such consequences are usually temporary, but repeated admission to hospital, especially in the early or middle years of childhood, may be followed by lasting emotional or behavioural disturbances. This result is more likely when there are poor family relationships or social problems. It is now general policy to encourage parents to visit their child in hospital frequently, to stay in hospital if the child is severely ill, and to take part in the child's care. General practitioners and hospital staff can prepare children for admission to hospital by explaining what will happen in terms appropriate to the child's age and by guiding the parents in how to do the same.

Disorders of adolescence

There are no psychiatric disorders specific to this period of life. Younger adolescents may develop the disorders of childhood, older adolescents may develop some of the disorders of adult life. For this reason, the subject will be considered briefly, drawing attention to the main conditions that are encountered at this age, but not repeating information presented elsewhere in this chapter and in other chapters in this book.

Emotional disorders

Anxiety disorders *Social phobia* often begins in early adolescence, and a few cases of agoraphobia begin in late teenage years. Some phobic disorders which started in childhood persist into adolescence. *Obsessional disorders,* which are rare in childhood, may begin in adolescence. *School refusal* and *truancy* are common between 14 years of age and the end of compulsory schooling.

Adjustment disorders with depressive symptoms are common in adolescence.

When **depressive disorders** occur at this age, they are characterized usually by loss of energy, difficult relationships at home, withdrawal from other social contacts, and underachievement at school. The typical adult picture with profound depressive mood with extreme guilt is less common; when present, these features suggest that the depressive disorder is the first phase of a manic-depressive disorder (which is discussed next).

Deliberate self-harm in children and adolescents is discussed on p. 255.

Manic-depressive disorder

Manic-depressive disorder is rare before puberty but increases in incidence during adolescence. The clinical features of the *depressive phase* are similar to those in adults (see p. 130) except that delusions and hallucinations are less frequent. At this age, *mania* presents most often with increased energy, reduced sleep, irritability, and disinhibited behaviour.

Treatment of manic-depressive disorder in adolescence resembles that given to adults (see p. 146) except that drug doses are lower according to age. Lithium is used less often than with adults but is occasionally necessary for recurrent disorders. ECT (electroconvulsive therapy) is very occasionally used in cases of very severe, drug-resistant depression in older adolescents.

Eating disorders

Bulimia nervosa and anorexia nervosa often begin in adolescence and are among the more common disorders at this age. These disorders are described on pp. 231 and 228.

Conduct disorders

Of the conduct disorders of adolescence, about half start in childhood. In adolescence the most common features of conduct disorders are truancy, offences against property, including the taking and driving of cars, abuse of alcohol and drugs and, among girls, promiscuity.

Schizophrenia

Schizophrenia may begin in adolescence, more commonly in boys than girls. The clinical picture is like that of schizophrenia in young adults (see p. 167). Treatment is also similar, though with reductions in drug doses according to age and an even greater emphasis on work with the family. The prognosis is poor.

Disorders of parent–child relationships

Child abuse (Table 19.16) results from the breakdown of the normal caring relationship between adults in the parental role and small children. The term *child abuse* refers to both *physical* and *sexual abuse*, and is sometimes used to include *emotional abuse* and *child neglect*. Two other forms of abuse are considered in this section. *Fetal abuse* is behaviour detrimental to the fetus, such as physical assault on the pregnant mother or the taking, by the mother, of substances likely to harm the fetus. In *Munchausen syndrome by proxy* a parent fabricates evidence to suggest, falsely, that the child is ill.

Physical abuse (non-accidental injury)

These terms refer to deliberate infliction of injury on a child, usually by one of the parents, a cohabitee of the mother or, occasionally, by a paid carer. Each year about 1 per 1000 children receive injuries of such severity that there is evidence of bone fracture or bleeding around the brain. Less severe injury is probably much more frequent, but does not always come to professional attention.

Detecting abuse Since parents seldom reveal the condition directly, the doctor has to be *alert to indirect indications*. Particular vigilance is needed when the family has features associated with a high risk for abuse (see below). The problem may become apparent when the parents bring a child to the doctor with an injury said to have been caused accidentally. Alternatively, relatives, neighbours, or other people may become concerned and report the problem to the police, social workers, or voluntary agencies. Suspicion of physical abuse should be aroused by:

- the *nature* of the injuries (see Table 19.17);
- *previous* suspicious *injury*;
- *unconvincing explanations* of the way in which the injury was sustained;
- *delay* in seeking help;

Table 19.16.
Forms of child abuse

- Physical abuse
- Sexual abuse
- Emotional abuse
- Fetal abuse
- Neglect
- Munchausen syndrome by proxy

Table 19.17.
Injuries caused by physical abuse

- Multiple bruising
- Abrasions
- Bites
- Burns
- Torn lips
- Fractures
- Retinal haemorrhage
- Subdural haemorrhage

- *incongruous reactions* to the injury by the parents or other carers;
- *fearful responses of the child* to the parents or carers;
- *other evidence that the child is distressed* such as social withdrawal, regression, low self-esteem, or aggressive behaviour.

Aetiology There are three sets of aetiological factors relating to the parents, the child, and the social circumstances. The common factor is a failure of the normal emotional bonding between the parent or other carer and the infant. These risk factors are summarized in Table 19.18. Knowledge of these factors assists in the detection of child abuse.

Management

Detection Doctors should be *alert to the possibility* of child abuse, and *aware of the risk factors* listed in Table 19.18. When abuse is suspected a specialist assessment should be arranged, giving a full account of the reasons for suspicion. Usually, the child will be admitted for assessment, which includes *photographs* of injuries and *radiological examination* which may show evidence of previous injury, or, occasionally, of a bone disorder such as osteogenesis imperfecta suggesting that fractures were caused accidentally. *Computerized tomography* is performed if subdural haemorrhage is suspected. All findings should be *documented fully* since evidence may be needed at subsequent legal proceedings.

Subsequent action When it has been decided that non-accidental injury is probable, an experienced senior doctor and social worker should *talk to the parents*. Arrangements should be made to *examine other children* without delay, to ensure their safety. The procedure varies with local administrative arrangements. In the UK social services play an important role. The general practitioner will be involved with the specialist team in the immediate and long-term plans for the child and the rest of the family.

Returning the child Sometimes the abused child can return home if support and close supervision are provided for the parents. When abuse has been severe or prolonged, however, the child may need to move to foster care while help is given to the parents. Sometimes permanent separation is necessary. These very difficult decisions are usually made by a paediatrician or child psychiatrist and a social worker, both experienced in such problems, after discussion with the family doctor. Since children returning to their parents may suffer further serious injury or even death, it is vitally important that a very careful assessment be made before a physically abused child is returned to the parents, and that there be close supervision of the child after return.

Prognosis Children who have been subjected to physical abuse are at high risk of subsequent emotional and behavioural disorder, delayed development, and learning difficulties. As adults, former victims of abuse may have difficulties in rearing their own children and some abuse them.

Sexual abuse

The term *sexual abuse* refers to the involvement of children in sexual activities to which they cannot give legally informed consent, or which violate generally accepted cultural rules, and which they may not fully comprehend. The term

Table 19.18.
Risk factors for physical abuse

In the parent
Very young age
Abnormal personality
Unsatisfactory or broken marriage
Social isolation
Former victim of abuse
Criminal record
Psychiatric disorder

In the child
Premature
Separated in early life
Needing special neonatal care
Congenital malformation
Chronic illness
Difficult temperament

Environmental
Poor housing
Family violence
Little feeling of community
Other stressful living conditions

covers various forms of sexual contact, sometimes involving violence, as well as activities such as posing for pornographic photographs or films. The abuser is usually known to the child and often a member of the family.

The **prevalence** of sexual abuse is difficult to determine; more cases have been reported to doctors in recent years but it is not certain whether this indicates a true increase in the problems, or more complete reporting.

Clinical features The children are more often female and the offenders usually male. Sexual abuse may be reported directly by the child or by a relative or other person. Children are more likely to report abuse when the offender is a stranger than when he is a family member. Sometimes, sexual abuse is discovered during the investigation of other conditions; for example, symptoms in the urogenital or anal area, behavioural or emotional disturbance, inappropriate sexual behaviour, or pregnancy. In adolescent girls, running away from home or unexplained suicidal attempts should raise the suspicion of sexual abuse. When abuse occurs within the family, marital and other family problems are common.

The immediate consequences of sexual abuse include anxiety, depression, and anger; inappropriate sexual behaviour; and unwanted pregnancy. Long-term effects include low self-esteem, mood disorder, self-harm, difficulties in relationships, and sexual maladjustment.

Assessment It is important to be alert to the possibility of sexual abuse, and to give serious attention to any complaint by a child of being abused in this way. It is also important not to make the diagnosis without adequate evidence from a thorough social investigation of the family, and from physical and psychological examination of the child. If the general practitioner suspects sexual abuse, he should obtain the advice of a child psychiatrist and a social worker experienced in these problems.

It is essential that information from children is obtained carefully. The child should be encouraged sympathetically to describe what has happened: drawings or toys may help younger children to give a description, but great care should be taken not to suggest answers to the child. When the circumstances make it appropriate a physical examination is carried out, including inspection of the genitalia and anal region. If intercourse may have taken place in the past 72 hours, specimens should be collected from the genital and any other relevant regions.

Management The initial management and the measures to protect the child are similar to those for physical abuse. In families where sexual abuse has occurred, the members may deny the seriousness of the abuse and the existence of other family problems. Sometimes a family member has engaged in other deviant sexual behaviour. The discovery of abuse may lead to family conflict that adds to the child's distress. Decisions about treatment and removal from home are taken only after the most careful consideration of all the implications. The sexual development of the abused child is often abnormal requiring help long after the event.

Late reports of sexual abuse Some adults report sexual abuse that occurred when they were children. Sometimes the adults have always been aware of the abuse but have been previously unable to confide in a doctor or other person. Reports of this kind indicate that childhood sexual abuse is a risk factor for emotional disorders in adult life. At other times adults report the recall of sexual abuse that they had not previously remembered. This latter experience usually takes place during a course of counselling and in some cases it transpires that the 'memory' is false and a response to repeated questioning or interpretations from the therapist ('false memory syndrome'). All such reports should be evaluated most carefully since false memories are, of course, highly distressing to the parents, or other supposed abuser, as well as to the patient.

Emotional abuse

The term *emotional abuse* refers usually to severe and persistent emotional neglect, verbal abuse, or rejection sufficient to impair a child's physical or psychological development. Emotional abuse often accompanies other forms of child abuse but may occur alone. Management resembles that for cases of physical abuse: the parents require help for their own emotional problems, the child needs counselling and, in severe cases, a period of separation from the parents.

Neglect

Child neglect includes neglect of the child's physical or emotional needs, upbringing, safety, or medical care, all of which may lead to physical or psychological harm. Child neglect is associated with adverse social circumstances, and is a common reason for foster care.

Neglect of a child's emotional needs and nutrition may lead to failure to thrive physically in the absence of a detectable organic cause. In children under 3 years, this condition is called *non-organic failure to thrive*; in older children it is called *deprivation dwarfism*. At both ages, there is reduction of height and usually weight, together with developmental delay. The children are irritable and unhappy. Given adequate care and nutrition most recover.

Munchausen syndrome by proxy

In this rare disorder, a parent (usually the mother) takes her child repeatedly to a doctor with false accounts of symptoms and sometimes with fabricated signs of illness such as haematuria. She seeks repeated investigations and treatment for the child. The parent has a personality disorder and sometimes a factitious disorder herself. She may be experiencing stressful circumstances but it is usually unclear why these should result in this unusual behaviour. Treatment is with general measures of counselling and help with social problems. The prognosis is poor for the child and the mother.

Further reading

Goodman, R. and Scott, S. (1997). *Child Psychiatry*. Blackwell, Oxford.
A clear account of child psychiatry which links research finding to practical advice about management.

Appendix: A comprehensive scheme for history taking and examination in child psychiatry

The format and extent of an assessment will depend on the nature of the presenting problem. The following scheme is taken from the book by Graham (1990), which should be consulted for further information. Graham suggests that clinicians with little time available should concentrate on items in **bold type**.

1. **Nature and severity of presenting problems(s). Frequency. Situations in which it occurs. Provoking and ameliorating factors. Stresses thought by parents to be important.**

2. *Presence of other current problems or complaints*
   (a) Physical. Headaches, stomach aches. Hearing, vision. Seizures, faints or other types of attacks.
   (b) Eating, sleeping, or elimination problems.
   (c) **Relationship with parents and siblings. Affection, compliance.**
   (d) Relationships with other children. Special friends.
   (e) Level of activity, attention span, concentration.
   (f) Mood, energy level, sadness, misery, depression, suicidal feelings. General anxiety level, specific fears.
   (g) Response to frustration. Temper tantrums.
   (h) Antisocial behaviour. Aggression, stealing, truancy.
   (I) **Educational attainments, attitude to school attendance.**
   (j) Sexual interest and behaviour.
   (k) Any other symptoms, tics, etc.

3. *Current level of development*
   (a) Language: comprehension, complexity of speech.
   (b) Spatial ability.
   (c) Motor co-ordination, clumsiness.

4. *Family structure*
   (a) Parents. Ages, occupations. **Current physical and emotional state**. History of physical or psychiatric disorder. Whereabouts of grandparents.
   (b) Siblings. Ages, presence of problems.
   (c) Home circumstances: sleeping arrangements.

5. *Family function*
   (a) **Quality of parental relationship. Mutual affection. Capacity to communicate about and resolve problems. Sharing of attitudes over child's problem.**
   (b) **Quality of parent–child relationship. Positive interaction: mutual enjoyment. Parental level of criticism, hostility, rejection.**
   (c) Sibling relationship.

(d) Overall pattern of family relationships. Alliance, communication. Exclusion, scapegoating. Intergenerational confusion.

6. *Personal history*

   (a) Pregnancy—complication. Medication. Infectious fevers.

   (b) Delivery and state at birth. Birthweight and gestation. Need for special care after birth.

   (c) Early mother–child relationship. Post-partum maternal depression. Early feeding patterns.

   (d) Early temperamental characteristics. Easy or difficult, irregular, restless baby and toddler.

   (e) Milestones. Obtain exact details only if outside range of normal.

   (f) **Past illnesses and injuries. Hospitalizations.**

   (g) Separations lasting a week or more. Nature of substitute care.

   (h) Schooling history. Ease of attendance. Educational progress.

7. *Observation of child's behaviour and emotional state*

   (a) **Appearance. Signs of dysmorphism. Nutritional state. Evidence of neglect, bruising, etc.**

   (b) **Activity level. Involuntary movements. Capacity to concentrate.**

   (c) **Mood. Expression or signs of sadness, misery, anxiety, tension.**

   (d) **Rapport, capacity to relate to clinician. Eye contact. Spontaneous talk. Inhibition and disinhibition.**

   (e) **Relationship with parents. Affection shown. Resentment. Ease of separation.**

   (f) Habits and mannerisms.

   (g) Presence of delusions, hallucinations, thought disorder.

   (h) Level of awareness. Evidence of minor epilepsy.

8. *Observation of family relationships*

   (a) Patterns of interaction—alliances, scapegoating.

   (b) Clarity of boundaries between generations: enmeshment.

   (c) Ease of communication between family members.

   (d) Emotional atmosphere of family. Mutual warmth. Tension, criticism.

9. *Physical examination of child*

10. *Screening neurological examination*

    (a) Note any facial asymmetry.

    (b) Eye movements. Ask child to follow a moving finger and observe eye movement for jerkiness, incoordination.

    (c) Finger–thumb apposition. Ask the child to press the tip of each finger against the thumb in rapid succession. Observe clumsiness, weakness.

    (d) Copying patterns. Drawing a man.

    (e) Observe grip and dexterity in drawing.

(f) Observe visual competence when drawing.

(g) Jumping up and down on the spot.

(h) Hopping.

(I) Hearing. Capacity of child to repeat numbers whispered two metres behind him.

Graham P. J. (1999) *Child Psychiatry: A Developmental Approach* (3rd edn). Oxford University Press.

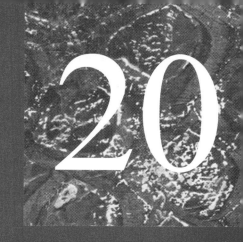

20

Mental retardation (learning disability)

- Terminology

- Epidemiology

- Clinical features

- Emotional and behavioural problems

- Physical disorders among people with mental retardation

- Effects of mental retardation on the family

- Causes of mental retardation

- Causes of behaviour problems

- Assessment of mental retardation

- Prevention and early detection

- Services for people with mental retardation

- Psychiatric disorder in mentally retarded people

- Treatment of psychiatric disorder

Mental retardation (learning disability)

The term *mental retardation* and the alternative term, *learning disability*, denote impairment of intelligence originating early in life (as opposed to dementia which develops later), with associated limitations of social functioning. Although not reversible, much can be done to enable people with this condition to live as normally as possible, usually outside hospital. To achieve this, the main requirements are educational and social rather than medical: special schooling, sheltered work and housing, support for the affected person and for the family. General practitioners provide general medical services for people with mental retardation. They are involved especially also in the early life of these patients working with paediatricians to help the family come to terms with the child's problems. Hospital doctors also see people with mental retardation among their patients.

All doctors need to be able to interview people with mental retardation, identify their physical and mental disorders, and understand how they react to stressful events. They need to know in general terms the range of causes of mental retardation and in more detail the two most frequent syndromes: *Down's syndrome* and *Fragile-X syndrome*. They need a broad understanding of the range of services available for these patients and when to refer to a psychiatrist.

Terminology

Several terms are used to describe people with intellectual impairment originating early in life. The term *mental retardation* is used in ICD-10 and DSM-IV. *Learning disability* is often used in the UK. Other terms used in the past for this condition include mental deficiency, mental subnormality, and mental handicap. In this chapter, we use the term *mental retardation* since it is used in international classifications and because the condition usually involves more than difficulty in learning.

Although the central feature of mental retardation is intellectual impairment, a definition solely in these terms is unsatisfactory. Social criteria need to be added for the practical purpose of distinguishing people who can lead a normal or near normal life, from those of the same intellectual level who cannot. Thus, the definition of mental retardation in DSM-IV includes, after the requirement for intellectual impairment, the phrase 'with concurrent deficits and impairments in adaptive behaviour, taking into account the person's age'. Nevertheless, degrees of intellectual impairment are important and subgroups are recognized within the international classifications based on IQ: mild (IQ 50–70); moderate (IQ 35–49); severe (IQ 24–34); profound (IQ below 20).

Epidemiology

Among the population aged 15–19 years, the *prevalence* of moderate and severe mental retardation is about 3 to 4 per 1000; 6 to 8 in a general practitioner's average list of 2000 patients. This prevalence has changed little since the 1930s even though the *incidence* of severe mental retardation has fallen by a third to a half as a result of improved antenatal and neonatal care, and other factors. The reason that the prevalence has not changed despite the lower incidence, is that mentally retarded people are living longer.

Clinical features

The general feature of all forms of mental retardation is low performance on all kinds of intellectual task including learning, short-term memory, the use of concepts, and problem solving. Sometimes, one specific function is impaired more than the rest; for example, the use of language. Clinical features are described best by reference to the subgroups of mild, moderate, severe, and profound disability. (See Table 20.1 and Fig. 20.1.)

Mild mental retardation (IQ 50–70)

About 80% of people with mental retardation fall into this group. They are usually unremarkable in appearance and any sensory or motor deficits are slight. Most develop more or less normal language abilities and social behaviour during the

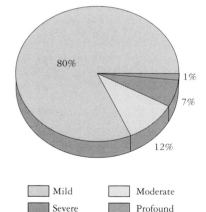

80%
1%
7%
12%

Mild · Moderate
Severe · Profound

Fig. 20.1 Degrees of retardation.

Table 20.1.
Levels of mental retardation

Mild
(IQ 50–70): 80% of all those affected
- Specific causes uncommon
- Many need practical help and special education
- Few need special psychiatric or social services

Moderate
(IQ 35–49): 12% of all those affected
- Most can manage some independent activities
- Require special education, sheltered occupation, and supervision

Severe
(IQ 20–34): 7% of all those affected
- Specific causes usual
- Social skills severely limited
- Require close supervision and much practical help

Profound
(IQ below 20): 1% of all those affected
- Specific causes usual
- Physical problems usual: severely disabled
- Require help with basic self-care

pre-school years, so that in the least severe cases the mental retardation may not be identified until the child starts school. In adult life most can live independently, although some need help with housing and employment, and when they are experiencing stressful events.

Moderate mental retardation (IQ 35–49)

Individuals in this group account for about 12% of those with mental retardation. Most have enough language development to communicate, and most can learn to care for themselves albeit with supervision. As adults most can find their way about and undertake simple routine work.

Severe mental retardation (IQ 20–34)

About 7% of the people with mental retardation have severe retardation. In the pre-school years their development is greatly slowed and, in later years, so is their learning in school. Eventually, many can be trained to look after themselves under supervision and to communicate in a simple way. As adults most are able to undertake simple tasks and limited social activities. Many have associated physical disorders (see below).

(A small number of these people have some highly specific cognitive ability of a kind normally associated with superior intelligence, such as the ability to carry out feats of mental arithmetic or memory. Such people are called *idiots savants*.)

Profound mental retardation (IQ below 20)

About 1% of those with mental retardation are in this group. Few learn to care for themselves completely. Only a few eventually achieve some simple speech and social behaviour. Physical disorders are very frequent.

Emotional and behavioural problems

Reactions to stressful events

People with mental retardation react to stress in the same way as people of normal intelligence. They are, however, more likely to display distress through their behaviour than through words. Signs of agitation, fearfulness, or irritability, or dramatic behaviours may indicate an acute stress disorder. Sometimes, the reaction is to an *undiagnosed physical illness*, and this possibility should be considered on every occasion.

Behaviour problems

As well as the direct effects of intellectual impairment, children with mental retardation may show any of the common behavioural problems of childhood (see Chapter 19). These problems tend to occur at a later age than in a child of normal intelligence, and to last longer, although they usually improve slowly with age.

Many children with mental retardation are *distractible, overactive,* and *impulsive.* More severe behaviour problems include *repeated self-injury and 'autistic' behaviours,* such as stereotyped repetitive and apparently purposeless activities such as rocking to and fro, head-banging, and mannerisms. These severe problems are more frequent among people with severe mental retardation, occurring in about 40% of children and 20% of adults.

In a minority of cases aggressive or uncontrolled behaviour is so severe as to threaten the well-being of the patient or the carers. Such severely disordered behaviour is referred to as *challenging behaviour*.

Sexual problems

Masturbation in public is the most frequent of these problems. Some people with mental retardation show a child-like curiosity about other people's bodies which can be misunderstood as sexual. Concern is sometimes expressed that people with mental retardation may have sexual intercourse and produce mentally retarded children. In fact, many of the causes of mental retardation are not inherited; and most of those that are heritable are associated with infertility. A more important concern is that, even if their children are of average intelligence, people with severe mental retardation are unlikely to be able to function well as parents. Contraceptive methods reduce the risk of unplanned pregnancy; when it occurs, difficult problems can arise and specialist advice is necessary if termination of pregnancy or sterilization are considered.

Physical disorders among people with mental retardation

Physical disorders are most frequent among those with severe and profound mental retardation, most of whom have problems such as sensory or motor disabilities, or epilepsy. Only a third of such people are continent and ambulant; a quarter are highly dependent on other people. Disorders of hearing or vision add an important additional obstacle to normal cognitive development. Motor disabilities, which are frequent, include spasticity, ataxia, and athetosis.

Effects of mental retardation on the family

When a newborn child is found to have mental retardation, it is inevitable the parents are distressed. Some reject the child at first although this rejection seldom lasts long. More often the diagnosis is not made until after the first year of life. When this happens, the parents have to make changes in their earlier hopes and expectations, and many parents experience prolonged depression, with guilt, shame, or anger. A few parents reject the child, while others become overinvolved in his or her care to the detriment of their other children. Most parents eventually achieve a satisfactory adjustment but however well they adjust psychologically, they are faced with the prospect of prolonged hard work, and difficult social problems. If the child also has a physical handicap, these problems are greater. For these reasons, the parents of a child with mental retardation need long-term support.

Causes of mental retardation

Mild mental retardation is usually due to a combination of genetic and adverse environmental factors, such as extreme prematurity and damage during birth. *Severe and profound mental retardation* is usually due to specific pathological conditions, most of which can be diagnosed in life and about two-thirds of which can be diagnosed before birth. The cause of moderate mental retardation are varied.

General causes

- **Genetic causes** Much mild mental retardation represents the lower end of the normal distribution curve of intelligence which is mainly determined by polygenic inheritance. Specific genetic abnormalities are responsible for many of the metabolic and other disorders which cause severe retardation. (Some of these causes are discussed further below.)

- **Antenatal damage** caused by *intrauterine infection* (such as rubella or syphilis), or toxic substances (such as *lead poisoning* or *excessive alcohol* use by the mother). In developing countries, *hypothyroidism* due to iodine deficiency is important.

- **Perinatal damage** This damage arises from birth injury, kernicterus, and intraventricular haemorrhage, and other less frequent conditions.

- **Postnatal damage** due to injury or resulting from child abuse, infections (encephalitis and meningitis), and lead intoxication.

- **Social factors** Mental retardation is associated with lower social class, poverty, poor housing, and an unstable family environment.

- **Malnutrition** is a common cause of mental retardation in developing countries. It is much less frequent in Western countries.

Specific causes

Many causes of mental retardation have been identified, including abnormalities of chromosomes or genes, some of which are associated with specific biochemical abnormalities. Because most of these causal conditions are rare they are not described in this chapter. A full account will be found in a textbook on paediatrics, and some basic information is given in the Appendix to this chapter (p. 444). (*The numbers in parenthesis in this section correspond to those in the Appendix.*)

Genetic causes

Genetic causes fall into five groups of which only two of the more frequent, Down's syndrome and Fragile-X syndrome will be are described here, basic information about the other genetic disorders will be found in *Additional information* and in the Appendix.

1. **Dominant conditions** Neurofibromatosis (9) and tuberose sclerosis (10) are examples of these rare conditions.

2. **Recessive conditions** This is the largest group of specific gene disorders. It includes most of the inherited metabolic conditions, such as phenylketonuria (3), homocystinuria (4), and galactosaemia (5).

3. **Chromosome abnormalities** The most common chromosome abnormality is Down's syndrome (described below). Abnormalities in the number of sex chromosomes as in Klinefelter's syndrome (XXY), and Turner's syndrome (XO) sometimes lead to mental retardation as well as to physical abnormalities.

4. **X-linked conditions** In males, up to a fifth of mental retardation has causes linked to the X chromosome. Specific genes on that chromosome cause rare

Additional information Causes of mental retardation

Genetic
- Dominant genes (causing gross brain disease)
  - Neurofibromatosis
  - Tuberose sclerosis
- Recessive genes causing metabolic disorder involving:
  - amino acids (e.g. phenylketonuria, homocystinuria)
  - the urea cycle (e.g. citrullinuria, aminosuccinic aciduria)
  - lipids (Tay–Sachs, Gaucher, and Niemann–Pick diseases)
  - carbohydrate (galactosaemia)
  - mucopolysaccaridoses (e.g. Hurler's syndrome)
- Chromosome abnormalities
  - Down's syndrome
  - Klinefelter's syndrome
  - Turner's syndrome
- X-linked disorders
  - Lesch–Nyhan syndrome
  - Fragile-X syndrome
  - Cranial malformations
  - Hydrocephalus
  - Microcephalus
- Polygenic factors
  - Influencing the normal distribution of intelligence

Antenatal damage
  - Infections
    rubella, cytomegalovirus, syphilis, toxoplasmosis
  - Intoxications
    lead, certain drugs, alcohol
  - Physical damage
    injury, radiation, hypoxia
  - Endocrine disorders
    hypothyroidism, hypoparathyroidism

Perinatal damage
- Birth asphyxia
- Kernicterus
- Intraventricular haemorrhage

Postnatal damage
  - Injury
    accidental, child abuse
  - Infections
    encephalitis, meningitis
  - Lead intoxication

Malnutrition

syndromes including the Lesch–Nyhan syndrome (8). In most cases, although the chromosome is demonstrably abnormal, no specific gene has been implicated. These latter cases are referred to as 'Fragile-X syndrome' (see below).

5. **Conditions known to be inherited but in a less well understood way** Anencephaly, microcephaly.

Down's syndrome (Table 20.2)

This condition is a frequent cause of mental retardation occurring in 1 of every 600–700 births. This incidence is decreasing because of prenatal detection of Down's syndrome fetuses by amniocentesis and, if the mother wishes, termination of pregnancy.

The **clinical picture** is made up of features any one of which can occur in a normal person. When four of these features occur together, there is strong evidence for the syndrome. The *external abnormalities* are:

(1)   head—the occiput is flat.

(2)   eyes—there are oblique palpebral fissures and epicanthic folds.

(3)   mouth—a small mouth and teeth, furrowed tongue, and high-arched palate.

(4)   hands—these are short and broad, with a curved fifth finger, and a single transverse palmar crease.

(5)   joints—these show hyperextensibility or hyperflexibility with hypotonia of the muscles.

Internal abnormalities, which are common, include *congenital heart disease,* especially septal defects (in about 20%), and *intestinal abnormalities*, especially duodenal obstruction. *Hearing* may be *impaired*.

In Down's syndrome the *degree of mental retardation* varies considerably; usually the IQ is between 20 and 50 but in 15% it is greater than 50. The *temperament* of children with Down's syndrome is usually affectionate and easygoing, and many show an interest in music. *Behaviour problems* are less frequent than in other forms of mental retardation.

In the past, many of those with Down's syndrome died in infancy but with improved medical care more survive into adult life, and about a quarter now live beyond the age of 50. Signs of ageing appear prematurely and, in the brain, *Alzheimer-like changes* develop in middle life.

Aetiology In about 95% of cases there is trisomy of chromosome 21 (i.e. three chromosomes 21 instead of the usual two). These cases, which result from *failure of dysjunction* during meiosis, are more frequent in the children of older mothers and the risk of recurrence in a subsequent child is about 1 in 100.

The remaining 5% of cases of Down's syndrome are attributable either to *translocation* involving chromosome 21. Translocation is often inherited and the risk of recurrence, about 1 in 10, is higher than that in the non-disjunction cases.

When non-disjunction takes places during a cell division after fertilization, normal and trisomic cells occur together in the same person, a condition known as *mosaicism*. In these cases, the effects on cognitive development are particularly variable.

Table 20.2.

Down's syndrome

External abnormalities

Flat occiput
Oblique palpebral fissures
Epicanthic folds
Small mouth, high-arched palate
Furrowed tongue

Short, broad hands
Single transverse palmer crease
Curved fifth finger

Hypotonia and extensive joints

Internal abnormalities

Congenital heart disease
Intestinal abnormalities

Impaired hearing

Fragile-X syndrome

In this condition, a break is seen in an X chromosome in a proportion of cells, when these are cultured in a medium deficient in folate. The disorder occurs in up to 1 in 1000 males and in a milder form in 1 in 200 females. The condition is the second most frequent cause of mental retardation (Down's syndrome is the first) accounting for about 7% of moderate and about 4% of mild mental retardation among males, and about 3% of moderate and mild mental retardation among females.

Affected children have *characteristic features*, none of which is diagnostic. These are: high forehead, prominent supraorbital ridges, and large ears. After puberty, the testes are enlarged. These children also have increased rates of abnormalities of speech and language, social impairment, and disorders of attention.

Since absence of these physical characteristics does not exclude the diagnosis it is appropriate to test for the disorder in all unexplained cases of mental retardation. The condition is due to an abnormal gene which contains an amplified CGG repeat sequence. Testing can identify heterozygous females who are clinically normal, and identify males who are carriers.

Causes of behaviour problems

The causes of behavioural problems among people with mental retardation fall into four groups:

- **Organic brain pathology** is a commonly associated with behaviour problems in people with severe mental retardation.
- **Epilepsy** is strongly associated with behaviour disorder, especially hyperkinetic behaviour. (Some behaviour disorder associated with epilepsy is caused by the anticonvulsant drugs.)
- **Psychological causes** account for some of the behavioural problems of people with mental retardation. These causes include frustration associated with communication difficulty, inability to acquire social skills, and educational failure.
- **Social factors** such as family tensions or bereavement are important causes of behaviour problems. An overstimulating environment may cause behaviour problems, while an understimulating one may lead to withdrawal and self-stimulation.

Assessment of mental retardation

Severe mental retardation is usually diagnosed in infancy, as it is often associated with physical abnormalities or with delayed motor development. It is more difficult to diagnose less severe mental retardation which has to be done on the basis of delays in psychological development. A full assessment includes history taking, interviewing, physical examination, behavioural assessment, developmental testing, and examination of the mental state.

This section is concerned mainly with the assessment of children since this is when assessment usually takes place. A similar scheme is used when adolescents or adults are assessed and the account includes advice on interviewing these people.

History taking

Particular attention is given to any *family history* suggesting an inherited disorder, and to *abnormalities in the pregnancy or delivery*. Dates of passing *developmental milestones* should be ascertained, and a full account obtained of any *behaviour disorders*. Adults with mental retardation who have reasonable language ability, can be interviewed as well as informants. When language is less well developed, the account has to be obtained mainly from informants.

Interviewing people with mental retardation

The procedures are generally similar to those described in Chapter 2, for interviewing patients of normal intelligence, but some special points should receive attention:

- Ask *simple questions* avoiding subordinate clauses, passive verb constructions, figures of speech, and other complexities of grammar.
- *Allow adequate time* for the patient to respond and do not appear impatient.
- *Check answers to closed questions* (e.g. 'do you feel sad?') which may have to be used because the patient cannot volunteer information. A positive answer can be checked by asking the opposite (e.g. 'do you feel happy?').
- *Check other answers.* Some learning disabled people repeat the interviewer's last words, and such responses should be checked. For example: Interviewer 'Do you feel sad?'; Patient: 'sad'.
- *Check with informant.* People with learning disabilities often find difficulty in timing the onset or describing the sequence of symptoms. Whenever possible these and other important points should be checked with an informant.

Physical examination

The physical examination should include the recording of *head circumference, height,* and *weight.* Abnormal physical signs may indicate one of the rare specific syndromes. The *neurological examination* should include attention to vision and hearing.

Behavioural assessment

This is based on the observations of the child's *ability to communicate, sensorimotor skills,* any *unusual behaviour* and, at an appropriate age, ability for *self-care* It is often useful to ask parents, teachers, and others involved to keep records of any problem behaviours.

Developmental testing

This is a complex procedure which is performed usually in a specialist unit. Clinical observation is combined with standardized measurements of *intelligence, language development, motor performance,* and *social skills.*

Overall assessment

This starts by distinguishing between mental retardation and other conditions, especially delayed maturation, blindness, deafness, childhood autism, and childhood psychosis. The last four may coexist with mental retardation and worsen the behaviour problems. A formulation is made of all the medical and social factors contributing to the overall handicaps, and the attitudes of people who may be involved in the patient's care.

Prevention and early detection

Prevention

Primary prevention depends mainly on genetic screening and counselling, together with good antenatal and obstetric care. In some developing countries, correction of iodine deficiency and malnutrition is important. *Secondary prevention* aims to reduce the effect of the primary disorder; for example by providing 'enriching' education.

Genetic screening and counselling Most parents seek advice only after a first mentally retarded child has been born. Those asking for advice before or during the first pregnancy usually do so because there is a mentally retarded person on one or other side of the family. Specialist advice is usually needed to assess the risk that an abnormal child will be born, and to explain this risk to the parents so that they can make their own decision whether to start or continue the pregnancy.

Antenatal care *Immunization against rubella* should be provided for girls who lack immunity, before the age at which they could become pregnant. Women already pregnant should be advised on the *harmful effects of excessive alcohol* consumption. *Improved care for premature and low birthweight infants* can prevent mental retardation in some infants who would otherwise have suffered brain damage. However, the same methods enable the survival of retarded children who, without these methods, would have died. (See Table 20.3.)

Early detection

Prenatal care *ultrasound scanning* of the fetus, *amniocentesis*, and *fetoscopy* can reveal disorders due to chromosomal abnormalities, most open neural tube defects, and about half of inborn errors of metabolism. Because amniocentesis carries a small but definite risk, it is usually offered only to women who have carried a previous abnormal fetus, women with a family history of congenital disorder, and those over 35 years of age.

Postnatal care Phenylketonuria, hypothyroidism, and galactosaemia can be detected by routine testing of infants.

Services for people with mental retardation

Principles of service provision (see Table 20.4)

Services for people with mental retardation should:

- provide a pattern of life that is as similar as possible to that of other people ('normalization');
- recognize that each person with mental retardation has individual needs;
- develop abilities as well as compensating for disability;
- offer a choice of services and involve the retarded person in the choice.

Table 20.3.
Prevention and early detection of mental retardation

1. **Prevention**
   - Before pregnancy
     – rubella immunization
     – genetic counselling
   - During pregnancy
     – avoid excess alcohol
   - After delivery
     – care of premature infants
2. **Early detection**
   - During pregnancy
     – ultrasound screening
     – amniocentesis
     – fetoscopy
   - After delivery
     Screening for:
     – phenylketonuria
     – hypothyroidism
     – galactosaemia

Most mental retardation is detected by family doctors and paediatricians. However, the wide range of needs of people with mental retardation can be met only be a care team that includes psychiatrists, psychologists, nurses, residential care staff, teachers, occupational therapists, physiotherapists, and speech therapists. Self-help groups for parents are useful, and volunteers can play a valuable part in the arrangements.

Care for people with mild and moderate mental retardation

Few people with mild mental retardation need specialist services. Most live with their families, cared for when necessary by the family doctor. When specialist treatment is needed it is usually for associated physical disability or illness, emotional disorder, or psychiatric illness. When placement away from home is needed it is usually because of difficulties in the family, or physical problems. In these cases fostering or boarding school placement for children or residential care for adults is arranged. Adults with mild mental retardation may need extra support when they are facing problems with housing and employment, or with the problems of growing old.

Help for families

Parents need help as soon as the diagnosis of mental retardation is made. It is seldom enough to give an explanation of the problem once; most parents need to hear the information several times before they can take in all its implications. Adequate time is needed to explain the prognosis, indicate what help can be provided, and discuss the part the parents can play in helping their child achieve his full potential. As explained above, parents need continuing psychological support and help with practical matters such as day care during school holidays, babysitting, or arrangements for family holidays. These provisions are needed especially at times of change for the patient, especially leaving school and at times when there are additional problems in the family such as the illness of another child.

Education

Education and training should begin early. Extra education and training before school age (*compensatory education*) helps children with mental retardation to realize their potential. When the normal school age is reached, the least disabled children can be educated in a special class in an ordinary school. More disabled children benefit more from attendance at a school for children with learning difficulties. For the intermediate levels of disability a choice has to be made between education in an ordinary school or a special school. The former offers the advantages of more normal social surroundings and greater expectations of progress; it has the disadvantages of lack of special teaching skills and the risk that the child may not be accepted by more able children. Since learning is slow, education needs to extend into adult life.

Leaving school

The period after leaving school is difficult for people with mental retardation and they need much help from their general practitioner and the specialist services. It

Table 20.4.
Principles of service provision

- 'Normalize' the person's life
- Recognize individual needs
- Develop abilities
- Offer choice

is important to review the prospects for employment, suitability for further training, and requirements for day care. At this stage of life, it may be difficult for the parents to look after a young person with severe mental retardation and residential care may be required. Wherever the person is living, there is a need for sheltered work or other occupation after leaving school.

Training and work

Most people with mild mental retardation are capable of work and benefit from appropriate training. However, except at times of full employment, suitable work may not be available and sheltered occupation is needed. Most school-leavers with moderately severe mental retardation need sheltered work or further training when they leave school. Most need these special provisions throughout their lives, although some do progress to normal employment.

Social activities

People with mental retardation need to develop leisure activities appropriate to their age, ability, and interests. Whenever possible these should be obtained by joining activities arranged for able people, but clubs and day centres for the disabled are also needed. For the most disabled, leisure activities need to be arranged as part of the programme of the training centres which provide sheltered work.

Accommodation

Many people with mental retardation live with their families. For the rest, a range of accommodation is required ranging from ordinary housing to staffed hostels. A useful intermediate level of supervision is provided in a 'core and cluster' system in which several group homes are sited near to a central staffed unit. When parents grow old and can no longer care for their disabled son or daughter, special accommodation is required. In most places the supply of such accommodation has not kept pace with the increasing life expectancy of people with mental retardation.

Help with financial and other problems

People with mental retardation may need help in managing their money, dealing with forms, regulations, and other problems of daily life.

General medical services

People with mental retardation sometimes receive substandard medical care because doctors do not detect their needs or do not provide the extra support needed to enable these patients to co-operate with treatment. It is good practice to keep a register of these patients and arrange regular health checks. (See Table 20.5.)

Care for people with severe mental retardation

A general practitioner with 2000 patients will care for, on average, only two children with severe mental retardation. In two of three cases, the severely disabled

Table 20.5.

Components of a service for people with mental retardation

- Support for family at home; respite admissions
- Education, training, and occupation
- Social activities
- Accommodation
- Help with financial and other problems
- General medical services

child can remain at home provided that the parents are helped to deal with behavioural problems, epilepsy, physical disability, or incontinence. This help may be day care, or respite care—short stays in residential care or hospital when the parents need a holiday, or when another member of the family is ill. When the child attends school, there is often a need for help with transport and for support in the school holidays. As well as these practical provisions, parents need information and psychological support.

The remaining one-third of severely retarded children need residential care, often because of physical disability, behavioural problems, or incontinence too great for the parents to manage.

Care for the elderly

As people with mental retardation live longer, provision is needed increasingly for the later years of their lives. At this stage, parents are no longer able to provide care and physical illness or dementia may add to the person's disability. It is important to recognize these problems when planning services.

Psychiatric disorder in mentally retarded people

Diagnosis

Diagnosis is often difficult because symptoms may be modified by low intelligence, and because patients need a minimum verbal fluency (corresponding to an IQ level of about 50) to describe their experiences. More emphasis has to be given to abnormalities of behaviour and less to reports of abnormal mental phenomena than would be the case in people of normal intelligence.

Psychiatric disorder in people with mental retardation is usually suggested by change in behaviour. It should be remembered that such a change can result also from *physical illness* or from *stressful events*, and both need to be excluded before the diagnosis of mental disorder can be made with confidence.

Prevalence of mental disorder

Among people with mental retardation the prevalence of mental disorder increases with the severity of the condition: with mild mental retardation the prevalence of mental disorder is similar to that among people of normal intelligence; among people with severe mental retardation it is greater. All types of mental disorder may occur at any level of mental retardation but the most frequent at the severe level are *autism, hyperkinetic syndrome, stereotyped movements, pica,* and *self-mutilation.*

Delirium dementia

These disorders are common among people with mental retardation. Sometimes, disturbed behaviour resulting from *delirium* is the first indication of physical illness. As with people of normal intelligence, delirium is more common among children and the elderly. *Dementia* causes a progressive decline in intellectual and social functioning from the previous level. Among the causes of dementia (see p. 318), Alzheimer's disease is more common in patients with Down's syndrome than in the general population (see p. 435).

Schizophrenia

In people with mental retardation delusions are less elaborate than in schizophrenics of normal intelligence, and hallucinations have a simple and repetitive content. 'First rank' and other typical symptoms are rarely present, and often the main features are a further impoverishment of person's already limited thinking, and an increased disturbance of behaviour and social functioning. When the IQ is below 45, it is difficult to make a definite diagnosis of schizophrenia. When the diagnosis of schizophrenia is likely but uncertain, a trial of antipsychotic drugs may be carried out to find out whether the patient's condition improves.

Affective disorder

When people with mental retardation develop a *depressive disorder* they are less likely than people of normal intelligence to complain of low mood or to express depressive ideas. Diagnosis has to be made mainly on an appearance of sadness, reduction of appetite and disturbance of sleep, and on behavioural changes of retardation or agitation. A severely depressed patient with adequate verbal abilities may describe depressive ideas or delusions, or hallucinations. A few of these patients make attempts at suicide although these are usually poorly planned. *Mania* has to be diagnosed mainly on overactivity and behavioural signs indicating excitement and irritability.

Other disorders

Stress-related and *adjustment disorders* occur commonly among people with mild and moderate mental retardation, especially when they are facing changes in the routine of their lives. *Anxiety disorders* are common, while conversion and dissociative symptoms are more conspicuous than in the corresponding disorders of people of normal intelligence. *Treatment* of all these conditions is directed to reducing stressors by effecting improvements in the patient's environment; if verbal skills are sufficient, counselling is used.

Personality disorder

Personality disorders are common among people with mental retardation and sometimes lead to greater problems in management than the learning problems. There is no specific treatment and management has to be directed to finding an environment as suitable as possible to the patient's temperament. If verbal skills are sufficient, counselling may be helpful.

Hyperkinetic syndrome

This syndrome occurs more commonly among children with mental retardation than among those of normal intelligence. The clinical picture and treatment are the same as those among children of normal intelligence (see p. 410).

Challenging behaviour

Challenging behaviour (that is, behaviour that threatens the safety of patient or other people) may be caused by psychiatric disorder but it has many other causes including:

- pain and discomfort due to associated physical conditions;
- frustration due to difficulty in communication;
- epilepsy;
- side effects of medication.

Treatment of psychiatric disorder

Treatment of mental disorder among people with mental retardation is similar to that of the same disorder in a patient of normal intelligence. Patients are less likely to report the side effects of drugs, and particular care is needed in adjusting dosage. In the more serious cases, admission to hospital is likely to be needed.

For challenging behaviour, the cause is treated if possible. If the behaviour persists, behavioural treatment may be tried, directed to changing any factors that appear to be reenforcing the behaviour.

Further reading

Bouras, N. (ed.) (1994). *Mental Health in Mental Retardation*. Cambridge University Press. *Reviews of the diagnosis and management of the psychiatric disorders and behaviour problems associated with mental retardation. See especially chapter 4: The inner world of people with mental retardation, Chapter 7: Psychiatric disorders in mental retardation and Chapter 22: Community services.*

Appendix: Notes on some causes of mental retardation

Syndrome	Aetiology	Clinical features	Comments
Chromosome abnormalities (For Down's syndrome and X-linked retardation see text)			
1. Triple X	Trisomy X	No characteristic feature	Mild retardation
2. *Cri du chat*	Deletion in chromosome 5	Microcephaly, hypertelorism, typical cat-like cry, failure to thrive	
Inborn errors of metabolism			
3. Phenylkentonuria	Autosomal recessive causing lack of liver phenylalanine hydroxylase. Commonest inborn error of metabolism	Lack of pigment (fair hair, blue eyes) retarded growth. Associated epilepsy, microcephaly, eczema, and hyperactivity	Detectable by postnatal screening of blood of urine. Treated by exclusion of phenylalanine from diet during early years of life
4. Homocystinuria	Autosomal recessive causing lack of cystathione synthetase	Ectopia lentis, fine fair hair, joint enlargement, skeletal abnormalities similar to Marfan's syndrome. Associated with thromboembolic episodes	Retardation variable. Sometimes treatable by methionine restriction
5. Galactosaemia	Autosomal recessive causing lack of galactose-1-phosphate-uridyl transferase	Presents after the introduction of milk into diet. Failure to thrive, hepatosplenomegaly, cataracts	Detectable by postnatal screening for the enzymic defect. Treatable by galactose-free diet. Toluidine blue test on urine

Syndrome	Aetiology	Clinical features	Comments
6. Tay–Sachs' disease	Autosomal recessive resulting in increased lipid storage (the earliest form of cerebromacular degeneration)	Progressive loss of vision and hearing. Spastic paralysis. Cherry red spot at macula of retina. Epilepsy	Death at 2–4 years
7. Hurler's syndrome (gargoylism)	Autosomal recessive affecting mucopolysaccharide storage	Grotesque features. Protruberant abdomen. Hepatosplenomegaly. Associated cardiac abnormalities	Death before adolescence
8. Lesch–Nyhan syndrome	X-linked recessive leading to enzyme defect affecting purine metabolism. Excessive uric acid production and excretion	Normal at birth. Development of choreoathetoid movements, scissoring position of legs, and self-mutilation	Can be diagnosed prenatally by culture of amniotic fluid and estimation of relevant enzyme. Postnatal diagnosis by enzyme estimation in a single hair root. Death in second or third decade from infection or renal failure. Self-mutilation may be reduced by treatment with hydroxytryptophan
Other inherited disorders			
9. Neurofibromatosis (Von Recklinghausen's syndrome)	Autosomal dominant inheritance	Neurofibromata, *café au lait* spots, vitiligo. Associated with symptoms determined by site of neurofibromata. Astrocytomas, meningioma	Retardation in a minority

Syndrome	Aetiology	Clinical features	Comments
10. Tuberose sclerosis (epiloia)	Autosomal dominant (very variable penetrance)	Epilepsy, adenoma sebaceum on face, white skin patches, shagreen skin, retinal phakoma, peri-ungual fibromata. Associated multiple tumours in kidney, spleen, and lungs	Retardation in about 70%
11. Lawrence–Moon–Biedl syndrome	Autosomal recessive	Retinitis pigmentosa, polydactyly, sometimes with obesity and impaired genital function	Retardation usually not severe
Infection			
12. Rubella embryopathy	Viral infection of mother in first trimester	Cataract, microphthalmia, deafness, microcephaly, congenital heart disease	If mother infected in first trimester, 10–15% infants are affected (infection may be subclinical)
13. Toxoplasmosis	Protozoal infection of mother	Hydrocephaly, microcephaly, intracerebral calcification, retinal damage, hepatosplenomegaly, jaundice, epilepsy	Wide variation in severity
14. Cytomegalovirus	Virus infection of mother	Brain damage. Only severe cases are apparent at birth	

Syndrome	Aetiology	Clinical features	Comments
15. Congenital syphilis	Syphilitic infection of mother	Many die at birth. Variable neurological signs. 'Stigmata' (Hutchinson teeth and rhagades often absent)	Uncommon, since routine testing of pregnant women. Infant's Wasserman reaction positive at first but may become negative
Cranial malformations			
16. Hydrocephalus	Sex-linked recessive. Inherited developmental abnormality (e.g. atresia of aqueduct, Arnold–Chiari malformation. Meningitis. Spina bifida)	Rapid enlargement of head in early infancy, symptoms of raised CSF pressure. Other features depend on aetiology	Mild cases may arrest spontaneously. May be symptomatically treated by CSF shunt. Intelligence can be normal
17. Microcephaly	Recessive inheritance, irradiation in pregnancy, maternal infections	Features depend on aetiology	Evident in up to a fifth of institutionalized mentally retarded patients
Miscellaneous			
18. Spina bifida	Aetiology multiple and complex	Failure of vertebral fusion. Spina bifida cystica is associated with meningocele or, in 15–20%, myelomeningocele. Latter causes spinal cord damage, with lower limb paralysis, incontinence, etc.	Hydrocephalus in four-fifths of those with myelomeningocele. Retardation in this group

Syndrome	Aetiology	Clinical features	Comments
19. Cerebral palsy	Perinatal brain damage. Strong association with prematurity	Spastic (commonest), athetoid and ataxic types. Variable in severity	Majority are below average intelligence. Athetoid are more likely to be of normal IQ
20. Hypothyroidism (cretinism)	Iodine deficiency or (rarely) atrophic thyroid	Appearance normal at birth. Abnormalities appear at 6 months. Growth failure, puffy skin, lethargy	Now rare in Britain. Responds to early replacement treatment
21. Hyperbilirubinaemia	Haemolysis, rhesus incompatibility, and prematurity	Kernicterus (choreoathetosis), opisthotonus, spasticity, convulsions	Prevention by antirhesus globulin. Neonatal treatment by exchange transfusion

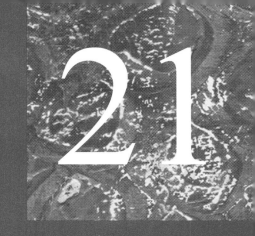

21

Psychiatry and the law

- Psychiatry and civil law

- Psychiatry and criminal law

Psychiatry and the law

The relationship of psychiatry to the law is of importance to all doctors for three reasons:

1. The law regulates the circumstances under which treatment can be given without patients' consent and the compulsory admission of psychiatric patients to hospital. Primary care practitioners and hospital doctors may encounter situations in which patients refuse essential treatment and may be involved in emergency decisions to invoke powers of compulsory admission (since the details of mental health law varies among countries only general principles are described in this chapter).

2. There are other situations in which doctors may be asked for reports used in legal decisions: capacity to make a will, to care for property, and claims for compensation for injury.

3. A minority of patients behave in ways which break the law. Doctors may be asked by the courts for advice about the relationship between the psychiatric disorder and the illegal acts.

The chapter ends with advice on the writing of reports for the courts and other medicolegal purposes.

Psychiatry and civil law

Laws concerning compulsory admission and treatment

Consent to treatment

In general, the law requires that patients cannot be treated unless they first consent. This consent must be given:

- **voluntarily**, without undue influence;
- **by the patient**; no one can consent on his behalf, although he may obtain advice from relatives or others whom he trusts;
- by the patient, who has been **informed** of the likely benefits, side effects, and possible adverse outcomes of the treatment.

Except for minor procedures, the patient's consent should be **documented**.

There are special problems about informed consent for treatment in those who are mentally ill. Some patients, by reason of their illness, are not capable of informed consent and some do not recognize that they are ill and require treatment. To be capable of consent, patients need to be able to:

- **understand** the information provided about the treatment;
- **retain** this information;
- **evaluate** the information to arrive at a decision.

Patients with delirium or dementia may be unable to consent to treatment *because they cannot understand, retain, or evaluate information*. (Dementia does not inevitably lead to these consequences and each patient should be evaluated carefully.)

Other psychiatrically ill people are capable of consent but *do not recognize that they are unwell or in need of psychiatric treatment*. This arises particularly with schizophrenia and manic-depressive disorders.

All countries have laws covering the circumstances in which compulsory psychiatric treatment can be given to patients with psychiatric disorder who do not consent. In general, compulsory treatment can be initiated only in hospital.

Compulsory treatment of mental illness

Mental health laws regulate the circumstances in which people with mental illness can be admitted to hospital and treated without their consent. These laws have three purposes which are shown in Table 21.1. They ensure essential treatment for mentally ill people who do not recognize that they are ill, and refuse treatment. Three criteria are used to decide whether treatment is essential; they are required to ensure:

(1) *the safety of the patient*—usually from suicidal impulses;

(2) *the safety of others*—for example, from the violent impulses of a paranoid patient;

(3) measures needed urgently to *prevent deterioration* which will lead to one of the two consequences listed above.

The details of mental health law vary in different countries; even within the UK, the laws in England and Wales differ in certain ways from those in Scotland and Northern Ireland. The most widely used sections of the Mental Health Act for England and Wales are shown in Table 21.2 as an illustration of the general principles discussed below. Readers working in countries other than England and Wales should ask their teachers about local legislation (the law in England and Wales is also summarized in the Appendix).

There are important general features of most systems of law:

Joint decisions The patient's refusal to have treatment cannot be overturned by a single doctor except in situations of extreme urgency. For example, in England and Wales two doctors and a social worker are required to agree about the decision.

Defined periods of detention The law sets strict limits on the period of involuntary detention and treatment. If longer periods of detention are needed, further orders must be made.

Appeal against detention An important safeguard against misuse of the power to detain is a system of independent review. The detailed arrangements vary in different countries; for example in England and Wales patients can appeal first to members of the board of management of the hospital to which they have been admitted. If this appeal fails, they can appeal to a mental health tribunal consisting of a lawyer, a doctor, and a layperson.

Table 21.2.

Mental Health Act 1983 for England and Wales: the most widely used sections

Section number	Order	Duration	Authorization
2	Assessment order	28 days	Recommendation of two doctors (one approved) plus application by nearest relative or social worker
3	Treatment order	6 months initially and renewable	As for Section 2
4	Emergency order	72 hours	Recommendation by one doctor plus application by nearest relative or social worker
5.1	Holding order	72 hours	One doctor
5.2	Holding order	6 hours	One registered mental nurse
58	'Hazardous treatment'		Consent or second opinion
136	Police order	72 hours	Police officer

Early discharge from detention Some patients recover so quickly that compulsory detention is no longer needed at a time before the original detention period has elapsed. In these circumstances the original order can be terminated.

Provision for detention of patients already in hospital The provisions described so far apply to patients who are not in-patients at the time when the order is made. Sometimes a patient enters hospital voluntarily and then demands to leave. Normally, he is free to do this but, in some circumstances, discharge would endanger his own life or health or endanger other people. If there is evidence of mental disorder, mental health laws provide that the patient can be held in hospital for a brief period sufficient to arrange a full assessment for detention.

Detention by the police Police officers sometimes encounter people apparently suffering from mental disorder. Mental health laws generally contain provision for the police to detain such persons until they can be assessed.

Consent to certain treatments Generally, the legal authority to detain the patient carries with it authority to give basic treatment even without the patient's consent (e.g. sedation). However, in some countries additional authority has to be obtained before certain treatments can be given without consent. In England and Wales, these treatments are electroconvulsive therapy and medication continued for more than three months for patients subject to mental health law orders.

Patients who have offended People with psychiatric illness who have been convicted of offences may need to be transferred to hospital either from the court or after a period in prison. Mental health laws contain provisions for the compulsory detention in hospital of such people, either on terms similar to those of detained patients who have not offended or with restrictions on the consultant psychiatrist's usual powers of discharge. These provisions, which are complex and mainly of concern to psychiatrists, are not detailed here.

Other aspects of civil law

Patients' ability to manage their affairs

Some patients, most often those who are demented, become incapable of managing their affairs by reason of mental disorder and are vulnerable to exploitation. When this happens, legal arrangements exist to enable another responsible person to act for the patient. The doctor should advise the close relatives when this circumstance arises, explain the risks to property, and outline the legal provisions. If the relatives decline to take action the doctor can initiate proceedings himself. In English law there are two procedures: power of attorney and receivership. Comparable procedures are available in other countries.

Power of attorney requires the person to give written authorization for someone else to act for him. It is, of course, essential that the person giving authority is able to understand what he is doing and be able to judge the suitability of the person chosen to act for him.

Receivership is a more complex procedure with the greater safeguards needed for a person who is unable to make the judgement required in authorizing a power of attorney. An application is made to a legal body (in England and Wales the Court of Protection) which decides for the patient whether to appoint someone (a 'receiver') to act on his behalf.

Making a will

Doctors are sometimes asked to advise whether a patient is capable of making a will; that is, whether he has 'testamentary capacity'. The requirements are that the person:

• understands what a will is;

• knows the nature and extent of his property (although not in detail);

• knows who are his close relatives and can assess their claims to his property;

• does not have any mental abnormality that might distort his judgement (e.g. delusions about the actions of his relatives).

Most patients with mental disorder are wholly capable of making a will.

Fitness to drive

Questions about fitness to drive arise quite often in relation to psychiatric disorder. Patients may drive recklessly if they are manic, depressed and suicidal, or aggressive; or if they abuse alcohol or drugs. Concentration on driving may be impaired in many kinds of psychiatric disorder, and also by the sedative side effects of drugs used in treatment. The issue should be considered in all cases in which the patient drives a motor vehicle. Advice to stop driving should be given if necessary and the patient reminded of his duty to report certain illnesses to the licensing authority. Particular caution is required for patients who drive public service vehicles or goods vehicles.

Compensation for personal injury

Doctors are often asked to write medical reports about disability following accidents or other trauma and in relation to claims of medical negligence. Such reports are concerned mainly with the nature and outlook of physical disability, but they should include any psychiatric consequences directly attributable to the trauma or induced by the physical disability. It may be necessary to comment on the possibility of exaggeration or even simulation.

The relationship between accidents and psychiatric disorder is considered on p. 213.

Psychiatry and criminal law

Few psychiatric patients break the law and when they do, it is usually in minor ways. Although serious violent offences by psychiatric patients receive much publicity, they are infrequent and committed by an extremely small minority of patients. It is, however, important that doctors are aware of the risk of criminal behaviour amongst those who are mentally ill. Threats of violence to self or to others should be taken seriously, as should the possibility of unintended harm resulting from disinhibited, reckless, or ill-considered behaviour. Specialist advice should always be sought where there is concern and doubt about appropriate action.

Apart from providing factual medical reports, doctors may be asked to advise on certain legal issues. Most are the province of the specialist psychiatrist but general practitioners and other doctors may be asked for advice.

- Advice to the police when they are deciding whether to proceed with charges against mentally ill people.
- Fitness to plead.
- Assessment of responsibility.
- Advice on sentencing.
- Treatment of offenders:
  - in a penal institution,
  - in hospital,
  - in the community.
- Assessment of dangerousness.

Fitness to plead

This term refers to a person's fitness to defend himself against the charges. A person judged unfit to plead is not tried but detained in a hospital until fit to plead, at which time (if it comes) the case is tried. To be fit to plead, a person must be able to:

(1) understand the nature of the charge;

(2) understand the difference between a plea of guilty and a plea of not guilty;

(3) instruct lawyers;

(4) challenge jurors;

(5) follow evidence presented in court.

A person can suffer from severe mental disorder and still be fit to plead.

Assessment of criminal responsibility

In deciding whether a person is guilty of an offence against the law emphasis is placed, in the legal system, on the person's intentions at the time of the offence and on his ability to control his actions at that time—the concept of **responsibility**.

For most offences, a person is not regarded as culpable unless he was able to chose whether or not to perform the unlawful action, and unless he was able to control his behaviour at the time. The doctor has to make a judgement about the mental state at the time of the offence but can base this only on the mental state at the time of a medical assessment made after (sometimes long after) the event, together with the offender's account and that of any witnesses. If the doctor was treating the person before the offence, he will have knowledge of their mental state at that time but can still only make a judgement about the mental state when the offence was carried out.

In English law, questions about **diminished responsibility** are most often raised in relation to a charge of murder: if the plea is upheld and the person is found guilty, it is of manslaughter not murder.

Advice relevant to sentencing

The court may ask for medical advice that will assist in deciding the appropriate sentence after a person has been found guilty. This advice may be about the prognosis of any mental disorder that is present, the likely effects of psychiatric treatment, and the probability of the person offending again.

Additional information Preparing a medical report

When a doctor is asked for a written medical report on a person he should avoid as far as possible technical language, he should explain any technical terms that are essential, and he should not use jargon. The report should be concise, have a clear structure, and be limited to matters relevant to the reason for the report. The following headings are recommended.

Report for criminal proceedings

1. *The doctor's particulars:* full name, qualifications, and present appointment.

2. *When the interview was conducted*; whether any third person was present.

3. *Sources of information* including any documents that have been examined.

4. Relevant points from the *family and personal history* of the defendant. Usually these can be brief, especially if a social report is available to the court.

5. The accused person's *account of the events of the alleged offence*; whether he admits to the offence or has another explanation of the events; if he admits to it, his attitude and expressed degree of remorse.

6. *Other relevant behaviour* such as the abuse of alcohol or drugs, the quality of relationships with other people, general social competence, behaviour indicating ability to tolerate frustration.

7. *Mental state at the time of the assessment*, mentioning only positive findings or specifically relevant negative ones.

8. A *diagnosis* in terms of relevant legal categories: in Britain the categories of *mental illness*, *mental impairment*, and *psychopathic disorder* are used in the Mental Health Act. A more specific diagnosis can be added (such as dementia or schizophrenia) but the court is unlikely to be helped by the finer nuances of diagnosis.

9. *Mental state at the time of the alleged offence* As explained above, this question is highly important in law but difficult to answer on medical evidence. A judgement is made on the points set out on p. 456: in summary, present mental state, diagnosis, the accused person's account, and accounts from any witnesses. If the person has a chronic mental illness (such as dementia) it is less difficult to infer his mental state at the time of the alleged offence than it is if he has a depressive disorder which could have been more or less severe at the former time than it was at the assessment. To add to the difficulty, the court does not simply require a general statement about the mental state at the time, but a specific judgement about the accused person's intentions.

10. *Fitness to plead* is referred to when this is relevant (see p. 455 for further advice on this point).

11. *Advice on further treatment* is likely to be particularly helpful to the court. Any recommendations should be feasible and to ensure this the person making the report will need to consult colleagues if he cannot himself carry out the whole of the recommended procedures. It is not the doctor's role to advise the court about sentencing, although sometimes it is helpful to indicate the likely psychiatric consequences of different forms of sentence that might be considered by the court (e.g. custodial vs. non-custodial).

Reports for compensation and other civil proceedings

The general principles are similar to those described above. It is essential to provide information about the circumstances of the event and the immediate and later reactions to it.

The conclusions should summarize the psychological and social consequences of the trauma and the extent to which they appear to be attributable to it. In many cases there is evidence that psychological problems or social difficulties preceded the event and it is important to decide how far the psychological and social changes found after the trauma are a continuation of these previous difficulties rather than new developments. Evidence from a close relative or other informant, interviewed separately, should be obtained whenever possible.

Acting as a witness

If the doctor is required to give verbal evidence in court, it is prudent to speak beforehand to a lawyer involved to find out what points are likely to be raised in court. The doctor should prepare by reading available documents including witness statements and any social report. If necessary, he should consult medical works of reference. Doctors should remember that their role is to use their special knowledge to assist the court to reach its own decision, not to tell the court what to do. When replying to questions in court, answers should be brief, clear, and restricted to the medical evidence. Speculation should be avoided.

Associations between particular offences and psychiatric disorder

Most offences have predominantly social causes and few are associated specifically with psychiatric disorder. Since categories of offence are defined for legal purposes, it is not surprising that there is no close correspondence between these categories and categories of psychiatric disorder. Any offence can be associated with several kinds of psychiatric disorder.

Crimes of violence

Homicide In the UK, between less than a third of homicides are by mentally disordered people. In countries with higher homicide rates the proportion is lower. The victims are usually family members or close acquaintances. The disorders most often associated with homicide are: schizophrenia, personality disorder, severe depressive disorder, and alcoholism; many murderers are intoxicated with alcohol at the time of the crime. Pathological jealousy, which may be associated with any of these conditions, is particularly dangerous.

Infanticide, the killing of a child below the age of 12 months by the mother, is of two kinds. When the killing is within 24 hours of birth, the baby is usually unwanted, and the mother is often young, distressed, and ill equipped to deal with the child, but not usually suffering from psychiatric disorder. When the killing is more than 24 hours after the birth, the mother usually has a puerperal psychosis. About a third of mothers in this second group try to kill themselves after killing the child.

Family violence short of homicide, is common but often undetected. It is strongly associated with excessive consumption of alcohol. It may affect children (child abuse is considered on p. 410), the spouse, or an elderly relative living in the house. Wife battering is associated with aggressive personality, alcohol abuse, and sexual jealousy. Marital therapy may be attempted to reduce factors provoking the violence, but often alternative safe accommodation has to be found for the woman and any children.

Sexual offences Most sexual offences are committed by men. The most frequent offences are indecent exposure, rape, and unlawful intercourse. The common sexual offence among women is prostitution.

Indecent exposure of the genitalia is mainly an offence of men between 25 and 35 years of age. The offence is usually a result of the psychiatric disorder known as exhibitionism (see p. 302), although in a minority exposure is a prelude to a sexual assault.

Rape is forceful sexual intercourse with an unwilling partner. The degree of force varies: in some cases force is threatened either verbally or with a weapon, in others there is extreme brutality. Few rapists have a psychiatric disorder.

Unlawful intercourse is sexual intercourse with a child under the age at which legal consent can be given. The sexual acts vary from minor indecency to seriously aggressive penetrative intercourse but most do not involve violence. The offence is common.

An adult who repeatedly commits sexual offences against children is known as a *paedophile*. Most are male. Some are timid and sexually inexperienced, some mentally retarded, and have difficulty in finding a sexual partner of their own age. Others prefer intercourse with children to that with adults. Although most offences do not involve major assault and most convicted offenders do not re-offend, an important minority persist in their behaviour and a few progress to more serious and damaging forms of sexual behaviour with children.

Incest is sexual activity between members of the same family, most often between father and daughter, or between siblings. Child sexual abuse is described in Chapter 19. When incest has been discovered the family needs much specialist support to deal with guilt and recriminations. *The effects of sexual abuse on children are described on p. 420.*

Other offences

Arson is setting fire to property, an act which may also endanger life. Most arsonists are male. Usually there is no obvious motive for the act and many arsonists are referred for a medical opinion. However, few have a psychiatric disorder.

Shoplifting Most shoplifters act for gain but a minority do so when mentally disordered. Patients with alcoholism, drug dependence, and chronic schizophrenia may shoplift because they lack money, and patients with dementia may forget to pay. Patients with depressive disorder or anorexia nervosa may shoplift with less obvious motives when they do not need what they have stolen. Among middle-aged women shoplifters it is common to find family and social difficulties and depression.

Repeated gambling ('pathological gambling') This term is used to describe a condition in which a person describes an intense urge to gamble and a preoccupation with thoughts about gambling. Gambling is not, itself, an offence but large debts can accumulate and may result in stealing or fraud. Some psychiatrists regard this condition as a disorder akin to addiction to alcohol, and offer treatment similar to that used for substance abuse. The results of such treatment are uncertain.

Associations between specific psychiatric disorders and types of offence

The associations between particular offences and psychiatric disorder are described above. However, in clinical practice it is sometimes necessary to review the associations also from the opposite standpoint; the offences most often carried out by patients with particular disorders. These associations are summarized in Table 21.3.

Treatment of mentally abnormal offenders

The courts take psychiatric evidence into account when sentencing mentally disordered offenders, and this evidence includes advice about psychiatric treatment. The treatment of mental disorder in an offender is not different from that of the

Table 21.3.

Associations between psychiatric disorders and offending

Schizophrenia	Crime is uncommon and usually minor. Persecutory delusion or hallucinations may lead to violent offences. Threats of violence should be taken seriously.
Depressive disorder	Some depressive delusions may lead to attempts at homicide to spare the victims from what is seen as an intolerable future. Infanticide within 12 months of birth.
Mania	Exuberant, unpredictable behaviour may result in fraud, theft or, rarely, violence.
Organic mental disorder	Dementia may result in shoplifting or disinhibited minor sexual offences.
Personality disorder	Common characteristic of serious offenders. Link between antisocial personality and violent offences.
Alcohol abuse	Common association, includes family and other violence, and dangerous driving.
Drug abuse	Particularly associated with theft to obtain or pay for drugs.
Mental retardation	Usually minor crimes by individuals lacking understanding of the legal implications of their actions.

same disorder in a person who has not offended but treatment may need to given in a more secure place.

Usually, appropriate treatment can be given within the ordinary psychiatric services, as an out-patient or as an in-patient. However, when there is a continuing risk to other people of aggression, arson, or sexual offences, treatment is arranged in a unit providing greater security to ensure the protection of society. Mental health legislation is generally used to detain these patients. Severe personality disorders are common among offenders but few are amenable to treatment.

Victims of crime

Doctors are sometimes asked to assist the victims of crime. Most of these people are suffering from one of the reactions to stress described in Chapter 6, and require the forms of treatment outlined there. A few develop a depressive disorder, anxiety disorder, post-traumatic stress disorder (see p. 93) in response to the stressful events and are treated in the ways described in the chapters dealing with these conditions.

Victims require immediate support and practical help from doctors in primary care or from emergency department staff. They also need to be told that they can obtain later help if required by consulting doctors or one of the police and community schemes which provide counselling and practical help.

Victims of rape and other sexual assault often suffer severe immediate distress, and many experience post-traumatic stress disorder and sexual dysfunction. In some regions, special services have been set up to help rape victims deal with the immediate psychological effects of the experience and to identify persistent symptoms which may require specialist treatment.

Further reading

Faulk, M. (1994). *Basic Forensic Psychiatry* (2nd edn). Blackwell, Oxford.
A comprehensive introductory text.

Gunn, J. and Taylor, P. (1992). *Forensic Psychiatry*. Butterworths, London.
A comprehensive work of reference.

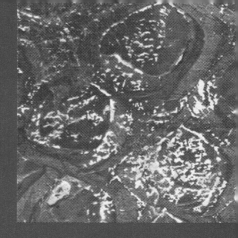

Appendix: The law in England and Wales

- The Mental Health Act

- Admission for assessment

- Treatment orders

- Admission to hospital of those appearing before the courts

- Discharge of patients

- Consent to treatment

- Children and the law

Appendix: The law in England and Wales

This appendix is an introduction to the principal sections of the law of England and Wales relating to psychiatric practice. It begins with a review of the Mental Health Act, and then outlines the law in relation to child and adolescent psychiatry. More detailed information can be obtained from the publications listed on p. 461 and, of course, from the Act itself. Psychiatrists practising elsewhere than in England and Wales will need to consult guides to their local legislation and its application in clinical practice.

The Mental Health Act

The Mental Health Act 1983 regulates the care of mentally abnormal persons. It consolidates the Mental Health Act 1959 and the Mental Health (Amendment) Act 1982, which made provisions for compulsory treatment and about consent to treatment. It also set up the Mental Health Act Commission, which is an independent multidisciplinary body appointed by the Secretary of State. The Commission has powers to safeguard the interests of detailed patients. Its duties are to visit such patients, investigate complaints, receive reports on patients' treatment, and appoint doctors and others to give opinions on consent to treatment.

Parts IV and V of the Mental Health Act provide the legal basis for compulsory admission and detention of psychiatric patients. Provision for compulsory detention is also made by the Criminal Procedure (Insanity) Act 1964, which relates to people found 'not guilty by reason of insanity' or 'unfit to plead' (see p. 455).

Under the Mental Health Act there are three main groups of compulsory order for assessment and treatment:

1   admission for assessment (Sections 2, 4, 5, 135, 136);

2   treatment orders (Sections 3, 7);

3   admission and transfer of patients concerned with criminal proceedings (Sections 37, 41, 47, 49).

The short-term orders listed in (1) above apply to any mental disorder, which need not be specified. For the long-term orders listed under (2) and (3), it must be stated that the patient suffers from one of four types of mental disorder: mental illness, psychopathic disorder, mental impairment, or severe mental impairment.

The Act does not define 'mental illness', but it states that no one should be 'treated as suffering from mental disorder by reason only of promiscuity, or other immoral conduct, sexual deviancy or dependence on alcohol or drugs'.

The Act gives the following definitions of the three other types of mental disorder.

a **Severe mental impairment** means a state of arrested or incomplete development of mind which includes severe impairment of intelligence and social functioning and is associated with abnormally aggressive or seriously irresponsible conduct on the part of the person concerned.

b **Mental impairment** means a state of arrested or incomplete development of mind (not amounting to severe mental impairment) which includes significant impairment of intelligence and social functioning and is associated with abnormally aggressive or seriously irresponsible conduct on the part of the person concerned.

c **Psychopathic disorder** means a persistent disorder or disability of mind (whether or not including significant impairment of intelligence) which results in abnormally aggressive or seriously irresponsible conduct on the part of the person concerned.

The Act also specifies the various people who may be involved in procedures for admission and treatment.

- *Responsible medical officer*: the doctor in charge of treatment.
- *Nearest relative*: nearest adult relative (in the order of spouse, son or daughter, father or mother, sibling, grandparent, grandchild, uncle or aunt, nephew or niece). The elder or eldest of relatives of the same kind (e.g. siblings) is preferred, and full siblings have precedence over half-siblings. Preference is also given to a relative with whom the patient lives or who cares for him. The definition includes cohabitees (who may be of the same sex as the patient) who have lived with the patient for a specified time. However, they come last on the list of relatives and cannot claim precedence over a husband or wife other than through agreement or under an Order of Court or by desertion.
- *Approved social worker* (formerly mental welfare officer): social workers approved by the local authority as having appropriate competence in dealing with mentally disordered persons.
- *Approved doctor*: a doctor approved under Section 12 of the Act by the Secretary of State as having special experience in the diagnosis or treatment of mental disorder.

The three main groups of compulsory order will now be reviewed in turn.

Admission for assessment

Although a full understanding of the proper use of compulsory admission can be gained only from clinical experience, the clinician needs to be aware of the following general conditions governing compulsory detention.

Section 2: Application for admission for assessment (28 days)

This is the usual procedure for compulsory admission when informal admission is not appropriate in the circumstances. Detention is for assessment, or for assessment followed by medical treatment. The following grounds must be satisfied.

1   The patient suffers from a mental disorder which warrants his detention in hospital for assessment (assessment followed by treatment).

2   Admission is necessary in the interests of the patient's own health or safety or for the protection of others.

The procedure requires the following.

1   *Application* by the patient's nearest relative, or an approved social worker who must have seen the patient within the last 14 days. The approved social worker should, as far as practicable, consult the nearest relative.

2   *Medical recommendations* by two doctors, one of whom must be approved under Section 12 of the Act. The two doctors should not be on the staff of the same hospital unless it would cause undesirable delay to find a doctor from elsewhere. There should not be more than 5 days between the examinations.

Section 4: Emergency order for assessment (72 hours)

This section allows a simpler procedure than Section 2 and provides power to detain patients in emergencies. It is usually completed in the patient's home by the family doctor but is also occasionally used in general hospital casualty departments. Section 4 should be used only when there is insufficient time to obtain the opinion of an approved doctor who could complete Section 2. The grounds are as for Section 2. It is expected that a Section 4 order will be converted into a Section 2 order as soon as possible after the patient has arrived in hospital. The procedure for a Section 4 order requires the following.

1   Application by an approved social worker, who must have seen the patient within the previous 24 hours, or the nearest relative.

2   Medical recommendation by one doctor, who need not be approved under Section 12 of the Act. The patient must be admitted within 24 hours of the examination (or of the application if made earlier).

Section 5: Change to compulsory detention (72 hours)

This is an order for the emergency detention of a patient who is already in hospital as a voluntary patient but wishes to leave, although the doctor believes that an application should be made for compulsory admission under the Act. It requires a single medical recommendation by the doctor in charge of the patient's care or by another doctor who is on the staff of the hospital and nominated by the doctor in charge. (This power applies to patient in any hospital.) It is usual to consider a change to a Section 2 or Section 3 order as soon as possible.

If a Section 5 order cannot be obtained immediately, a registered mental nurse or registered nurse for the mentally subnormal may invoke a 6-hour **holding order**. The nurse must record that the patient is suffering from mental disorder such that, in the interests of the patient's health or safety or for the protection of others, he should be restrained from leaving the hospital. The holding order applies only when the patient is already under treatment for a mental disorder. It lapses as soon as the doctor signs Section 5. (This power applies only to a patient in a psychiatric ward.)

Section 115: Powers of entry and inspection

An approved social worker can enter and inspect any premises (within the area of the local authority in which the patient lives) if he has reason to believe that a mentally disordered patient is not under proper care. This social worker must be able to provide authenticated documentation of his status.

Section 135: Warrant to search for and remove patients

Any approved social worker who believes that someone is suffering from a mental disorder and is unable to care for himself or is being ill-treated or neglected may apply to a magistrate for a warrant for that person's removal to a place of safety.

Section 136: Mentally disordered person found in a public place

Any police constable who finds in a public place someone who appears to be suffering from a mental disorder may take the person to a place of safety (which usually means a police station or a hospital) if the person appears to be in immediate need of care or control, of if the police constable thinks that it is necessary to do so in the person's interest, or for the further protection of other persons. The person is detained so that he can be examined by a doctor and any necessary arrangements can be made for his treatment or care. The authority under Section 136 expires when these arrangements have been completed or within 72 hours, whichever is the shorter.

Treatment orders

Section 3: Admission for treatment (6 months)

The grounds for this longer-term order as follows.

1   The patient is suffering from mental illness, severe mental impairment, psychopathic disorder, or mental impairment, that is, a mental disorder of a nature or degree which makes it appropriate for him to receive medical treatment in a hospital.

2   In the case of psychopathic disorder or mental impairment, such treatment is likely to alleviate or prevent a deterioration of his condition.

3   It is necessary for the health or safety of the patient or for the protection of other persons that he should receive such treatment and that it cannot be provided unless he is detained under this section.

The procedure is as follows.

1   *Application.* This is made by the patient's nearest relative or an approved social worker. If practicable, the latter must consult the nearest relative before making an application and cannot proceed if the nearest relative objects.

2   *Medical recommendation.* As for Section 2 with the addition that the recommendations must state the particular grounds for the doctor's opinion, speci-

fying whether any other methods of dealing with the patient are available and, if so, why they are not appropriate. The doctor must specify one of the four forms of mental disorder.

3   *Renewal.* The order must be renewed on the first occasion for a further 6 months and subsequently for 1 year at a time.

Section 7: Reception into guardianship

Guardianship is more appropriate than the provisions of Section 3 for the long term treatment of patients living in the community. The application, medical recommendation, duration, and renewal procedure are similar to those for Section 3. The guardian, who is usually but not always the local social services department is given authority (Section 8) for supervision in the community, including the following powers:

1   to require the patient to live at a place specified by the guardian;

2   to require the patient to attend places specified by the guardian for medical treatment, occupation, training, or education;

3   ensure that a doctor, social worker, or other person specified by the guardian can see the patient at his home.

Admission to hospital of those appearing before the courts

These sections of the Mental Health Act allow the court to order psychiatric care for those charged with or convicted of an offence punishable by imprisonment. Medical recommendations are required together with an assurance that a hospital place is available.

Remands to hospital and interim hospital orders

1   Persons on remand (but not in custody) may be treated as voluntary patients. Sometimes, psychiatric care may be made a condition of the granting of bail. In addition, the Mental Health Act 1983 gave the courts the following powers:

2   to remand an accused person to a hospital for medical reports (Section 35);

3   to remand an accused person to hospital for treatment (except for murder cases) (Section 36);

4   to make an interim hospital order on a convicted person to assess suitability for a hospital order (Section 38).

Procedure (1) requires a medical recommendation by an approved doctor that there is reason to suspect mental disorder. Procedures (2) and (3) require medical recommendations by two doctors (one of whom must be approved) that the person is suffering from mental disorder.

Section 37: Hospital order

A court may impose a hospital order, which commits an offender to hospital on a similar basis to that of a patient admitted for treatment under the civil provisions of Section 3 of the Act (see above). The duration of the order is 6 months.

Medical recommendation: two doctors, one of whom must be approved.

Section 41: Restriction order

When a Section 37 hospital order is made by a Crown Court, the court may also make an order under Section 41 of the Act restricting the person's discharge from hospital. The restriction order may be either without limit of time or for a specified period. If it is for a fixed term; once that term expires or otherwise ceases to have effect, the patient will still be detained under a hospital order but without restriction, that is, Section 37.

Section 47: Transfer to hospital from prison

This section authorizes the Home Secretary to transfer a person serving a sentence of imprisonment to a local National Health Service hospital or special hospital (Section 48 covers other prisoners not serving sentences for criminal offences). A direction for transfer has the same effect as a hospital order. The patient's status changes to that of a notional Section 37 at the time of the 'earliest date of release'.

The Home Secretary can make the direction with or without special restriction on discharge (Section 49).

Medical recommendation: two doctors, one of whom must be approved.

Discharge of patients

Patients on emergency orders (Sections 4, 5, 135, 136) can be discharged by the responsible medical officer. Patients on a Section 2 order can be discharged by the responsible medical officer, the hospital managers, the nearest relative, or a mental health review tribunal. The same applies to patients on Section 3, except that the responsible medical officer may register an objection to discharge by relatives if he considers that the patient is a danger to himself or others. Patients under guardianship are in the same position as patients on Section 3 except that the local health authority replaces the hospital managers.

The nearest relative has no rights to discharge patients on Section 37 or Section 47 orders. Patients on Section 41 and Section 49 restriction orders can be discharged only by the responsible medical officer with the consent of the Secretary of State for Home Affairs, or by a mental health review tribunal.

Mental health review tribunals

These are regional tribunals that provide an appeal procedure for patients subject to longer-term orders. They hear appeals against compulsory orders and automatically review certain patients under Section 3 and 37 (see list below). Review tribunals may order immediate or delayed discharge. The members of a panel are appointed by the Lord Chancellor and include a lay member, a doctor, and a lawyer who is the chairman. When the patient is subject to a restriction order, the chairman of the panel is a judge. Patients are entitled to be provided with legal representation.

For the various sections of the Act, the timing of application for appeal is specified:

Section 4 and 5	No appeal.
Section 2	Application must be made within 14 days.
Section 3	Application can be made in the first 6 months, the second 6 months, and then annually; review is automatic if there has been no appeal either in the first 6 months or in any 3-year period.
Section 37 (with or without Section 41)	Application can be made in the second 6 months and then annually; review is automatic if there has been no appeal in any 3 year period.
Guardianship	An application can be made in each period of detention; no automatic review.

Consent to treatment

Under common law, no treatment can be given to a voluntary patient without his valid consent. This requires that the patient voluntarily (i.e. without being subjected to coercion or unreasonable influence) agrees to the treatment and is capable of making that decision. Doctors should not give treatment without such consent unless the treatment is essential to safeguard the health or preserve the life of the patient.

The Mental Health Act 1983 introduced provisions to serve two purposes: to give authority for certain treatments to be given without consent, and to safeguard psychiatric patients' interests in relation to treatment procedures.

The Act specifies certain emergency conditions under which treatment can be given without consent to a detained patient. Any treatment (provided it is not irreversible or hazardous) can be given to such a patient without his consent if it is immediately necessary to save the patient's life, to prevent a serious deterioration in his condition, to alleviate serious suffering, or to prevent violence or danger to the patient himself or to others.

The Act also defines various groups of treatments according to the type of consent required for them. The allocations of particular treatments to these groups are specified in the Act, in Regulations (which are compulsory) and in a Code of Practice (which is advisory). Certain patients are excluded from the stipulations concerning consent to treatment, namely those detained under Sections 4, 5, 135, and 136, those remanded to hospital for reports, and those subject to Section 41 orders but conditionally discharged by the Home Secretary. For these patients the doctor has only common-law rights and duties when giving treatment.

For other patients, three groups of treatments are stipulated, of which all three apply to detained patients and only the first to voluntary patients.

1   *Treatments which give rise to special concern.* This group applies to both voluntary and detained patients. It includes psychosurgery and other treatments which are yet to be specified, but does not include ordinary medication or electro-

convulsive therapy (ECT). The patient must consent to treatments included in this group, and there must be a second opinion provided by an independent doctor who will be required to consult two people (one a nurse, one neither a doctor nor a nurse) who have been professionally concerned with the patient's treatment. He considers both the treatment proposed and the patient's ability to give consent. In addition, two independent people must certify as to the patient's ability to give consent. Approval of treatment by the second opinion procedure may cover a plan of care including more than one form of treatment.

2   *Other treatments listed in Regulations.* This group applies to detained patients. It consists of other treatments specified in the Act or in Regulations. It includes some forms of medication and ECT. For these treatments, a second opinion must be obtained as in (1) if the patient does not consent, cannot give consent, or withdraws consent. Again, the second opinion may cover a plan of treatment. However, for most forms of medication these procedures do not apply during the first 3 months of treatment.

3   *Other forms of treatment.* Treatments not referred to in (1) or (2) can be given to detained patients without their consent. It should be noted that, according to the act, medical treatment 'includes nursing and also includes care, habilitation and rehabilitation under medical supervision'.

The Court of Protection

This court has a very long history and is responsible for the mentally ill or impaired. Most of its functions are carried out by the Master and other officers appointed by the Lord Chancellor. They are assisted by medical, legal, and general panels of Lord Chancellor's Visitors, who visit patients to review their capacities and the implementation of procedures approved by the Court. Applications to the Court may be made by the nearest relative or any interested party. They should include a medical certificate from a doctor concerned in the patient's care and an affidavit of the patient's family and property. After considering the evidence, the judge may appoint a receiver to administer the patient's affairs and also to 'do or secure the doing of all such things as appear necessary or expedient'. During the management of a patient's affairs by the Court, medical opinion may be sought about the patient's ability to make a will and about any application to end the Court management.

Children and the law

Parental consent is normally required for the medical care of children under the age of 16. There are some uncertainties about the occasions on which parents need not be notified when children aged 15 or 16 consult doctors. When in doubt it is sensible to seek further advice from an experienced child psychiatrist, a medical defence society, or another authority.

Compulsory admission under the Mental Health Act is hardly ever used for children under the age of 16 for two reasons. First, there are alternatives such as care proceedings or an application for the child to be made a ward of court. Secondly, parents have powers up to the age of 16, or up to the age of 18 if the child is not capable of consent.

Index

Page numbers in *italics* refer to tables or boxes. vs. in sub-entries denotes 'differentiation from'.